Language and Health in Action

Edited by

Lynnette Arnold
Jennifer R. Guzmán
Emily Avera
Anna I. Corwin

OXFORD
UNIVERSITY PRESS

OXFORD
UNIVERSITY PRESS

Great Clarendon Street, Oxford, OX2 6DP,
United Kingdom

Oxford University Press is a department of the University of Oxford.
It furthers the University's objective of excellence in research, scholarship,
and education by publishing worldwide. Oxford is a registered trade mark of
Oxford University Press in the UK and in certain other countries.

Published in the United States of America by Oxford University Press
198 Madison Avenue, New York, NY 10016, United States of America

British Library Cataloguing in Publication Data
Data available

Library of Congress Control Number: 2025938782

ISBN 9780198933915
ISBN 9780198933922 (pbk.)

DOI: 10.1093/9780198933953.001.0001

The manufacturer's authorized representative in the EU for product safety is
Oxford University Press España S.A. of Parque Empresarial San Fernando de Henares,
Avenida de Castilla, 2 – 28830 Madrid (www.oup.es/en or product.safety@oup.com).
OUP España S.A. also acts as importer into Spain of products made by the manufacturer.

About the Companion Website

Oxford University Press has created a website to accompany *Language and Health in Action*. For each chapter, the website lists additional resources, including further reading and multimedia materials such as short videos, longer films, and podcasts, that may be helpful in teaching the chapter. The reader is encouraged to consult this resource in conjunction with the chapters.

The companion website can be accessed www.oup.com/LanguageandHealth.

Editors' Welcome

Language and Health in Action started with conversations. In hallways at conferences, on listserv threads, in personal emails, we and many of our colleagues asked each other, "What readings are you assigning in your language and health courses?" Over and over we heard similar answers. It was hard to find teachable texts. Although we remained convinced that scholarship at this intersection was of profound importance for students, it tended to be written for specialists. Existing texts were challenging, particularly for students who were encountering linguistic and medical anthropology for the first time. We wanted to harness the tremendous potential for language-focused research on health issues to impact our students, and so the idea for this book was born.

Our vision for *Language and Health in Action* has also been shaped by our own research. We, the editors of this book, have investigated the role of language in health issues that include aging, cross-cultural medicine, blood transfusion services, and family care. We have worked in settings ranging from the Americas to Africa. We find this work's real-world applications and consequences most compelling. Together with the contributing authors of this book, we aim to reinvigorate scholarship at this intersection with a new sense of purpose by demonstrating the relevance of language-health research for many current issues. We see teaching as a key means for ensuring that insights from this scholarship reach not only future clinicians, but also policy makers, voters, and educators, as well as individuals, family members, and communities as they deal with critical matters of health and wellbeing.

With this inspiration in mind, we have worked to create a book that introduces readers to the complex interrelationship between language and health and invites readers to enact this knowledge in their personal and professional lives. While we have designed the book for teaching, we hope that the clear definitions, examples, and accessible style will encourage scholars and practitioners from a range of medical and health-related disciplines to explore how attention to language might enhance their work. Likewise, we hope that this volume will encourage teachers and researchers in linguistic anthropology and related fields to leverage health issues as an exemplar for why attention to language matters.

Following the book's Foreword, which outlines the theoretical and methodological foundations of language-health research, we have written an introduction that centers key concepts for readers who may be new to anthropological writing and thinking about language and health. The original research that makes up the core of the volume is organized into five thematic sections, starting where readers might expect, with a focus on clinical interaction, including nursing, medical training, and non-biomedical settings. The second section explores access to healthcare in multilingual and multicultural contexts, encouraging readers to consider global diversity and grassroots health education. The third section examines processes of health communication, exploring its historical roots, the role of the media, and how people build community in the face of stigma and disease. Building on these insights, the fourth section explores language and the environment, looking deeply at people's stories to understand how social and natural environments shape health (in)equities. The final section of the book focuses on healing, examining how language serves as a critical resource in cases of addiction, amputation, and terminal diagnosis. The book concludes with an Afterword that illuminates how attention to language is vital to ethical medical care.

In support of instructors and students, we have provided a series of questions at the conclusion of each chapter. The "reflection questions" can be used to guide individual student responses, while the "small group" questions are close reading prompts designed to help students understand specific pieces of each chapter's argument. The "large group" questions are designed to help students understand the overarching claim of each chapter and consider how it connects to other cases or topics in language and health. In addition, an "Explore More" list for each chapter can be found on the companion website. These lists include relevant scholarship and multimedia resources that we have found useful for teaching with *Language and Health in Action.*

We are glad you have found this book and are joining the conversation. We hope that the stories and insights here will inspire future conversations in your life as you navigate the many dimensions of health and wellbeing that come with being human.

Contents

List of Contributors

Lynnette Arnold PhD is Associate Professor, Department of Anthropology, University of Massachusetts Amherst, Amherst, MA, USA.

Emily Avera PhD is Assistant Professor, Department of Sociology and Anthropology, Colgate University, Hamilton, NY, USA.

Steven P. Black PhD is Professor, Department of Anthropology, Georgia State University, Atlanta, GA, USA.

Charles L. Briggs PhD is Distinguished Professor, Department of Anthropology, University of California, Berkeley, Berkeley, CA, USA.

Mara Buchbinder PhD is Professor and Chair, Department of Social Medicine, University of North Carolina at Chapel Hill, Chapel Hill, NC, USA.

Anna I. Corwin PhD is Associate Professor and Chair of the Women's Spirituality Program, California Institute of Integral Studies, San Francisco, CA, USA.

Mario Deng MD is Professor, David Geffen School of Medicine at UCLA, Los Angeles, CA, USA.

Paja Faudree PhD, MFA is Associate Professor, Department of Anthropology, Brown University, Providence, RI, USA.

Margarita Francisco is Ark City Community Liaison for Alce su Voz Wichita State University, Witchita, KS, USA.

Marjorie Harness Goodwin PhD is Distinguished Research Professor, Department of Anthropology, University of California, Los Angeles, Los Angeles, CA, USA.

Jorge Tibor Gutiérrez BA, Lic. is a member of RENPO (Red Nacional de Pueblos Originarios en Respuesta al VIH/SIDA), Chile.

Jennifer R. Guzmán PhD is Professor, Department of Anthropology, State University of New York at Geneseo, Geneseo, NY, USA.

T. S. Harvey PhD is Associate Professor, Department of Anthropology, Vanderbilt University, Nashville, TN, USA.

Stephanie Keeney Parks PhD is University of California Chancellor Postdoctoral Fellow, Department of Anthropology, University of California, Los Angeles, Los Angeles, CA, USA.

Daniel W. Krugman MSPH is PhD Student, Department of Anthropology, Brown University, Providence, RI, USA.

Hyemin Lee PhD is Postdoctoral Associate in East Asian Studies and Lecturer in Anthropology, Council on East Asian Studies, MacMillan Center for International & Area Studies, Yale University, New Haven, CT, USA.

Abby Mack PhD is Assistant Professor, Department of Anthropology, University of Kentucky, Lexington, KY, USA.

Xochitl Marsilli-Vargas is Associate Professor, Department of Spanish and Portuguese, Emory University, Atlanta, GA, USA.

Claudia Morales PhD is Assistant Professor, Department of English and Creative Writing, Dominican University of California, San Rafael, CA, USA.

Hannah S. Noblewolf PhD(c) MA is Doctoral Candidate, Department of Anthropology, State University of New York at Albany, Albany, NY, USA.

Mohamed Yunus Rafiq PhD is Assistant Professor, Department of Anthropology, New York University, Shanghai, China.

Federica Raia PhD is Associate Professor, Department of Education and David Geffen School of Medicine at UCLA, Los Angeles, CA, USA.

Raúl Rangel Fernández MA is PhD student, Department of Modern and Classical Languages and Literatures, and Graduate Student Assistant, Alce Su Voz at Wichita State University, Witchita, KS, USA.

Paula F. Saravia PhD is Assistant Teaching Professor, Department of Anthropology, University of Washington, Seattle, WA, USA.

Insa M. Schmidt MD, MPH is Assistant Professor, Department of Medicine, Boston University Chobanian & Avedisian School of Medicine, Boston Medical Center, Boston, MA, USA.

Merav Shohet PhD is Associate Professor, Department of Anthropology, Boston University, Boston, MA, USA.

Rachel Showstack PhD is Associate Professor of Spanish, Department of Modern and Classical Languages and Literatures, Wichita State University, Wichita, KS, USA.

Lissie Wahl PhD is an independent researcher of global health, social medicine, and interpreter studies, Boston, MA, USA.

Lisa Wolf PhD, RN is Associate Professor, Elaine Marieb College of Nursing, University of Massachusetts, Amherst, Amherst, MA, USA.

Acknowledgments

The final form of this volume has benefitted from the labor and care of many people. We are, first and foremost, grateful to the chapter authors, who accepted our invitation to contribute and graciously responded to our many editorial suggestions and requests throughout the writing process. We have learned enormously from your work and our conversations.

We are indebted to Charles L. Briggs and Mara Buchbinder, whose respective work is foundational to the innovative scholarship that is happening today at the intersection of linguistic and medical anthropology. We appreciate that your contributions to this volume provide historical context and forward-looking suggestions for the kinds of research that can continue to advance understanding.

Thanks to the students in Emily's fall 2023 and fall 2024 Language and Medicine classes at Colgate University who helped evaluate and source some of the multimedia "Explore More" resources located on the companion website. Thanks also to the students in Lynnette's spring 2024 Language and Health class at University of Massachusetts, Amherst. Your reading, discussion, and thoughtful feedback on early versions of each chapter have helped to enhance the readability and usefulness of every part of the book.

Thank you, Ashley McGraw, for your assistance with compiling student feedback, bringing continuity to the pedagogical materials across the book, and keeping track of such things as word counts, image quality, and copyright information. Your work has been vital in finalizing this manuscript.

Important interlocutors as we conceptualized the book included Elinor Ochs, Sonya Pritzker, Baili Gall, and attendees at the "Teaching at the Intersection of Linguistic and Medical Anthropology" roundtable at the 2023 joint meetings of the American Anthropological Association, and the Canadian Anthropology Society / Société Canadienne d'Anthropologie in Toronto. We are grateful for the incisive suggestions made by Sherine Hamdy, Jessica Hardin, Steve Black, and Jonathan Rosa on the first draft of our chapter "Key Concepts in Language and Health". And we are indebted to the anonymous reviewers for their feedback on the book proposal and complete manuscript.

We have been fortunate to work with talented and supportive editors at Oxford University Press including Meredith Keffer, Julia Steer, Jade Dixon, and Mhairi Bennett. Thanks to Lavanya Sathiamurthy for guiding the production process. Deep appreciation to Allison Adelman of Silver Academic Editing for your careful and detailed work on the index.

Financial support for our work on this project came from a New York State/United University Professionals Individual Development Award, a sabbatical award, and faculty incentive grant from SUNY Geneseo, professional meetings and research start-up funds from Colgate University, and start-up funds from UMass Amherst and support from the Department of Anthropology at UMass. The wonderful staff at the Highlights Foundation writing retreat center at Boyds Mills provided a welcoming space for us to meet in person for a few precious days in spring 2023 and summer 2024. We could not have asked for a more beautiful space in which to write, talk, walk, and think.

This book has been a collaborative undertaking from start to finish. We are deeply indebted to our families and communities for their support, to our colleagues from whom we have learned so much, and to our students who inspired this project.

Foreword

Beyond Linguistic and Medical Anthropology Divides: The Emergence of Critical Synthetic Perspectives

Charles L. Briggs

Introduction

Becoming an ethnographer can involve surrendering oneself to unforeseen futures. My research in a Venezuelan rainforest, which began in 1986, seemed destined to forge new links between linguistic and medical anthropology. I was an ethnographer conducting research in a place where around a third of children died before reaching the age of 5, tuberculosis was common, and outbreaks of malaria, measles, and whooping cough were not infrequent. Illness, curing, and death thus dominated everyday conversation. Then a short November 1992 visit found me unexpectedly surrounded by hundreds of frightened friends. Focused on a new loanword, cholera, their stories came at me like a tropical downpour, telling of an unknown disease that killed healthy adults in as little as eight hours. Healers reported failing utterly; several prominent practitioners, including one of my teachers, died after treating patients. I could not dodge the responsibility to support people who had treated me so generously. I collaborated for fifteen months with a Venezuelan public health practitioner, Clara Mantini-Briggs, establishing small medical stations, treating hundreds of patients in areas that had never seen a doctor, and giving cholera-prevention talks night and day. Once cholera deaths ended, we accepted residents' challenge to figure out why so many people died, share their stories of the epidemic, and join them in affirming that their lives should matter as much as anyone else's. These experiences forced me to see how tightly medical and linguistic profiling were entwined, thereby creating inequities based on constructing populations as deficient in their perceived inability to master dominant languages and to understand biomedical knowledge. Witnessing the fatal effects of what I came to call health/communicative inequities pushed me to propose a new goal: a struggle for communicative justice in health.

Accepting this challenge as a scholar entailed finding tools in linguistic and medical anthropology and connecting them. I found myself doing so at a time when distanced, purportedly "objective" scholarship was increasingly giving way to new forms of collaboration. Many researchers were shifting their focus from race to racisms, from documenting purportedly silent, suffering populations to analyzing

Charles L. Briggs, *Beyond Linguistic and Medical Anthropology Divides*. In: *Language and Health in Action*. Edited by: Lynnette Arnold et al., Oxford University Press. © Charles L. Briggs (2026). DOI: 10.1093/9780198933953.002.0001 structural factors that produce inequities. Now many researchers build on their own experiences of structural violence in challenging dominant theories, research strategies, and rhetorics of scholarly authority. Scholarship is viewed as part of forces that produce inequities and resist change. Even as a conservative backlash currently attempts to undermine diversity, equity, and justice in universities, struggles continue to challenge how white supremacy, ableism, and heteropatriarchy shape undergraduate and graduate education, faculty recruitment and tenure, and who gets published by prestigious journals and presses. Time-worn characterizations of linguistic and medical anthropology as too specialized and technical have lost currency as practitioners develop unique perspectives on issues of vital scholarly and public concern.

Integrating linguistic and medical anthropology is crucial for analyzing and confronting inequities. Linguistic anthropologists have mapped communicative inequities and identified structural forces that produce them. Extending debates about white supremacy and racism, scholars carved out a field of raciolinguistics to "enhance our understanding of the processes of racialization by highlighting language's central role in the construction, maintenance, and transformation of racial and ethnic identities" (Alim, Rickford, and Ball 2016:7). Rosa and Flores focused on how language and race "have been co-naturalized in particular societal contexts" (2020:90). They drew on Inoue (2003) in analyzing a "white listening subject" that constitutes its racial privilege by imagining subjects and communicative practices judged to violate communicable norms and examine how "raciolinguistic ideologies" stigmatize the linguistic practices of racialized populations (Rosa and Flores 2020:93). Raciolinguistic research seeks to confront white supremacy and promote justice.

Hill (2008) sparked research on linguistic racism, drawing attention beyond overt discrimination, which many whites would condemn, to covert forms that invisibly reproduce stereotypes. She analyzed a dominant ideology that imagines language as 1) referential, tied to stable relationships between sound and meanings, and 2) personalistic, purportedly expressing individual beliefs and intentions. Insidiously, this ideology directs attention away from the harm racist speech inflicts on persons and populations. Graham (2011), Kroskrity (2015), Meek (2006, 2013), and Perley (2011) demonstrated how centrally "language ideological processes of racialization" (Kroskrity 2021:180) shape denigrating constructions of Indigenous people, documenting white scholars' complicity.

Within medical anthropology, scholars have extensively documented health inequities. Farmer (2004) analyzed how racism, wealthy nations, multilateral organizations, public health policies, and capital-driven structures of healthcare inflict "structural violence" on poor and racialized populations. Scheper-Hughes (1992) scrutinized how state policies produce astronomically high rates of child mortality in Northeastern Brazil, providing coffins but not adequate food, potable water, or life-saving treatments. Davis (2019) sensitively documented how medical racism positions Black female professionals—despite their apparent class privileges—as more likely to face maternal and infant mortality than white females. Benton (2015) and Nguyen (2010) traced how global health and development schemes exported Euro-American agendas, thwarting health needs of low-income Africans. Biehl (2005) and Han (2012) analyzed how care provided by family members and neighbors can enforce unhealthy health policies (Castro and Singer 2004).

Much work has analyzed diseases of inequity, including human immunodeficiency virus (HIV) / acquired immunodeficiency syndrome (AIDS) (Farmer 1992; Sangaramoorthy 2014), diabetes (Doucet-Battle 2021; Moran-Thomas 2019), sickle cell anemia (Rouse 2009), tuberculosis (Farmer 1999), cholera (Briggs and Mantini-Briggs 2003), and the destruction of farmworkers' bodies (Holmes 2013). Singer and colleagues (2017) argued that health inequities emerge in syndemics, where poverty and racism intersect with multiple illnesses. Hansen, Netherland, and Herzberg (2023) examined how racialization enabled pharmaceutical companies to market opioids, trapping white, middle-class, US residents in avalanches of overdose deaths.

Despite this impressive work, research is often still guided by entrenched (sub)disciplinary boundaries that limit anthropological contributions to studying both communicative and health inequities. Two fundamental problems here are that these inequities are co-produced by many of the same structural factors and that their interaction amplifies effects and hides underlying causes. Researchers demonstrated that Black and Latinx patients receive lower quality healthcare than white patients (Smedley, Stith, and Nelson 2003). Analyzing medical profiling, Van Ryn and Burke (2000) showed that US physicians sometimes assumed that Black patients abused drugs and alcohol more frequently, were less educated and intelligent, less attentive to medical guidance, and less likely to follow treatment guidelines. Systemic health inequities are thus often individualized as questions of communicative incompetence, bad behavior, ignorance, or non-compliance.

By weaving together work on linguistic and medical inequities, my goal is to demonstrate that the reach of analysis can be extended by exploring their synergistic—and sometimes lethal—effects. We can also go beyond witnessing them to join struggles for communicative justice in health. I begin by highlighting precedents for contemporary efforts to bring linguistic and medical anthropological perspectives into dialogue and reviewing some important current scholarship at this intersection (see Briggs 2024 for a more comprehensive discussion). I close by laying out different tactics for moving across (sub)disciplinary boundaries, suggesting ways that this process can become transformative.

Locating Precedents: How Scholars Have Forged Links between Linguistic and Medical Perspectives

Tracing previous efforts to link research on language and health, I begin this section with two remarkable scholars who might not always come to mind in this regard: Gregory Bateson and Frantz Fanon. Bateson was a British-American social scientist who, after initial training in the natural sciences, studied anthropology, linguistics, and psychology. He framed his work as interdisciplinary, using analogies from physics and biology in rethinking social sciences (Harries-Jones 2016). In the mid-1950s, Bateson collaborated with psychiatrists to develop new family therapy techniques. In a classic article, "Toward a Theory of Schizophrenia," Bateson suggested that a root cause of schizophrenia was patients' inability to learn everyday processes of metacommunication, which he defined as "the ability to communicate about communication, to comment upon the meaningful actions of oneself and others" (Bateson 1972:215). Like much contemporary linguistic anthropology, this work focused on close analysis of face-to-face interactions. Bateson attempted to resolve schizophrenia's "puzzling" nature by tracing it to contradictory metacommunicative signals given to children by their mothers who, through words and bodily signals, promised intimacy and love but then withdrew. This "double bind" developed as the child was punished by the mother for accurately interpreting contradictions between messages and metamessages and for failing to do so; the latter course led the child to misinterpret "his [sic] own internal messages" (214). Schizophrenia emerged as "the double bind structure comes to be a habitual expectation" (206).

Lempert (2024:63) suggests that Bateson's interest in close empirical work on psychiatry was oriented toward producing "broader lessons about human interaction." Indeed, rather than applying the structural linguistics of the day, Bateson used systems thinking in redefining communication. Shifting the focus away from referential content to form, he emphasized context, not as given but as constructed through metacommunication. Bateson's interdisciplinary team combined psychiatry, linguistics, and anthropology, enabling them to rethink biomedical and communicative perspectives simultaneously. Nevertheless, the work isolated and universalized "communication" in granting it causal status. Bateson similarly universalized models of schizophrenia, interaction, and "the family" even as he blamed women and specifically mothers for individual pathologies and social problems. It was simply assumed that "the family" was heterosexual and that "the mother" was the primary caregiver, extracting this seemingly basic unit from broader contexts of race, class, and—central to Deleuze and Guattari's (1977) reanalysis—double binds engendered by logics of capital.

A more sociopolitically informed understanding of these issues can be found in the work of a contemporaneous revolutionary psychiatrist working in France and Algeria, Fanon ([1952]2008). Even as Fanon similarly linked psychopathologies among Black and white patients to "the family," Fanon distanced himself from universalizing models by analyzing how colonialism, race, and racism shaped family patterns. Rather than emphasizing parent-child psychosexual conflicts, Fanon focused on how denigrating images of Black and Native American characters in children's literature affected children's socialization. Interaction also figured in his analysis in terms of what takes place when Black children experience racist encounters with whites, finding themselves equated with denigrating Black figures, not white heroes.

Of particular relevance to the history of research on the co-production of linguistic and health inequities is Fanon's trenchant account of the role of colonialism in structuring how white French physicians treated non-white patients, which provides a remarkably prescient model for thinking about health/communicative inequities and for doctor-patient interaction in general. He X-rayed contrastive ways doctors addressed European patients—politely, using the formal, *vous* address form, versus using the subordinating *tu* form and a speech style he called "pidgin" with Black and Arab patients. Although white French physicians who treated non-whites in France and its colonies asserted that this speech style matched their patients' way of speaking, Fanon argued that "pidgin" constituted a denigrating stereotypic language that no one spoke. Doctors justified this practice instrumentally as maximizing communicability: "Speaking to black people in this way is an attempt to reach down to them, to make them feel at ease, to make oneself understood and reassure them" ([1952]2008:15). Fanon's analysis instead suggested that it produced what I call incommunicability, constructing racialized subjects as communicationally defective and thus incapable of becoming rational actors (Briggs 2024:57).

Fanon presaged what would become one of the most visible arenas in which scholars address interfaces between communication and medicine through investigations of "doctor-patient interaction" (Heritage and Maynard 2006b). This research is analytically centered in Conversation Analysis (CA), focusing on "actual occurrences" of social interaction using "materials collected from *naturally occurring* occasions of everyday interaction by means of audio- and video-recording equipment or film" (Atkinson and Heritage 1984:2). Published texts present segments of these recordings in the form of transcripts prepared in a format designed to emphasize features of interaction.

A central focus has been on analyzing phases of clinical interactions, identified as Opening, Presenting Complaint, Examination, Diagnosis, Treatment, and Closing (Heritage and Maynard 2006a). Different types of talk and specific forms of interaction emerge in each segment. CA researchers have identified characteristics recurrent in most doctor visits as well as features associated with medical specialties, such as general practitioner encounters, gynecology, pediatrics, and cancer care. Researchers have argued that subtle changes in question wording can make a significant difference in provider-patient conversations. Heritage and Maynard (2006b:365) suggested, for example, that using the word "some" in the question "Do you have some/any other concerns you want to address today?" will cut in half the number of patient concerns that remain unaddressed.

Crucially, some contributors to the literature on clinical interaction are either practicing physicians or faculty members in medical schools. Based on his experience at Harvard Medical School, Mishler (1984) suggested that physicians use their control over questions to direct attention away from patients' "lifeworlds" and toward doctors' perspectives, thereby augmenting their authority and emphasizing technical biomedical frames. Physician-sociologist Waitzkin suggested that standardized clinical routines enable doctors to "convey ideologic messages under the rubric of scientific medicine" (1991:19). By scrutinizing a random sample of recorded interactions, Waitzkin looked closely at how physicians drew attention away from employment, family life, gender, aging, ways of coping with stress, economic insecurity, and racial and other inequities. He thus concluded that clinical encounters reproduce broader patterns of racism and other inequalities. Having practiced as a physician for over fifty years enabled him to analyze how problematic interactional features thwarted adequate care and how profit orientations, bureaucratic structures, and the power of insurance and governmental regulators thwarted the goals of doctors and patients alike (Waitzkin 2000). Another medical school faculty member, Buchbinder, explored the complex relational communicative practices used by adolescent patients, clinicians, and parents in grappling with pain (2015) and has analyzed how assisted-dying debates and practices often hinge on linguistic as much as medical ideologies (2021). Trained in the professional practice field of social work, Carr (2011) documents how clinical addiction treatment imposes dominant discursive practices as a means of producing rehabilitated subjects.

Teaching in sociology and cognitive science departments and the UC San Diego Medical School, Cicourel was a major influence on linguistic anthropology. While he shared a strongly empirical orientation and similarly recorded and closely analyzed conversations, Cicourel (1992) challenged CA practitioners' assertions that conversational recordings can be analyzed without investigating broader contexts. Rather than viewing clinical interactions as isolated artifacts, Cicourel studied, for example, how patients' interactions with nurses and physicians were successively recontextualized in physicians' notes, their conversations with other specialists, and subsequent inscriptions in charts, laboratory reports, and other documents. In this classic article, Cicourel demonstrated the impossibility of analyzing a conversation between three medical school physicians without knowing their medical specialties, the setting (a hospital microbiology lab), the activities undertaken in association with the conversation (examining laboratory specimens), previous conversations about the case, and the social and bureaucratic organization of the medical school. Cicourel asserted the need for ethnographic evidence, including observations of broader social and institutional contexts and interviews with patients, physicians, and technicians. Guzmán (2020) similarly suggested that interpreting conflict in pediatric visits between Mapuche Indigenous families and non-Indigenous physicians in Chile required ethnographically exploring the broader work required by families to access biomedical care, including their arduous process of arranging transportation.

Researchers have also used close analysis to demonstrate the interactional work that patients, family members, and other caregivers do in cases of chronic illness. Goodwin (2018) extensively videotaped interactions with his father, Chil, after a stroke had restricted his vocabulary to three words: *yes*, *no*, and *and*. Goodwin's detailed analyses showed how Chil used prosody, gesture, and the co-production of discourse with family members to remain an active participant in conversations. Rather than emphasizing his conversational and cognitive limitations as a speaker, Goodwin analyzed Chil's participation in "a distributed multiparty system organized through co-operative action" (59). Ochs studied autism spectrum disorder and agoraphobia (Capps and Ochs 1995; Ochs 2015). The autism research involved initial ethnographic observations, video recording children at school and home, and audio recordings made by the parents. Ochs and her collaborators suggested that accurately analyzing the speech of children diagnosed with high-functioning autism involved complementing CA-style analyses with ethnographic explorations of "socio-cultural dimensions of perspective-taking" (Ochs and Solomon 2004:141). Corwin (2021) assessed how older Catholic nuns used interactional strategies to support peers exhibiting symptoms of dementia in sustaining their cognitive and social engagement.

Studies of medical translation similarly direct attention to language/medicine connections. US patients who do not share a language with their providers are legally guaranteed qualified interpreters. Although designed to promote communicability, research suggests that translation can rather increase health/communicative inequities (Briggs 2017). Professional interpreters are expected to provide communicability across language differences between patients and providers. Given that they are usually more identified with the perspectives of medical professionals, however, interpreters sometimes obscure how patients question or resist professionals' efforts to control clinical interactions (Davidson 2001). Such decisions can withhold evidence that patients are displaying signs of active engagement, thereby jeopardizing their classification as good, cooperative patients and increasing the likelihood that they will be deemed incommunicable. When bilingual children are pressed into service as informal interpreters, they must deal with "managing a synchronous, multiparty interaction" (Reynolds and Orellana 2009:215) and navigating medical terminology in two languages. It is common for providers and parents alike to repay their complex efforts with "critiques of their linguistic, cognitive, social, and behavioral competencies" (221). Stepping out of the biomedical realm, Pritzker (2014) analyzes discourse practices used for translating Chinese medicine as it circulates between the United States and China.

Although research on narratives has been an important focus for linguistic anthropologists, much research on their crucial role in medicine and healing has come from medical anthropologists. Kleinman (1988) classically emphasized the importance of attuning physicians to the "illness narratives" of their patients, thereby learning not simply about the events surrounding a particular case but patients' "explanatory models" that shape how they understand them. Mattingly (1998) argued that narratives go beyond reflecting illness experiences to shape how treatment unfolds. Her sensitive work on occupational therapy analyzed how coordinated movements involving patients' and therapists' bodies act out narratives. A robust body of literature on medical education documents the central role of learning to transform patients' accounts, physical examinations, and laboratory results into brief narratives that "en-case" (Holmes and Ponte 2011) biomedical perspectives, designed to index diagnostic hypotheses and satisfy the expectations and time constraints of medical faculty (Good and DelVecchio Good 2000).

Narrativization also enters centrally into constructing epidemics. Wald (2008) traced recurrent elements of "outbreak narratives" that feature projections of a point of origin and a communicable trajectory of contagion, thereby constructing Others as threatening a vulnerable body politic. Scholars analyzed how health professionals and journalists constructed an "AIDS epidemic" narrative that stigmatized gays, Haitians, and drug users (Farmer 1992; Patton 1990). Avera (2023) showed that forms of racial violence can lead complex afterlives in biomedical practices through her analysis of how linguistic and biological projections of personal and national identity shaped epidemiological determinations as to whose blood was used for transfusions by a post-apartheid South African blood service. Briggs and Mantini-Briggs (2003) traced how public health officials and journalists created a dominant narrative around cholera cases in the Delta Amacuro rainforest of Eastern Venezuela in 1992–1993. Drawing attention away from public health authorities' failure to provide potable water, sewage facilities, and adequate healthcare, a faux narrative of "Indigenous culture" blamed Indigenous residents for spreading the disease. Many rainforest residents told narratives that pinpointed anti-Indigenous racism and governmental actions as explaining why some 500 people died from an easily prevented and treated bacterial infection. Subsequently, an outbreak of an unknown disease persisted over a year and killed thirty-eight children and young adults but remained undiagnosed by clinicians or epidemiologists. Stereotypes honed during the earlier cholera epidemic undermined professionals' willingness to listen to parents who had lost as many as three children in this new epidemic. Ultimately, a series of collective events in which parents and other residents provided detailed narrative accounts, along with clinical examination, enabled physician Mantini-Briggs to pinpoint the cause as bat-transmitted rabies (Briggs and Mantini-Briggs 2016). Attempting to sort out the catastrophic scale of the US COVID-19 pandemic and its lasting social and political effects could be aided by joining linguistic anthropologists' detailed techniques for analyzing the poetics of narratives with medical anthropologists' attunement to heterogeneous perspectives and practices emerging from complex, uncertain patterns of microbial transmission and infection (Briggs 2024).

Research has also focused on clinical encounters in non-biomedical contexts. I published two essays that studied healer-patient encounters in Delta Amacuro, Venezuela, including the treatment for a painful laceration by a stingray and a 6-year-old's severe respiratory infection (Briggs 1994, 1996). Having worked with the healers and their families for years, I was able to observe the events from the initial presentation of symptoms, the healer's conversations with patients and family members, the aftermath of the treatment, and the broader context in which they unfolded, in addition to recording the interventions and transcribing and discussing them with healers, patients, and family members. Although the exchanges about diagnosis and treatment took place in the everyday language, Warao, the healing songs themselves used a "healer's language" understood only by invisible pathogenic agents and healers. Rather than revolving narrowly around comprehension of the practitioner's words, the impact of treatment on the patients involved the effects of poetic or formal features, such as grammatical parallelism and musical features (including use of a rattle), therapeutic touch, and the transformation of the healer's body and voice into a complex bridge between human and more-than-human worlds. In these examples, poetic and referential dimensions reached beyond specific provider-patient dyads and specific illnesses to trace the effects of broader ecological, social, and political relations. I later argued that rather than simply projecting features of "Western medicine" onto non-biomedical interventions to render them intelligible, becoming attentive to the poetics of healing can provide new ways of appreciating the poetics of biomedical practice (2024:102–103).

Another important subject involves the massive shift toward digital health, including cell phones, websites, telemedicine, digital records, and social media. A couple of examples: Arnold (2020) analyzed cell phone calls through which members of a transnational family coordinated their collective emotional and practical response to a relative's terminal diagnosis. Friend (2022) documented how modesty, sex, and desire travel digitally through digital health education programs and online pornography in Senegal. Her work points to research on the role of health education and communication in global health. Anthropological research has focused on how health education and communication programs create global and local hierarchies of knowledge and the imposition of discursive and bodily practices purportedly designed to erase ignorance and "misinformation" (see for example Bulled 2015; Nguyen 2010).

The US dynamics during the COVID-19 pandemic provides a striking example. Health authorities imposed two roles on residents: 1) to passively assimilate shifting and uncertain knowledge about the new virus, faithfully adhering to official guidelines; and 2) undertake a vast burden of care, not just caring for themselves and family members (in all but severe cases) but individually devising ways to reorganize domestic spaces, education, parenting, social relations, labor, and consumption. This vast attempt to impose a unilinear, hierarchically structured health/communicative model floundered by virtue of how it contradicted decades of promoting active patient-consumers who were empowered to seek heterogeneous sources of health advice and use them in formulating self-interested strategies to improve their health and wellbeing. Conservative whites particularly resented being demoted from the active, individualist position, while the historical experiences of medical inequity and abuse sometimes led racialized communities to distrust authorities who promised, once again, to tell their members what was good for their health. Rejecting these health/communicative directives, including by attempting to participate in producing knowledge about COVID-19, became synonymous with spreading "misinformation"—and thus becoming a threat to public health (Briggs 2024; Briggs and Hallin 2024).

Conclusion: The Challenges of Boundary Crossing

In sum, despite a long-standing separation between linguistic and medical anthropology, the work I have briefly outlined has shown why it is so valuable to bring communicative and health-based perspectives into dialogue. The following chapters demonstrate how research conducted by scholars seeks to combine perspectives based in linguistic and medical anthropology and other fields in profound and exciting ways. I hope that this book will inspire new topics and perspectives. Before beginning, some readers may be new to the idea that disciplines (and subdisciplines) carve up research topics in very different ways and often defend the perspectives in which scholars have been trained as privileged ways of knowing the world. Others may view crossing these boundaries as easy and unproblematic. Moving between fields and carving out new ways of thinking is exciting and productive but also complex and challenging. I would like to contrast three types of strategies in suggesting why this type of work can sometimes generate obstacles and what can make it particularly rewarding.

Some researchers attempt to fly over (sub)disciplinary boundaries like a jet traversing different countries. To extend the metaphor, the resulting perspective promises to provide a distanced, comprehensive view of scholarly landscapes, projecting a sense of ease in moving between them and combining their professional languages and modes of inquiry. Nevertheless, this approach does not effectively engage with or tell readers much about the people who live down below. (Sub)disciplines have their own sets of presuppositions, meaning basic assumptions about what constitutes knowledge. Their members share ideas about what techniques are appropriate for conducting research, analyzing data, and assessing the validity and reliability of conclusions. As Latour (1987) and other science-and-technology scholars have demonstrated, these features are never homogeneous: disciplines are also constituted by debates and shifts over time regarding which approaches are deemed most appropriate, and they are populated by networks of scholars who support one position or another. Doing transdisciplinary research well involves learning how each (sub)discipline operates and engaging with how its practitioners not only conduct research but write about it, that is, scrutinizing its rhetorics. Claiming the privilege to use multiple disciplines without learning what makes them tick leaves these presuppositions, research methods, and textual features intact. Moreover, this mode of boundary crossing generally leads practitioners in each (sub)discipline to either look the other way or react negatively, given that such research is likely to be judged to ignore how they go about their work.

A second common approach is the pick-and-mix technique. Here researchers grab A theory and B method from X (sub)discipline and a seemingly corresponding C and D from Y field. Diverse elements are then juxtaposed to form a seemingly novel approach that ideally combines the advantages of each (sub)discipline. The result, I fear, is often a set of bad bedfellows. Component theories and research techniques involve implicit assumptions that enable them to operate and constrain their use.

Unless these differences are taken into account, the value of amplifying perspectives can be undermined by contradictions between their associated assumptions and methods, much like ordering parts manufactured for a variety of different cars and trucks and trying to use them to build an engine. Such juxtapositions make it challenging to construct a coherent and convincing argument.

A third way of doing things is more productive. Here a researcher takes the time to learn two or more (sub)disciplines thoroughly before attempting to combine them. Grasping their presuppositions and research techniques enables scholars to do more than make their work recognizable to practitioners who share them. People who operate solely within one field tend to internalize its basic assumptions and methods, coming to take them for granted. When learning two or more sets, however, their conceptual infrastructures are likely to be more consciously accessible, and it is easier to scrutinize the historical trajectories in which they came to be adopted and to evaluate their affordances, the sorts of operations they make it easier to perform, as well as their limitations. This third style of transdisciplinary research involves using this sort of critical scrutiny to transform aspects of each (sub)disciplinary infrastructure in juxtaposing them. The result can go beyond combining established fields to transform them in ways that will produce new perspectives and potentially change how scholars in each (sub)discipline do their work. I believe that this sort of work is most effective when it addresses theoretical issues head-on, often as tightly interwoven with in-depth research on specific worlds built on connections between humans and non-humans (Haraway 2008; Latour 2004).

I suggest that this is a particularly fruitful way of undertaking work that moves between linguistic and medical anthropology. As I noted, each has been characterized by forms of training and largely mutually exclusive bibliographic patterns and professional networks that make it more difficult to carry on conversations across them, let alone conduct path breaking work that spans them. These subdisciplinary conventions limit not just collaboration but research within each.

This book passes this challenge along to readers in three ways. One is by providing examples of work that moves in the direction, often implicitly, of pushing at the borders of existing modes of inquiry by examining how particular, situated phenomena are co-produced as linguistic/communicative and health/medical dimensions unfold. Another is that some chapters analyze how forms of inequity become more toxic and intractable as linguistic and medical inequities are imbricated. Beyond deepening scholarly perspectives, this type of analysis can greatly assist practitioners, policy makers, activists, and community leaders who desire health/communicative justice, that is, real change. Finally, this collection presents itself not as the final word on how this kind of work should be undertaken but as an invitation, especially addressed to students and emerging scholars, to develop the required skills and boldly launch research projects that will advance it. I have tried to play a small part here, and I will be anxiously waiting to learn how readers push it forward.

References

Alim, H. Samy, John R. Rickford, and Arnetha F. Ball, eds. 2016. *Raciolinguistics: How Language Shapes Our Ideas about Race*. New York: Oxford University Press.

Arnold, Lynnette. 2020. Cross-Border Communication and the Enregisterment of Collective Frameworks for Care. *Medical Anthropology* 39(7): pp. 624–637. https://doi.org/10.1080/01459740.2020.1717490.

Atkinson, J. Maxwell, and John Heritage. 1984. Introduction. In *Structures of Social Action*, ed. J. Maxwell Atkinson and John Heritage, pp.1–15. Cambridge: Cambridge University Press.

Avera, Emily. 2023. "Blood Has No Colour": Racialized Donor In/Ex-clusion in the South African Blood Service. *Medical Anthropology* 42(3): pp. 207–221.

Bateson, Gregory. 1972. *Steps to an Ecology of Mind*. New York: Ballantine.

Benton, Adia. 2015. *HIV Exceptionalism: Development through Disease in Sierra Leone*. Minneapolis: University of Minnesota Press.

Biehl, Joáo. 2005. *Vita: Life in a Zone of Social Abandonment*. Berkeley: University of California Press.

Briggs, Charles L. 1994. The Sting of the Ray: Bodies, Agency, and Grammar in Warao Curing. *Journal of American Folklore* 107(423): pp. 139–166.

Briggs, Charles L. 1996. The Meaning of Nonsense, the Poetics of Embodiment, and the Production of Power in Warao Shamanistic Healing. In *The Performance of Healing*, ed. Carol Laderman and Marina Roseman, pp. 185–232. New York: Routledge.

Briggs, Charles L. 2017. Towards Communicative Justice in Health. *Medical Anthropology* 36(4):287–304.

Briggs, Charles L. 2024. *Incommunicable: Toward Communicative Justice in Health and Medicine*. Durham, NC: Duke University Press.

Briggs, Charles L., and Daniel C. Hallin. 2024. *Making Health Public: How News Coverage Is Remaking Media, Medicine, and Contemporary Life*. Second edition. London: Routledge.

Briggs, Charles L., and Clara Mantini-Briggs. 2003. *Stories in the Time of Cholera: Racial Profiling during a Medical Nightmare*. Berkeley: University of California Press.

Briggs, Charles L., and Clara Mantini-Briggs. 2016. *Tell Me Why My Children Died: Rabies, Indigenous Knowledge, and Communicative Justice*. Durham, NC: Duke University Press.

Buchbinder, Mara. 2015. *All in Your Head: Making Sense of Pediatric Pain*. Oakland: University of California Press.

Buchbinder, Mara. 2021. *Scripting Death: Stories of Assisted Dying in America*. Oakland: University of California Press.

Bulled, Nicola. 2015. *Prescribing HIV Prevention: Bringing Culture into Global Health Communication*. Walnut Creek, CA: Left Coast Press.

Capps, Lisa, and Elinor Ochs. 1995. *Constructing Panic: The Discourse of Agoraphobia*. Cambridge, MA: Harvard University Press.

Carr, E. Summerson. 2011. *Scripting Addiction: The Politics of Therapeutic Talk and American Sobriety*. Princeton, NJ: Princeton University Press.

Castro, Arachu, and Merrill Singer, eds. 2004. *Unhealthy Health Policy: A Critical Anthropological Examination*. Walnut Creek, CA: AltaMira.

Cicourel, Aaron V. 1992. The Interpenetration of Communicative Contexts: Examples from Medical Encounters. In *Rethinking Context: Language as an Interactive Phenomenon*, ed. Alessandro Duranti and Charles Goodwin, pp. 291–310. Cambridge: Cambridge University Press.

Corwin, Anna I. 2021. *Embracing Age: How Catholic Nuns Became Models of Aging Well*. New Brunswick, NJ: Rutgers University Press.

Davidson, Brad 2001. Questions in Cross-Linguistic Medical Encounters: The Role of the Hospital Interpreter. *Anthropological Quarterly* 74(4):170–178.

Davis, Dána-Ain. 2019. *Reproductive Injustice: Racism, Pregnancy, and Premature Birth*. New York: NYU Press.

Deleuze, Gilles, and Féliz Guattari. 1977. *Anti-Oedipus: Capitalism and Schizophrenia*. New York: Viking.

Doucet-Battle, James 2021. *Sweetness in the Blood: Race, Risk, and Type 2 Diabe*tes. Minneapolis: University of Minnesota Press.

Fanon, Frantz. [1952]2008. *Black Skin, White Masks*, transl. Richard Philcox. New York: Grove Press.

Farmer, Paul. 1992. *AIDS and Accusation: Haiti and the Geography of Blame*. Berkeley: University of California Press.

Farmer, Paul. 1999. *Infections and Inequalities: The Modern Plagues*. Berkeley: University of California Press.

Farmer, Paul. 2004. An Anthropology of Structural Violence. *Current Anthropology* 45(3): pp. 305–325.

Friend, Juliana. 2022. "Don't Watch this Video!" Online Privacy, Porn, Sutura, and Health among Senegal's Digital Dissidents. Unpublished Ph.D. Dissertation, Department of Anthropology, University of California, Berkeley.

Good, Byron J., and Mary-Jo DelVecchio Good. 2000. "Fiction" and "Historicity" in Doctors' Stories: Social and Narrative Dimensions of Learning Medicine. In *Narrative and the Cultural Construction of Illness and Healing*, ed. Cheryl Mattingly and Linda C. Garro, pp. 50–69. Berkeley: University of California Press.

Goodwin, Chuck. 2018. *Co-Operative Action*. Cambridge: Cambridge University Press.

Graham, Laura. 2011. Quoting Mario Juruna: Linguistic Imagery and the Transformation of Indigenous Voice in the Brazilian Print Press. *American Ethnologist* 38(1): pp. 164–183.

Guzmán, Jennifer R. 2020. Time Discipline and Health/Communicative Labor in Pediatric Primary Care. *Medical Anthropology* 39(7): pp. 609–623.

Han, Clara. 2012. *Life in Debt: Times of Care and Violence in Neoliberal Chile*. Berkeley: University of California Press.

Hansen, Helena, Jules Netherland, and David Herzberg. 2023. *Whiteout: How Racial Capitalism Changed the Color of Opioids in America*. Oakland: University of California Press.

Haraway, Donna J. 2008. *When Species Meet*. Minneapolis: University of Minnesota Press.

Harries-Jones, Peter. 2016. *Upside-Down Gods: Gregory Bateson's World of Difference*. New York: Fordham University Press.

Heritage, John, and Douglas W. Maynard, eds. 2006a. *Communication in Medical Care: Interaction between Primary Care Physicians and Patients*. Cambridge: Cambridge University Press.

Heritage, John, and Douglas W. Maynard. 2006b. Problems and Prospects in the Study of Physician-Patient Interaction: 30 Years of Research. *Annual Review of Sociology* 32: pp. 351–374.

Hill, Jane H. 2008. *The Everyday Language of White Racism*. Chichester: Wiley-Blackwell.

Holmes, Seth M. 2013. *Fresh Fruit, Broken Bodies: Migrant Farmworkers in the United States*. Berkeley: University of California Press.

Holmes, Seth, and Maya Ponte. 2011. En-case-ing the Patient: Disciplining Uncertainty in Medical Student Patient Presentations. *Culture, Medicine, and Psychiatry* 335(2): pp. 163–182.

Inoue, Miyako. 2003. The Listening Subject of Japanese Modernity and His Auditory Double: Citing, Sighting, and Siting the Modern Japanese Woman. *Cultural Anthropology* 18(2): pp. 156–193.

Kleinman, Arthur. 1988. *The Illness Narratives: Suffering, Healing and the Human Condition*. New York: Basic.

Kroskrity, Paul V. 2015. Discursive Discriminations in the Representation of Western Mono and Yokuts Stories: Confronting Narrative Inequality and Listening to Indigenous Voices in Central California. In *The Legacy of Dell Hymes*, ed. Paul V. Kroskrity and Anthony K. Webster, pp. 135–163. Bloomington, IN: Indiana University Press.

Kroskrity, Paul V. 2021. Covert Linguistic Racisms and the (Re-)Production of White Supremacy. *Journal of Linguistic Anthropology* 31(2): pp. 180–193.

Latour, Bruno. 1987. *Science in Action: How to Follow Scientists and Engineers through Society*. Cambridge, MA: Harvard University Press.

Latour, Bruno. 2004. *Politics of Nature: How to Bring the Sciences into Democracy*. Cambridge, MA: Harvard University Press.

Mattingly, Cheryl. 1998. *Healing Dramas and Clinical Plots: The Narrative Structure of Experience*. Cambridge: Cambridge University Press

Meek, Barbra. 2006. And the Injun Goes How! Representations of American Indian English in (White) Public Space. *Language in Society* 35(1): pp. 93–128.

Meek, Barbra. 2013. The Voice of (White) Reason: Enunciations of Difference, Authorship Interpellation, and Jokes. In *Confronting the Past and Constructing the Present: Language Ideology and Identity. Papers in Honor of Jane H. Hill*, ed. Shannon T. Bischoff, Debbie Cole, Amy V. Foundation, and Mizuki Miyashita, pp. 339–363. Amsterdam: John Benjamins.

Mishler, Elliot. 1984. *The Discourse of Medicine: Dialectics of Medical Interviews*. Norwood, NJ: Ablex.

Moran-Thomas, Amy. 2019. *Traveling with Sugar: Chronicles of a Global Epidemic*. Oakland: University of California Press.

Nguyen, Vinh-Kim. 2010. *The Republic of Therapy: Triage and Sovereignty in West Africa's Time of AIDS*. Durham, NC: Duke University Press.

Ochs, Elinor. 2015. Corporeal Reflexivity and Autism. *Integrative Psychological and Behavioral Science* 15(2): pp. 275–287.

Ochs, Elinor, and Olga Solomon. 2004. Introduction: Discourse and Autism. *Discourse Studies* 6(2): pp. 139–146.

Patton, Cindy. 1990. *Inventing AIDS*. New York: Routledge.

Perley, Bernard C. 2011. *Defying Maliseet Language Death: Emergent Vitalities of Language, Culture and Identity in Eastern Canada*. Lincoln: University of Nebraska Press.

Pritzker, Sonya. 2014. *Living Translation: Language and the Search for Resonance in U.S. Chinese Medicine*. Oxford: Berghahn Books.

Reynolds, Jennifer F., and Marjorie Faulstich Orellana. 2009. New Immigrant Youth Interpreting in White Public Space. *American Anthropologist* 111(2): pp. 211–223.

Rosa, Jonathan and Nelson Flores. 2020. Reimagining Race and Language: From Raciolinguistic Ideologies to a Raciolinguistic Perspective. In *The Oxford Handbook of Language and Race*, ed. H. Samy Alim, Angela Reyes, and Paul V. Kroskrity, pp. 90–107. New York: Oxford University Press.

Rouse, Carolyn Moxley. 2009. *Uncertain Suffering: Racial Health Care Disparities and Sickle Cell Disease*. Berkeley: University of California Press.

Sangaramoorthy, Thurka 2014. *Treating AIDS: Politics of Difference, Paradox of Prevention*. New Brunswick, NJ: Rutgers University Press.

Scheper-Hughes, Nancy. 1992. *Death without Weeping: The Violence of Everyday Life in Brazil*. Berkeley: University of California Press.

Singer, Merrill, Nicola Bulled, Bayla Ostrach, and Emily Mendenhall. 2017. Syndemics and the Biosocial Conception of Health. *The Lancet* 389(10072): pp. 941–950.

Smedley, Brian D., Adrienne Y. Stith, and Alan Nelson, eds. 2003. *Unequal Treatment: Confronting Racial and Ethnic Disparities in Health Care*. Washington, DC: National Academies Press.

Van Ryn, Michelle, and Jane Burke. 2000. The Effect of Patient Race and Socio-Economic Status on Physicians' Perceptions of Patients. *Social Science and Medicine* 50(6): pp. 813–828.

Waitzkin, Howard. 1991. *The Politics of Medical Encounters: How Patients and Doctors Deal with Social Problems*. New Haven, CT: Yale University Press.

Waitzkin, Howard. 2000. *The Second Sickness: Contradictions of Capitalist Health Care*. Lanham, MA: Rowman and Littlefield.

Wald, Priscilla. 2008. *Contagious: Cultures, Carriers, and the Outbreak Narrative*. Durham, NC: Duke University Press.

Key Concepts in Language and Health

Lynnette Arnold, Jennifer R. Guzmán, Emily Avera and Anna I. Corwin

Why Language and Health?

At first glance, the relationship between language and health may seem straightforward. After all, language is a human universal. All people use language to communicate and do so every day. Similarly, people everywhere navigate health challenges, whether their own or those of loved ones, from minor ailments like a scraped knee to more significant concerns, including chronic and life-threatening diseases. The connections between these two pan-human experiences of language and health include clinical interaction, medical interpretation, and public health messaging but are also deeper and more far-reaching, as illustrated by the following examples from classic research in this area.

Many health problems involve the deterioration of language capacities. Language difficulties can be a telltale sign of cognitive change and may lead people to seek creative new ways of communicating (Goodwin 2010).

Familiar storylines, such as that of a detective sleuthing for clues, are pervasive in medicine and help doctors to explain, for example, the need for testing when a diagnosis is elusive (Mattingly 2010). Relatedly, metaphors play a critical role in how people conceptualize what happens to the body in illness and in treatment (Buchbinder 2015). Infections are imagined as invasions to be fought. Bodies are imagined as machines that can be fixed by installing new parts.

The ways that people narrate their experiences of illness can also hold clues about how a disease works. For example, patterns in the stories told by an agoraphobic woman revealed the sorts of circumstances that were triggering her panic attacks (Capps and Ochs 1997). In other contexts, personal storytelling can be an essential component of recovery (Carr 2011).

For many individuals and communities, sacred texts and prayer practices are critical healing resources. Ritual healing differs greatly across religious traditions and may involve practices such as laying on of hands, prayer, incantation, and divination (Csordas 1997; Dein 2002; Perrino 2002).

Even the incidence of disease can be impacted by the ways that particular kinds of stories circulate. Hong Kong saw a sudden rise in anorexia cases following the widely publicized death of 14-year-old Charlene Hsu Chi Ying from the disease (Watters 2010).

Lynnette Arnold et al, *Key Concepts in Language and Health*. In: *Language and Health in Action*. Edited by: Lynnette Arnold et al., Oxford University Press.
DOI: 10.1093/9780198933953.002.0002

And when certain people's medical knowledge is treated as authoritative and others' is ignored or silenced, this can determine who receives medical care and who is viewed as culpable during epidemics (Briggs and Mantini-Briggs 2016, 2004).

This book explores a broad range of ways that language matters for health, care, and healing. We examine **health/communicative inequities** (Briggs 2017), or the ways that language is implicated in patterns of illness and death that reflect and exacerbate social inequalities. The chapters relate richly descriptive and powerful stories of individuals and communities, revealing how they use language to grapple with structural inequities in their everyday lived experiences of navigating ill-health and seeking wellbeing.

How Does This Book Define and Approach Language?

The examples above reveal that language does things in the world. Language is more than simply a means of communicating information from one person to another. Language is a tool for acting in the world in multiple—and sometimes contradictory—ways. People use not only written, spoken, or signed words, but also gestures, facial expressions, tone of voice, images, emojis, and more, all of which we consider to be part of language. Language acts in specific contexts, and these social actions are negotiated in the immediate moment between interlocutors as well as over longer time spans and across communities as the meanings of language change.

To understand the remarkable flexibility of language, this section lays out a thought experiment, taking on the perspective of Carlos, a 4-year-old boy in Southern Chile who was feeling sick. On the day when the interaction below was recorded, Carlos's mother, Mariana, had brought him from their family farm to see a doctor, Delia, at the nearest public clinic (see Guzmán 2015 for a description of the study). Example 1 is a transcription, translated from Spanish, of the start of Carlos's doctor visit. To identify how much knowledge is required to make sense of this interaction, we begin by focusing on the details of the immediate interaction and then add more layers of cultural and historical context to develop deeper understandings.

Example 1

(01) Dr Delia:	Cuente nomás. ¿Qué le pasa a su bebé?	Just tell [me]. What's going on with your little one?
(02) Mariana:	El Carlos está con una tos. Eh ayer del- del jardín volvió así como decaído.	Carlos has a cough. Um yesterday from- from preschool he returned looking kind of fatigued.
(03) Dr Delia:	Ya.	Alright.

(04) Mariana:	Y en la noche estuvo con mucha mucha tos y-	And at night he was coughing a whole lot and-
(05) Dr Delia:	Ya. ¿Pero la tos sequita? ¿O tos como con desgarro?	Alright. But a dry cough? Or a cough like with phlegm.
(06) Mariana:	Claro. Con desgarro.	Right. With phlegm.
(07) Dr Delia:	Ya. ¿Fiebre tuvo o no?	Alright. Did he have a fever or not?
(08) Mariana:	Eh:, estaba- tenía la carita toda coloradita.	Um, he was- his little face was all flushed.
(09) Dr Delia:	Eso. ¿Pero no tiene termómetro en la casa?	Sure. But don't you have a thermometer at home?
(10) Mariana:	No. Se le quebró el termómetro-	No. The thermometer broke-
(11) Dr Delia:	Hay que tener un termómetro por los niñitos chicos. La única forma de objetivar la fiebre es con la temperatura.	One needs to have a thermometer for little kids. The only way to objectively identify a fever is with the temperature.

This dialogue is likely familiar to anyone who has consulted a doctor. But how might Carlos, who is just learning to use language in this context, make sense of this interaction? He might notice that the doctor asked about him but posed the question to his mother. He might wonder why his mother's answer was only about his cough. Why didn't she mention to the doctor that Carlos was in charge of sweeping the floor at home? He might also wonder why his mother didn't ask the doctor how she was doing. Wasn't that the polite thing to do? Through his participation in this and future doctor's visits, Carlos is learning norms of medical encounters. For instance, in this kind of activity, questions are medically focused and shaped by unspoken but powerful rules about who knows what, who should talk about what and when, and how each person should behave (cf. Stivers 2012). These implicit rules of language use are critical to how care is accomplished in a clinical setting.

Notably, language often does more than one thing at a time. Some functions may be explicit, while others are not. For instance, asking someone "what's going on" elicits an answer but also signals that the question asker has the right to ask the question and to expect an answer. In a clinical encounter, doctors are expected to ask such things of a patient or patient's caregiver, but not vice versa. This asymmetry in question asking is one of the communicative dimensions through which medical authority is maintained (Wilce 2009). A language user need not intend or even be aware of a particular consequence in order for it to happen. When doctors ask their patients "what's going on", they likely do not intend to reproduce power imbalances, but their patterned ways of using language nevertheless have this consequence.

People thus use language to accomplish work in the world that goes far beyond simply conveying information. Indeed, as we see in this example where a simple question is not merely a medical inquiry but also encodes hierarchy, the implicit meanings that language conveys are often far more consequential for the ways language acts in the world. Moreover, this work of language is collaboratively accomplished. For instance, unspoken rules in clinical encounters require participation from both doctors and patients. If Mariana had asked Dr Delia, "How are you doing?", the doctor might respond to the unusual question (perhaps after a brief pause) with a perfunctory answer ("I'm fine"), and then turn the interaction back to the medical task at hand. And if Mariana had told Dr Delia that Carlos was in charge of sweeping at home, the doctor might briefly acknowledge this but would surely return to discussing symptoms, as she did with her series of questions about Carlos's cough and the likelihood of fever. Saying that "language does things" means that people do things together with language.

Focusing only on people's roles in a given activity (for example as patients, parents, or doctors) does not fully capture the work language is doing. To illustrate this, we bring more detail to the thought experiment about Carlos's medical visit. Carlos and Mariana are Mapuche (the largest Native/Indigenous group in the Southern Cone of South America). At home their family speaks both Spanish and Mapuzungun, the Mapuche language. Dr Delia is Chilean but not Mapuche, and speaks only Spanish. Carlos might notice that his mother refrains from using Mapuzungun with the doctor. He is learning about bilingualism, the social power of different languages, and the strategic practice of code switching.

At 4 years old, Carlos may be only starting to notice the discriminatory stereotypes that circulate in Chile about Mapuche people, but Mariana is certainly aware of them. She likely tailors her talk with Dr Delia very carefully, doing her best to demonstrate that she speaks Spanish well and is a responsible caregiver to her son. In this way Mariana may hope to avoid the kind of implicit criticism underlying Dr Delia's question, "Don't you have a thermometer at home?".

Understanding the ideal of objectivity in biomedicine and the historical context of this interaction can also help illuminate why Dr Delia insisted on the importance of having a thermometer at home. This visit was recorded in July of 2009, during the height of the influenza A (H1N1) pandemic. In Chile, official diagnostic criteria for the disease included a fever of 38.5 degrees Celsius, a threshold that supported differential diagnosis, distinguishing potential cases of influenza A (H1N1) from more common respiratory diseases. By raising the issue of temperature taking, Carlos's doctor was attempting to comply with public health protocols to identify possible outbreaks.

As this thought experiment about Carlos's medical care illustrates, many contextual and historical factors shape talk about health. In addition to medical ideals, clinical protocols, and public health policies, socially significant differences such as race, ethnicity, gender, sexuality, class, ability, and neurodiversity also influence how health practitioners interact with patients. For instance, those who present as female and of reproductive age may routinely be asked "are you pregnant or might you be pregnant?" regardless of whether they have a uterus or engage in heterosexual intercourse. In the United States, physicians are more likely to dismiss the pain of Black women because of racist and dehumanizing stereotypes about their strength and fortitude (Davis 2019; Fabien 2017; Hoffman et al. 2016; Owens 2017), and gay men from communities of color are far less likely to be prescribed life-saving pre-exposure prophylaxis (PrEP) treatment for HIV than their white counterparts (Sullivan 2024). Attending to these multiple, often intersecting differences is important, because the unspoken rules that shape language use are informed by underlying beliefs about social difference that are held in a given community, region, or nation at a particular moment in time.

These rules are simultaneously conventional and variable. For instance, if five people were asked to explain how to properly talk to a doctor, they would likely come up with five different answers. Similarly, communities often develop their own specific ways of using language in relation to health, as illustrated in this chapters 9 and 8 by Black and Marsilli-Vargas. Notwithstanding these differences, doctors expect patients and their caregivers to conform to norms for talk in clinical settings. Patients who fail to do so may be misunderstood, rebuked, or denied care (Guzmán 2020).

Language is everywhere, working in patterned and variable ways that often escape notice, actively building the world. In the remainder of this section, we outline five key concepts that together can reveal the sometimes subtle but always powerful ways that language acts: history, perception, categories, intersectionality, and contestation (Rosa and Flores 2017). This framework comes from research on race and language, and we adopt it here because racialized people—like Carlos, Mariana, and other Mapuche people—often face serious health disparities. Applying these concepts to thinking about language and health can help to develop greater awareness about where, when, and among whom racial inequities—and indeed inequalities of all kinds—shape experiences of illness and wellbeing.

The first important concept is **history**. It is easy to be pulled in by the immediacy of language, the fact that it is unfolding in a particular moment in time. But the unspoken rules that shape how language is used emerged from specific historical conditions rife with inequalities. For instance, in this volume, Krugman and Rafiq (Chapter 7) discuss how different terms used to refer to cancer in Tanzania reflect colonial history as well as the contemporary dominance of English in biomedicine.

A historical understanding of language also draws attention to a second important dimension: that of **perception**. Discussions of language tend to focus on its production in speech, texts, signs, and so on. Focusing on perception highlights the different sorts of filters, or taken for granted beliefs, that shape how particular instances of language are interpreted. For instance, as Lee demonstrates (see Chapter 2) clinicians can have different beliefs about the extent to which patients themselves can or should articulate pain and symptoms in words. These ideas about the linguistic expressibility of illness shape how healers listen to patients' words and how they interact with their bodies.

It is not only individuals who perceive language through the filters of these beliefs. Institutions also perceive particular forms of language use as evidence of illness. For instance, trans and non-binary individuals who wish to access gender-affirming care are often required to first be diagnosed with gender dysphoria. To be diagnosed, an individual must meet specific criteria that are laid out in the *Diagnostic and Statistical Manual of Mental Disorders*. These criteria include that the person articulates particular kinds of distress related to their body and gender identity. This diagnostic process categorizes trans and non-binary gender expressions as pathology.

While the beliefs that guide perception of language use may appear just to be about language, ultimately, they are always rooted in beliefs about people, revealing the third concept: **categories**. One of the primary ways that language acts in the world is by making it seem like people naturally and inherently belong to certain groups, spanning racial or ethnic designations to nationality, to categories such as 'addict' or 'cancer survivor'. People can use this categorizing power explicitly by claiming particular identities or by ascribing them to others, as Noblewolf and Wolf show (see Chapter 1).

But language creates categories in far more subtle ways than this, often through implicit assumptions that are associated with particular ways of speaking. For instance, research in France found that when a patient's speech suggested they were from a lower socioeconomic class or might lack formal education, clinicians disclosed less to them about their prognoses (Fainzang 2015). Such perceptions are pervasive but occur mostly below the threshold of conscious awareness. Categorization thus often happens without explicit intent or even awareness on the part of the people who are interacting with one another.

Language can sort people into more than one category at once, with each category shaping how individuals experience other categories. The fourth key concept, **intersectionality**, emerges from the work of Black feminist scholars and activists in the United States (Combahee River Collective 1977; Crenshaw 1991). They pushed against the exclusion of Black women from conversations about gender, which historically focused on the experiences of white women; and from conversations about race, which focused on men's experiences. Instead, they emphasized that people encounter the world from a complex positionality that involves intersecting forms of oppression and privilege, shaped by deeply historical systems of oppression. For instance, as Keeney Parks demonstrates (see Chapter 3), in US clinical contexts, there are strong expectations for how patients should respond to clinician's questions that are based on neurotypical ways of interacting and white cultural norms. The linguistic practices of neurodivergent patients and patients of color may therefore be misunderstood, stigmatized, or even viewed as a marker of disease. Because these perceptions are encoded in diagnostic manuals and socialized in medical training, they work in aggregate and over time to reproduce intersectional inequalities.

Although language is often used in ways that shore up inequalities, it is also a resource for **contestation**. This fifth concept spotlights how language is used to resist discrimination, stigmatization, and inequities. This is not to say that language alone can remediate systemic injustices, but rather that looking through the lens of language can reveal patterns of resistance and resilience that might otherwise go unnoticed. For instance, in Chapter 10, Shohet and Schmidt's analysis of the personal narratives told by a Black man living with chronic kidney disease highlights his subtle but strong criticism of the role of racism in his illness experience.

While each of the chapters in this volume introduces additional ways of thinking about language in health-related contexts, these five key concepts can always be incorporated as additional analytics to gain deeper insights into how language is involved in care and healing.

How Does This Book Define and Approach Health?

Health is a phenomenon that exists on multiple scales, from the microscopic to the planetary. It is simultaneously larger and smaller than any individual. At one level, health is situated in the body. Over a lifetime, a person grows through developmental stages, sustains injuries, contracts illnesses and recovers from them, makes choices and engages in activities that impact these processes, and ultimately dies. Yet this is not the whole story. Human bodies are microcosms where populations of bacteria flourish. These are in turn sustained by plants and animals that are eaten and become part of the body, blurring the boundaries of what constitutes the individual. Health is also constituted through networks of social relations that include kin and friends but also many others who play integral roles: scientists researching new drugs, regulators working to limit air pollution, workers across the food system, legislators writing laws that shape access to resources, and the many nonhuman beings whose flourishing impacts and is impacted by humans. Because of these many interdependencies, health can be investigated multidimensionally and at many scales, including family, community, nation-state, ecosystem, and global society.

Just as health is a broad phenomenon, so too there are multiple dimensions and scales of ill-health. **Disease** is a term that refers to any pathological condition of the body. Observable and measurable with techniques such as palpation and with tools that include thermometers, stethoscopes, x-rays, and blood tests, diseases are diagnosable according to characteristic symptoms. The term **illness** refers to an individual's subjective experience of being unwell, regardless of whether they have been diagnosed with a disease. Because illness is a universal human experience, communities in every part of the world and at every time in history have come up with explanatory models to make sense of illness experiences. Although they do not necessarily align with particular diseases, models of illness are important because they shape how people experience, respond, and behave when they feel they are ill. A third important term, **sickness**, refers to the ways that ill-health constitutes a social problem. Scholars use the term to talk about the social interruptions that are caused by ill-health, including the ways that a given community handles these disruptions. **Stigma**, the social blame or shaming that is associated with having certain diseases or illness, is a common social response to sickness. For example, people may be judged for their behaviors when they have a sexually transmitted infection or diseases that are associated with diet or smoking (Brewis and Wutich 2019).

Healing practices, medical treatments, and other therapies generally address one or more aspects of disease, illness, or sickness. A given intervention may aim to determine the nature of a health problem, to identify its cause, to cure a disease or stop its spread across the population, to alleviate symptoms or minimize an individual's suffering, or to address the disruption that the health problem causes to a family or community. As a result, measures and perceptions of efficacy vary, depending on how well the intervention accomplishes particular goals, even if it does not resolve every aspect of the health problem. Language is crucial to these healing processes, as shown in chapters in this volume by Mack, Morales Ramirez, and Goodwin and colleagues.

The achievement of good health and the resolution of health problems are social accomplishments that generally require **care**. Care is enacted by people from family members to professionals and takes place across highly diverse settings, from homes to rehabilitation centers to hospitals. Care can be multidirectional, for example involving multiple parties attending to each other's needs; or unidirectional, when one person provides care and another person receives care (Corwin 2020). Requiring time and attention for the needs of others, care is fundamentally a form of labor. This labor includes not only physical tasks such as bathing or giving injections but also the communicative work involved in providing care and in maintaining the relationships that form the basis of care (Arnold 2021, 2024). It also requires access to resources which are often distributed in ways that are tied to hierarchical social structures. Surgeons and other physicians, for example, are often well paid and benefit from high social prestige. By comparison, others who perform critical care work such as nurses, medical interpreters, and home care workers, are less well paid and do not enjoy the same social prestige. Their vital contributions often go unrecognized, as does the necessary but unpaid care work of relatives and friends. Language is central to the ways that some forms of care are recognized and valued, while others are ignored or actively erased (Arnold and Black 2020).

In caring for the sick, across time, people everywhere have developed remarkably diverse ways of cultivating health and treating illness. For example, communities have learned about the medicinal properties of plants and have kept that knowledge alive across generations (see Chapter 12 by Faudree) as well as developing diverse forms of expertise for collaboratively addressing such universal human experiences as childbirth, injury, and aging (Corwin 2021).

The contemporary world is thus characterized by **medical pluralism**, the coexistence of many, diverse systems for healing. One consequence of the globalization of formerly localized medical traditions is a need for novel forms of translation, not only of words but of medical concepts, models of the human body, and practitioner training (Pritzker 2014). Notably, not all medical traditions are viewed as legitimate. In a given setting, the practice of some forms of medicine may be considered indispensable, while others are illegalized, stigmatized, or viewed as superstition.

One particular tradition has gained greater dominance and prestige than any other on a global scale. This system of medicine is rooted in the invention of science as an ostensibly objective means of studying the world, and gained a strong foothold in Europe in the nineteenth century when approaches to diagnosis and treatment became more standardized and effective. This medical system has been referred to with many names, including Western medicine, allopathic medicine, conventional medicine, scientific medicine, and **biomedicine**. The conventionalization of this medical tradition involved the emergence of new institutions, the hospital and the clinic, which have become the primary places many people go for treatment.

The primary goal of biomedicine is to treat and cure disease, and astounding achievements have been made toward eradicating diseases and ameliorating human health, thanks to the work of biomedical science. Notably, however, the invention and global dominance of biomedicine is also closely tied to histories of colonial domination and capitalism. **Colonialism** describes a nation-state or empire's establishment and maintenance of political control and exploitation of another territory and its population. Historically, colonial and imperialist projects intensified global commerce, as colonizers made settler claims to land, resources, and human societies to extract raw materials using enslaved and indentured labor forces and to open new markets for trade and consumption. All of these processes laid the groundwork for the global expansion of **capitalism**, a term that refers to the organization of an economy around the generation of profit by privatizing the ownership of property and the means of production, and through free market exchange of goods and services. Today, profit-driven medical industries are among the most lucrative in the world.

While it is important to remember that early science was not solely a European pursuit, and the development of biomedicine has led to many life-saving technologies, it is useful to understand that many of the cultural practices from the scientific revolution and the development of early European biomedical practices were closely tied to colonial rule. For example, from the seventeenth century onward, as Europeans encountered different groups of people in newly colonized provinces, they tried to make sense of contrasts in appearance and practices. Hypotheses emerged positing that people in different parts of the world were actually distinct subspecies or races of humans. Purported evidence for this bogus idea came from observed distinctions concerning arbitrary physical and biological features. At the same time, European scholars of language took interest in the linguistic diversity that characterized colonial frontiers. They wrongly assumed that Indigenous languages were unsophisticated and concluded that speakers of these languages were therefore less evolved. These invented hierarchies of racial superiority and inferiority were then leveraged to justify conquest and colonial domination. Racial classifications, buttressed by spurious linguistic theories, were used to argue that certain groups' vulnerability to disease signaled inherent biological weakness and inferior knowledge. This rationale obscured the fact that colonizing settlers themselves often transmitted infections, as when Europeans brought smallpox, measles, and typhus to the Americas, triggering epidemics of massive proportions.

Even today, harmful narratives that arose from colonial domination persist in stereotypes that associate impoverished and racialized communities with incommunicability, immorality, and unhygienic practices, implying that they are to blame for the spread of disease (Avera 2023; Briggs 2024; Briggs and Mantini-Briggs 2004; Chun 2020; Farmer 2001). These characterizations often inform public health campaigns and reinforce misleading perceptions about the former colonies of the Global South as dependent upon medical expertise from the Global North.

On the contrary, however, all communities historically developed knowledge about health and healing from their participation in a given ecosystem. Over time and through careful observation and experimentation, people learned to manage illnesses that were endemic where they lived, helping community members to recover and survive. This knowledge often circulated in spoken or written form relatively freely among kin and (often female) friendship networks (Gevirtz 2024). The invention of laboratory science radically altered these communicative chains, shifting the locus of expertise from family and community into the rarified professional and academic realm, where medicines came to be treated as trade secrets. The case of anti-malarial medications is illustrative. From long before colonization, Indigenous communities in what is now Peru used cinchona tree bark as an effective fever treatment. They shared this knowledge with Jesuit missionaries, who conveyed the information back to Europe, where laboratory scientists isolated quinine (an alkaloid) from cinchona. As the first effective anti-malarial drug, quinine helped to expand imperial projects from the Americas to tropical Africa, where colonial administrators and soldiers were now able to survive the disease. Discursively, the development of quinine as a novel biomedical product also served to rationalize colonization as a benevolent and civilizing force (Greene et al. 2019).

Ethical standards have been developed in contemporary times to minimize harm related to the development and testing of new drugs. For example, bioethical safeguards concerning the risks of experimental medications are managed in part by regulated language practices of disclosure and informed consent in clinical trials. Alongside these protective efforts, however, the circulation of information about medications and medical technology is also heavily regulated, by patents for example, and most drugs (many derived from plants) are commodities, produced by pharmaceutical companies that generate profits from their sale. In this system, the knowledge of Indigenous communities about medicinal plants is still frequently exploited (see Chapter 12), and commodified medical treatments are distributed not according to need but according to wealth.

Nearly everywhere in the world today, healthcare providers serve diverse populations, posing another challenge to equitable care. This diversity stems from human migration, accelerated by geopolitical conflict, climate change, and the globalized economy. Health organizations utilize a range of strategies to provide care and disseminate information under these circumstances. Some approaches involve the provision of medical interpretation (see Chapter 5) and multilingual health information (see Chapter 4). Other strategies have been developed under the model of cross-cultural medicine, often involving language-centered interventions such as multilingual signage, bilingual intercultural facilitators (see Chapter 6), and cultural competency training for staff (Guzmán 2024). While well intentioned, cultural competency programs can reinforce stereotypes, marking certain kinds of patients as deviating from the unmarked norm of the presumably culture-less patient (Jenks 2011). Following critiques, some programs now focus on unpacking how institutional medicine's "culture of no culture" is, in fact, deeply cultural, characterized by a particular set of values, norms, and ways of using language (Metzl and Hansen 2014; Taylor 2003).

Ultimately, both wellbeing and ill-health emerge from constellations of social and environmental factors that impact who is more or less likely to enjoy good health, become sick, receive care, access treatment, and recover. These factors, often referred to as **social determinants of health**, include such things as working conditions, pollution, and access to shelter, water, food, and vaccines. They also include matters of social distribution such as access to health information, medical care, and interpretation. Some scholars use an alternative term, **structural determinants of health**, to emphasize the interlocking, institutionalized, and historical patterns of oppression that shape health outcomes and determine the distribution of health resources. For example, chronic diarrheal disease, which plagues populations around the world, is a health problem that stems not from residents' identity or beliefs but from structural systems, including access to clean water and communication about water safety (see Chapter 11). Epidemiological patterns like this illustrate the workings of **structural violence**, forms of harm that result from the ways that economies, public policies, and social institutions are organized.

Ultimately, considering the many ways that structural forces impact how people flourish, live, age, experience illness, and die raises important questions about health (in)equity and health justice. The chapters in this volume explore these issues across scales and in different settings, giving dedicated attention to the ways that language and communication impact how people pursue health, address illness, and care for one another.

What Is an Ethnographic Approach to Language and Health?

This book brings together perspectives from researchers working on questions of language and health in a range of contexts around the globe. While the approaches taken in each chapter vary, the book as a whole demonstrates the importance of combining close attention to language use with the broader insights from **ethnography**. Along with other methods, such as interviewing, ethnographers spend an extended time at a research site, getting to know people and accompanying them in their lives through **participant observation**.

While the goal of research is to generate knowledge, it is important to reiterate that there is no view from nowhere (Black and Riner 2022). All research is the result of specific decisions made in the design and conduct of the investigation. This is as true for **qualitative** studies, such as those that characterize this volume, as it is for **quantitative** studies that are based on epidemiological statistics (population-level data on disease patterns) or other kinds of big data. While it is tempting to imagine quantitative approaches as more **objective**, these studies are shaped by researchers' decisions about what to count, how to count it, what to leave uncounted, and what to compare once things are counted. Once correlations are identified, making sense of these correlations is also an exercise in interpretation. Every one of these decisions involves **subjective** processes in which researchers' perspectives shape their findings in ways that are seldom acknowledged. Ethnographic research, on the other hand, aims to make researchers' decisions and perspectives transparent by including information about researchers' identities, their involvement in the community, their research objectives, and the sources of evidence on which their findings rest.

For those unfamiliar with ethnography, this approach may seem anecdotal, relying too much on single case studies. But ethnographic analysis, when conducted systematically, is a method that enables the identification of social patterns. The particular examples provided in written reports such as the chapters of this book are representative examples that illustrate these patterns. Through rigorous and sustained observation, documentation, recording, and careful analysis, ethnography can capture nuance and advance explanations about the social negotiation of health and illness that quantitative approaches cannot. Statistical analyses can capture correlations, but not the "how" or "why" of such correlations, questions that are at the heart of ethnographic research.

Ethnographic studies of language and health connect individual and community experiences with larger historical and social processes. These approaches illuminate how people act individually and together, while also showing how social institutions from governments and religious organizations to hospitals and medical schools shape encounters and experiences. In these ways, language-based ethnographies provide a window into how patterned moments are connected to people's lives, broader histories, structures of oppression, and medical cultures.

This book presents a collection of new research by scholars who are advancing understanding of how language shapes illness experience, medicine, care, and wellbeing. We aim to equip readers with tools and examples to better understand the intersections of language and health that they will encounter throughout life, whether as healthcare professionals or scholars, as familial or paid caregivers, or simply as individuals navigating what it means to be alive in a human body.

Questions for Reflection and Discussion

Reflection Question

1. Reflect on the two key terms of this book: language and health. Which of these terms do you feel that you know more about at this moment? Where does your knowledge come from? Be sure to include both formal education as well as life experiences that may have shaped what you know.
2. This chapter introduces many examples illustrating complex interactions between language and health. Which examples resonate most with you and why? What stands out about these cases and makes them interesting?

Looking In: Small Group Discussion Questions

1. Consider the example from the chapter of the first few minutes of a medical consultation for Carlos, a young boy from Southern Chile. What norms of clinical interaction were at play? How did the participants' roles shape their interaction? How did their social identities shape the interaction? In what ways did events in global health shape how the visit unfolded?
2. What are the five key concepts (adapted from raciolinguistics) that help us to understand how language acts in the world? For each key concept, give an example from the reading or elsewhere about how this concept leads to insights about language and health?
3. Health problems can be divided into matters of disease, illness, and sickness. What does each of these terms refer to? In what ways might they overlap? What differentiates them?
4. The authors of this chapter argue that understanding matters of health and language requires attention to colonialism and capitalism. Explain why this is the case. In your answer, identify two examples from the chapter that illustrate how those historical processes have shaped disease, medicine, or care.
5. What is medical pluralism? Which medical system is used most widely today? What are some of the factors that led to the global dominance of this system?

6. The approach to language and health that these authors present emphasizes attention to inequities. Choose the two terms from the chapter that you find most useful for thinking about inequities related to language and health. Explain why you chose these two concepts.
7. The authors suggest that ethnographic approaches can reveal different kinds of insights than quantitative studies do. What are the possibilities and limitations of each of these approaches?

Looking Out: Large Group Discussion Question

1. Why is it useful to think about language and health together? What might change if more workers in healthcare, parents, policy makers, voters, religious and community leaders, journalists, and people experiencing illness thought about language and health together?

References

Arnold, Lynnette. 2021. Communication as Care across Borders: Forging and Co-Opting Relationships of Obligation in Transnational Salvadoran Families. *American Anthropologist* 123(1): pp. 137–149. http://dx.doi.org/10.1111/aman.13517.

Arnold, Lynnette. 2024. Living Together across Borders: Communicative Care in Transnational Salvadoran Families. Oxford Studies in the Anthropology of Language. Oxford: Oxford University Press.

Arnold, Lynnette, and Steven P. Black. 2020. How Communicative Approaches Enrich the Study of Care. *Medical Anthropology* 39(7): pp. 573–581. https://doi.org/10.1080/01459740.2020.1814285.

Avera, Emily. 2023. "Blood Has No Colour": Racialized Donor In/Ex-clusion in the South African National Blood Service. *Medical Anthropology* 42(3): pp. 207–221. https://doi.org/10.1080/01459740.2023.2187295.

Black, Steven P., and Robin Conley Riner. 2022. Care as a Methodological Stance: Research Ethics in Linguistic Anthropology. In *Research Methods in Linguistic Anthropology*, ed. Sabina M. Perrino and Sonya E. Pritzker, pp. 97–123. London: Bloomsbury Academic.

Brewis, Alexandra A., and Amber Wutich. 2019. *Lazy, Crazy, and Disgusting: Stigma and the Undoing of Global Health*. Baltimore: Johns Hopkins University Press.

Briggs, Charles L. 2017. Towards Communicative Justice in Health. *Medical Anthropology* 36(4): pp. 287–304. doi: 10.1080/01459740.2017.1299721.

Briggs, Charles L. 2024. *Incommunicable: Toward Communicative Justice in Health and Medicine*. Durham, NC: Duke University Press.

Briggs, Charles L., and Clara Mantini-Briggs. 2004. *Stories in the Time of Cholera: Racial Profiling during a Medical Nightmare*. Berkeley, CA: University of California Press.

Briggs, Charles L., and Clara Mantini-Briggs. 2016. *Tell Me Why My Children Died: Rabies, Indigenous Knowledge, and Communicative Justice*. Durham, NC: Duke University Press.

Buchbinder, Mara. 2015. *All in Your Head: Making Sense of Pediatric Pain*. Berkeley, CA: University of California Press.

Capps, Lisa, and Elinor Ochs. 1997. *Constructing Panic: The Discourse of Agoraphobia*. Cambridge, MA: Harvard University Press.

Carr, E. Summerson. 2011. *Scripting Addiction: The Politics of Therapeutic Talk and American Sobriety*. Princeton, NJ: Princeton University Press.

Chun, Christian W. 2020. The Return of the "Yellow Peril." *Language, Culture and Society* 2(2): pp. 252–259.

Combahee River Collective. 1982. *A Black Feminist Statement [1977]. "All the Women are White, All the Blacks are Men, but Some of Us are Brave,"* ed. Gloria Hull, Patricia Scott, and Barbara Smith, pp. 13–22. New York: The Feminist Press.

Corwin, Anna I. 2020. Care in Interaction: Aging, Personhood, and Meaningful Decline. *Medical Anthropology* 39(7): pp. 638–652.

Corwin, Anna I. 2021. *Embracing Age: How Catholic Nuns Became Models of Aging Well*. New Brunswick, NJ: Rutgers.

Crenshaw, Kimberlé Williams. 1991. Mapping the Margins: Intersectionality, Identity Politics, and Violence against Women of Color. *Stanford Law Review* 43(6): pp. 1241–1299.

Csordas, Thomas J. 1997. *The Sacred Self: A Cultural Phenomenology of Charismatic Healing*. University of California Press.

Davis, Dána-Ain. 2019. Obstetric Racism: The Racial Politics of Pregnancy, Labor, and Birthing. *Medical Anthropology* 38(7): pp. 560–573. https://doi.org/10.1080/01459740.2018.1549389.

Dein, Simon. 2002. The Power of Words: Healing Narratives among Lubavitcher Hasidim. *Medical Anthropology Quarterly* 16(2): pp. 41–63.

Fabien, Vanessa. 2017. My Body, My Pain: Listen to Me and All Black Women. *The Root*. April 16. https://www.theroot.com/my-body-my-pain-listen-to-me-and-all-black-women-1794332651.

Fainzang, Sylvie. 2015. *An Anthropology of Lying: Information in the Doctor-Patient Relationship*. London: Routledge.

Farmer, Paul. 2001. *Infections and Inequalities: The Modern Plagues*. Berkeley: University of California Press.

Gevirtz, Karen Bloom. 2024. *The Apothecary's Wife: The Hidden History of Medicine and How It Became a Commodity*. Oakland: University of California Press.

Goodwin, Charles. 2010. Constructing Meaning through Prosody in Aphasia. In *Prosody in Interaction*, ed. Dagmar Barth-Weingarten, Elisabeth Reber, and Margaret Selting, pp. 373–394. Amsterdam: John Benjamins.

Greene, Jeremy, Marguerite Thorp Basilico, Heidi Kim, and Paul Farmer. 2019. Colonial Medicine and Its Legacies. In *Reimagining Global Health*, ed. Paul Farmer, Arthur Kleinman, Jim Yong Kim, and Matthew Basilico, pp. 33–73. Berkeley: University of California Press.

Guzmán, Jennifer R. 2015. The Epistemics of Symptom Experience and Symptom Accounts in Mapuche Healing and Pediatric Primary Care in Southern Chile. *Journal of Linguistic Anthropology* 24(3): pp. 249–276.

Guzmán, Jennifer R. 2020. Time Discipline and Health/Communicative Labor in Pediatric Primary Care. *Medical Anthropology* 39(7): pp. 609–623.

Guzmán, Jennifer R. 2024. Pursuit of Health/Communicative Justice through an Intercultural Health Model in Indigenous Chile. In *Language and Social Justice: Global Perspectives*, ed. Kathleen C. Riley, Bernard C. Perley, and Inmaculada M. García-Sánchez, pp. 392–411. London: Bloomsbury Academic.

Hoffman, Kelly M., Sophie Trawalter, Jordan R. Axt, and M. Norman Oliver. 2016. Racial Bias in Pain Assessment and Treatment Recommendations, and False Beliefs about Biological Differences between Blacks and Whites. *Proceedings of the National Academy of Sciences* 113(16): pp. 4296–4301. https://doi.org/10.1073/pnas.1516047113.

Jenks, Angela C. 2011. From "Lists of Traits" to "Open-Mindedness": Emerging Issues in Cultural Competence Education. *Culture, Medicine, and Psychiatry* 35(2): p. 209. https://doi.org/10.1007/s11013-011-9212-4.

Lempert, Michael. 2024. *From Small Talk to Micro Aggression: A History of Scale*. Chicago: University of Chicago Press.

Mattingly, Cheryl. 2010. *The Paradox of Hope: Journeys through a Clinical Borderland*. Berkeley, CA: University of California Press.

Metzl, Jonathan M., and Helena Hansen. 2014. Structural Competency: Theorizing a New Medical Engagement with Stigma and Inequality. *Social Science and Medicine* 103: pp. 126–133.

Owens, Deirdre Cooper. 2017. *Medical Bondage: Race, Gender, and the Origins of American Gynecology*. University of Georgia Press.

Perrino, Sabina. 2002. Intimate Hierarchies and Qur'anic Saliva (Tëfli): Textuality in a Senegalese Ethnomedical Encounter. *Journal of Linguistic Anthropology* 12(2): pp. 225–259.

Pritzker, Sonya E. 2014. *Living Translation: Language and the Search for Resonance in U.S. Chinese Medicine*. New York: Berghahn.

Rosa, Jonathan, and Nelson Flores. 2017. Unsettling Race and Language: Toward a Raciolinguistic Perspective. *Language in Society* 46(5): pp. 621–647. https://doi.org/10.1017/S0047404517000562.

Stivers, Tanya. 2012. Language Socialization in Children's Medical Encounters. In *The Handbook of Language Socialization*, ed. Alessandro Duranti, Elinor Ochs, and Bambi B. Schieffelin, pp. 247–267. Malden, MA: Wiley-Blackwell.

Sullivan, Patrick S., Stephanie N. DuBosea, Amanda D. Castelb, Karen W. Hoover, Marta Juhaszd, Jodie L. Guesta, Gordon Lea, Shamaya Whitbya, and Aaron J. Sieglera 2024. Equity of PrEP Uptake by Race, Ethnicity, Sex and Region in the United States in the First Decade of PrEP: A Population-Based Analysis. *The Lancet* 33: p. 100738. https://doi.org/10.1016/j.lana.2024.100738.

Taylor, Janelle S. 2003. Confronting "Culture" in Medicine's "Culture of No Culture." *Academic Medicine* 78(6): pp. 555–559. https://doi.org/doi.org/10.1097/00001888-200306000-00003.

Watters, Ethan. 2010. *Crazy Like Us: The Globalization of the American Psyche*. New York: Simon and Schuster.

Wilce, James M. 2009. Medical Discourse. *Annual Review of Anthropology* 38: pp. 199–215.

SECTION 1
CLINICAL INTERACTION
Editors' Introduction

Starting with the invention of the modern clinic or hospital, people have increasingly sought treatment for health problems in dedicated institutional settings. In clinical settings today, medical professionals effectively treat many diseases. Examining how these institutions are organized, including how language works in these settings, is therefore critical to understanding contemporary experiences of illness and healthcare.

Clinical medicine is organized around several key principles. One is the unidirectionality of care. As opposed to other contexts where people may provide mutual care for one another, in clinics medical professionals provide care for patients and are paid for this work. A second principle is that care in clinical settings focuses on individual health; medical efforts center on understanding and treating each patient's particular health problems. Finally, perhaps the most important principle is that of medical authority. Doctors, surgeons, therapists, nurses, and other clinicians receive specialized training in order to carry out their work. This expertise means they wield authority not only over treatment but also over talk.

Care relationships in hospitals and clinics are forged in large part through interaction. Talk in these settings is shaped by the fact that each person occupies a role—doctor, patient, caregiver, etc.—that comes with norms and expectations. These norms are tied to the values of the given medical system and structured around accomplishing specific medical goals, typically diagnosis and treatment. For patients, learning to follow these norms and speak effectively in clinical settings happens through **language socialization**, a process of learning through repeated participation in an activity (Clemente 2015; Schieffelin and Ochs 1986). Medical professionals also experience language socialization, but additionally are taught how to enact their roles through years of formal instruction and close supervision. Training in how to perform medicine and how to talk happens in tandem (Good and DelVecchio Good 2000).

Yet people are never "just" doctors or patients when they meet with one another and try to figure out the nature of a health problem and how to treat it. Studies of clinical interaction reveal that perceptions of people's identities, including discriminatory stereotypes, systematically shape how friendly or unfriendly clinical interaction may be and, even more consequentially, the quality of information, care, resources, and options that are provided to patients.

In terms of thematic domains, where language and health are entangled, perhaps most has been written about clinical interaction. The chapters in this section contribute to this important area of research by challenging presumptions and biomedical norms about the dynamics of clinical interactions and even what the clinic itself should be. Hannah Noblewolf and Lisa Wolf find that many emergency room nurses apply the label "mom" to any patient who is pregnant. They explore how this language practice reflects and reproduces gendered expectations that can be harmful. Hyemin Lee explores how the experience and expression of pain is handled in traditional Korean medicine. Stephanie Keeney Parks shows how medical students in psychiatry are trained to perceive Black patients' ways of speaking as pathological, reproducing the clinic as white public space.

References

Clemente, Ignasi. 2015. *Uncertain Futures: Communication and Culture in Childhood Cancer Treatment.* Oxford: Wiley-Blackwell.

Good, Byron, and Mary-Jo DelVecchio Good. 2000. "Fiction" and "Historicity" in Doctors' Stories: Social and Narrative Dimensions of Learning Medicine. In *Narrative and the Cultural Construction of Illness and Healing*, ed. Cheryl Mattingly and Linda Garro, pp. 50–69. Berkeley: University of California Press.

Schieffelin, Bambi, and Elinor Ochs. 1986. Language Socialization. *Annual Review of Anthropology* 15: pp. 153–191.

1

Everyone is "Mom"

Speaking Maternalism in US Emergency Departments

Hannah S. Noblewolf and Lisa Wolf

Author's Note

Throughout this chapter, the terms **pregnancy-capable people** or **pregnant people** are used to describe people who can become pregnant or who are pregnant. The exception to this is when another author's work is being referenced or quoted. The difference in language is important; language shapes the way we as humans perceive the world around us. Using gender-neutral terms acknowledges that some people who do not self-identify as women are able to get pregnant. This includes transgender men as well as non-binary people who were assigned female at birth. Oftentimes in obstetrics and gynecology, the default is to use language that assumes that pregnant people are cisgender women; such assumptions may lead to misgendering and negatively impact the wellbeing of trans and non-binary individuals (Zimman 2017). Protecting the wellbeing of all patients by using respectful language is an important form of inclusion that prevents negative mental health impacts.

Introduction

Cara and her partner (both white, middle class, in their mid-30s) came to their local emergency department (ED) for help after Cara had a seizure. She was quickly given a bed, but she and her partner have been waiting for hours to see someone who can do something about her situation. They know what the issue is—Cara is ten weeks pregnant, and pregnancy makes the medication she takes for her seizure disorder less effective. This problem could be solved by a change in her prescription. The situation feels straightforward to both Cara and her partner. The emergency medical team does not agree.

The medication that she takes to manage her seizures is considered to have an excellent safety profile. However, medications are not tested specifically on pregnant patients in clinical trials so there is not as much data on the effects on pregnant patients. Physicians tend to be cautious about prescribing anything at all to pregnant people, citing potential risks to the fetus.

Hannah S. Noblewolf and Lisa Wolf, *Everyone is "Mom"*. In: *Language and Health in Action*. Edited by: Lynnette Arnold et al., Oxford University Press. © Hannah S. Noblewolf and Lisa Wolf (2026). DOI: 10.1093/9780198933953.003.0001

Cara is depending on the decision that the physician in the ED makes. She and her partner recently moved to the area, so they have no established care. Their previous OBGYN (obstetrics and gynecology service) provider is 300 miles away and Cara's partner isn't comfortable driving her across the state for care when she may have another seizure. The local hospital closed their birthing center three months ago, meaning there are no OBGYN providers in the hospital that could explain to the ED doctor that the medication Cara is taking is considered reasonably safe for her as a pregnant woman.

As Cara is recovering from her seizure, the ED doctor informs them he is not comfortable with writing an updated prescription. They try to explain their situation, but he is unwilling to change his mind. "There's too much risk to the baby, I'm just not comfortable. Mom understands, right?"

Frustrated, they have no choice but to leave and seek care elsewhere. Regardless of how the couple decides to navigate their next steps, the doctor's focus on the risks to the pregnancy to the exclusion of Cara's health will result in a delay of care for Cara and increases the risk of her having another seizure before the time when she can see another provider.

Pregnancy and Language in the Emergency Room

As in Cara's case, the local ED is the closest place for an increasing number of pregnant people in the United States to seek care. This phenomenon is a result of expanding obstetric deserts (counties with no obstetric providers). The causes of obstetric deserts are varied, but often self-reinforcing. For example, common justification for shutting down obstetric services include "low birth volumes and staffing challenges" (Sonenberg and Mason 2023). When obstetric centers close, obstetricians, labor and delivery nurses, and nurse-midwives move to areas where they can find employment. This presents additional staffing challenges, further expanding these obstetric deserts.

In this context, how ED staff react to pregnant patients informs decisions about the health and safety of an increasing number of pregnant people. This chapter therefore explores how clinical staff interact with and respond to pregnant patients, tracing how professional obligations to care for pregnant patients as autonomous individuals are understood.

Our chapter suggests that the language healthcare workers use for, about, and with patients matters. It can change how patient symptoms and concerns are interpreted, the urgency with which patients are treated, and how patients themselves respond to the encounter. It may determine how likely they are to adhere to a treatment plan and how reliably they may return for care for the same or other concerns. Language use, no matter how insignificant it may at first seem, can impact the care provided to patients by healthcare professionals.

To explore the language of care for pregnant patients in EDs, this chapter draws on Lisa Wolf's clinical experience in emergency care, which included incidents like Cara's. Dr Wolf has thirty years of experience in ED clinical practice and twenty years' experience as a nursing educator and researcher. Hannah Noblewolf is a doctoral candidate in cultural medical anthropology with a background in linguistic anthropology. Her dissertation work focuses on abortion activism in West Texas. Both authors are white, middle-class women raised and educated on the east coast of the US. In addition to drawing on each author's individual expertise and experience, we analyze interviews collected by both authors as part of a joint study on the impacts of abortion bans on emergency healthcare.

Addressing Individual Patients as "Mom"

In the opening example, the avoidable delay to care that Cara experienced was related to the lack of access to obstetric care beyond the ED. But it was also underpinned by an ideology of maternalism that was exposed when the ED doctor addressed Cara as "mom."

Maternalism is an ideology (an often unspoken set of ideas shared by a social group) that a woman performing gender in an acceptable way is able and willing to become pregnant, carry the pregnancy to term, and raise a child or children. In short, the ideology of maternalism sees all women as current or eventual mothers. Indeed, any pregnancy-capable person is often subject to the consequences of this ideology regardless of their gender identity, sexuality, or any actual desire or capacity for children or parenthood.

Self-sacrifice is often synonymous with motherhood in western culture (Ginsburg 1989: 99; Lewin 1996: 111). By addressing Cara as "mom," the ED doctor projects expectations about how Cara should properly perform motherhood. In this environment, that means demonstrating that she possesses traits like self-sacrifice, nurturance, and selflessness through the choices she makes throughout her hospital stay. Though he may not have intended it in this way, the doctor's language use assumes that Cara, as a pregnant person, would consider *any* risk to the health of her pregnancy to be unacceptable. In the framework of maternalism, a "good" mother would avoid even the smallest risk of negative outcomes for a pregnancy, even at the cost of her own health. Maternalist ideologies make women's personhood inextricable from motherhood, making reproductive willingness essential both to be perceived as a full person and to be perceived as the ideal expression of a woman's personhood. Reproductive autonomy, including abortion, is challenged in this framework. This is partially because of the ideological underpinnings that a) abortion is understood to prolong the inevitable as all women will eventually become mothers; and b) to reject a pregnancy is to reject women's ascribed gender roles. This ideology exists in conjunction with the belief that there is a "right" type of mother; namely, a married, able-bodied, cisgender, white woman in her 20s or early 30s. Notes in medical charts about patients who are unmarried, female, racialized as non-white, or dependent on government assistance have been found to affect future care by biasing providers (Sun 2022). In challenging the validity of the reproductive decisions of pregnancy-capable people, maternalism challenges their status as women and thus their personhood.

By addressing Cara as "Mom," a category label, rather than using her name, the doctor fails to acknowledge her individual personhood. He also calls on her to embody the maternal trait of self-sacrifice, risking Cara's health by sticking with the lower dosage of her medication and, ironically, risking the health of the pregnancy as well. This is called **interpellation**.

Interpellation is the idea that words, phrases, social settings, and interactions can serve as a "call" for an individual to embody a specific subject, or a specific type of person. Through interpellation, specific behavior can be elicited based on the audience's cultural understanding of how to properly embody a role by fulfilling unspoken expectations. The use of terms like "Mom" and "Momma" can function as calls to embody the traits associated with motherhood (compassion, purity, self-sacrifice, nurturance) and to fulfill the role of "mother" throughout the social interaction.

People who are aware of how they may be perceived will, at times, demonstrate a preemptive response to interpellation by answering that call in advance of the interaction. Through this strategy, they try to gain control over how they are seen in an attempt to fit into a "more socially and ethico-morally acceptable form[s] of personhood" (Dick 2018). For instance, in the case above, a pregnant person might demonstrate such a preemptive response to interpellation by refusing a higher dose of medication to control their seizures, thereby maintaining that their primary concern is for the health of the fetus and demonstrating the self-sacrifice that is expected of mothers. If Cara had done so, she would have been seen as more socially obedient, performing her role as a woman in a way that would be satisfactory to the medical team responsible for her care.

Maternalist ideology and interpellation it produces therefore influence how pregnant people interact with their medical team. It can impede their ability to advocate for themselves if they fear being viewed and treated as "bad mothers." Poor women and women of color are already at a disadvantage—their reproduction is not only devalued, but actively discouraged through social pressures and public policy (Andaya 2019; Davis 2019; Mullings 1995). In addition, when a doctor addresses a pregnant patient as "Mom," this calls for the other members of the care team to treat the patient as an expectant mother—thus placing the weight of maternalist ideologies onto the patient's shoulders. Due in part to interpellation, the use of maternalist language can both define and determine the meaning and urgency of patient presentations.

Maternalism in Healthcare and the Law

How does maternalism inform healthcare? If we understand maternalism as a pervasive ideology, like a computer program that is always running in the background, then the tacit assumption that every pregnancy-capable person is pregnant or desires pregnancy affects who it is that healthcare workers see their patients to be and what their priority needs are. When everyone is "mom," the needs and agency of individuals may get lost, which is then a real challenge in clinical evaluation and decision making. Knowing she is pregnant, Cara's doctor may assume she would place the risks to her pregnancy above risks to herself. He did not offer to increase her medication as he might with any other patient presenting to the ED with breakthrough seizures. However, when making decisions to "take care" of their fetus, any pregnant person must also, of course, take care of themselves to ensure the health of the fetus (Mahmoud and Romanis 2023). The ideas of self-sacrifice embedded in maternalism erase this medical fact. This is due in part to the perception of healthcare providers that the fetus is a separate patient with different needs from the pregnant person.

Maternalism as a cultural ideology has far-reaching impacts in healthcare. "Preconception health" emerged as a public health strategy in the early 2000s (Waggoner 2013). In this aspect of maternalism, "women's health" is conflated with "maternal health" in a new way, elevating women as mothers, not as individuals. Waggoner uses the term **anticipatory motherhood** to refer to a framework that positions all cisgender women of childbearing age as "prepregnant" and exhorts them to minimize health risks to phantom fetuses and future pregnancies. A public health specialist explained the reality this policy reflects: "[Legislators] have very little support for uninsured women until they get pregnant because then it's about the baby. It's not about the mother ... But, you know, there's just no general primary care money for women ... because [women] don't have value unless they got [sic] a belly" (Waggoner 2013). This changed the burden of pregnancy and had the social effect of treating all non-pregnant pregnancy-capable people as potentially pregnant, reducing women's healthcare concerns to their reproductive capacity. This approach becomes a problem in healthcare because it leads public health policy makers and medical providers to lose sight of the very real person in front of them and focus on a potential pregnancy to the exclusion of anything else. Such frameworks can result in a reluctance to prescribe medications that treat depression, seizures, acne, and rheumatoid arthritis to pregnancy-capable people for fear of harm to a non-existent, but projected, future fetus (Shepherd and Sellers 2022).

In the case presented at the beginning of this chapter, maternalism is demonstrated in the way the provider decides to not adjust the anti-seizure medication due to the patient's pregnancy. This decision was made despite clinical practice guidelines that emphasize the importance of therapeutic drug monitoring and medication dosage adjustment during pregnancy and postpartum to mitigate the risk of increased seizure activity (Patel and Pennell 2016). The doctor's language use reflects the underlying maternalist ideologies through which the doctor fails to acknowledge Cara's individual personhood, while also calling on her to embody the maternal trait of self-sacrifice by accepting the personal risk her seizure disorder confers, rather than a much smaller risk of fetal abnormalities.

Maternalist Labels and Minimizing Health Concerns

The language of maternalism in clinical interactions, as shown in the opening vignette, demonstrates the pragmatic function of language, or its ability to impact the world. Language is not neutral. Maternalist language has immediate consequences for care, whether it is used to directly address patients, as in the case of Cara, or whether it is used to label and categorize pregnant patients. This labeling and categorization reveal underlying thought patterns and ideologies, and can also push both the patient and care team to fulfill set roles. In our research with ED nurses, we have found that such maternalist categorization is far-reaching. We conducted interviews with thirteen emergency nurses working in states with abortion restrictions, including Texas, Alabama, and Kentucky (Wolf et al. 2023). We asked nurses about their experiences with obstetric emergencies in this legal context.

In reporting their experiences, seven out of thirteen participants used the terms "Mom," "Momma," or "Mother" to refer to either hypothetical patients or past actual patients who had been experiencing obstetric emergencies. The situations discussed included non-viable pregnancies, pre-viable pregnancies, unwanted pregnancies (including patients actively seeking an abortion or who were in the ED with concerns post-abortion), and pregnancy loss. The initial focus of the study was the clinical decision making by nurses for patients with pregnancy emergencies, not the language that our nurse participants used. However, we were struck by the fact that over half of our participants referred to their obstetric patients as some variation of "Mom."

It may seem that these labels are simply a shorthand method of referring to a pregnant person, but referring to patients as representing a category obviates the individuality of each person's concerns and circumstances. Even in instances where the pregnancy wasn't wanted or wasn't viable, patients were referred to as "Mom."

> I would say that my experience in the emergency department has not been with my **mothers** seeking abortion care. (Participant 9)

In this quote Participant 9, despite referring to a context in which the *only* information they have about a hypothetical patient is that they are pregnant and trying to terminate that pregnancy, still refers to the hypothetical patient as a mother.

> [radio alert from EMS, assumed to be an unwanted pregnancy or attempted self-managed abortion] a **mother** coming in ... (Participant 4)

In this instance, Participant 4 is recounting an experience from her time in emergency medical services (EMS). When describing the situation, she talks about receiving a call for what was believed at the time to be an unwanted pregnancy that the patient may have tried to end on their own. Even in a context where the information she had at this point was that this person likely had ended a pregnancy intentionally, the patient is referred to as a mother.

This finding is striking in part because our participants universally put the pregnant person first in their anecdotes and hypotheticals—while still using terms like "mother" and "baby." For example, Participant 2 reflected:

> But you know, in my opinion you gotta protect the Momma, I mean the Momma is first. I mean, that's just that's just me ... I don't know what I would do until I'm in that situation. I, I like to think I know what I would do. But I don't. If it were me, and it was my body? You know, you don't even know that baby. You know, take care of that Momma first, but not everyone may feel that way. I don't know, I haven't been, I haven't been in that situation yet.

These examples demonstrate how deep-seated maternalist ideologies are. Having to explicitly state that the patient is the pregnant person demonstrates that they are pushing back against an assumption that the fetus is equally, if not more so, their patient. Close attention to regular patterns of language use can reveal how maternalism is spoken, even by people, like Participant 2, who explicitly oppose many aspects of maternalism. The use of maternalist language does not necessarily involve a conscious thought process, nor does it necessarily reflect an intentional decision in which a provider *decides* to change the way they provide care. The insidiousness of maternalist ideology and language is what makes it so difficult to address.

Nevertheless, this tendency to use maternalistic language reveals how the nurses implicitly understand their patients and assume their concerns in this context. But how does this framing affect patient care, the actual medical practice? Initially, maternalism can cause providers to dismiss legitimate health concerns ("well of course your back hurts, you're pregnant"), instead of looking for other causes of back pain such as a kidney infection or gallstones, or even pregnancy-related causes such as premature labor. There is a maternalist assumption here that pregnancy commonly involves discomfort and that there is an element of sacrifice inherent in pregnancy.

One participant described an incident where a pregnant patient came in under twenty weeks' gestation. She presented with lower pelvic cramping and spotting. Due to the "common" nature of that presentation and the fact that she was under twenty weeks pregnant, she was sent to a less urgent care area in the ED instead of the obstetrics (OB) floor of the hospital. At some point during her stay, the patient began to hemorrhage, and the emergency room (ER) staff found her "laying in a pool [of her own blood]." Despite this, it took approximately forty minutes for her to be seen by an OB nurse who determined that she needed to be brought upstairs to their department. The delay happened because every time the ED staff called to ask for assistance the OB nurses assumed it was a "normal" amount of bleeding for a pregnant patient and that the ED staff was overreacting.

As in this example, when maternalist ideologies are projected onto the healthcare encounter there can be an expectation of self-sacrifice, impacting the management of concerns around pain. The perception of the patient's acuity was incorrect, due at least in part to the maternalistic assumption that the correct performance of gender and pregnancy is to bear pain without complaint. The underlying assumption that pain is part of pregnancy and the postpartum phase and so can be dismissed or undermanaged ("it's not uncommon") leads to the dismissal of symptoms that would be considered a cause for concern in people who couldn't get pregnant. There are similar expectations about enduring pain without any pharmacological relief during pregnancy and after delivery due to an aversion toward the risk (no matter how small) that painkillers might pose to a fetus or breastfeeding infant, again drawing on the maternalist ideal of self-sacrifice.

Conclusion

We don't often think of the ED as a place to receive obstetric care, but due to expanding obstetric deserts and care-limiting legislation around abortion care, more and more pregnant people seek care in this setting. Because patients seen in the ED are often unknown to the clinical staff, the language that practitioners use to, about, and with patients matters in terms of how symptoms are perceived, documented, and managed.

Language has consequences for care; considering the pragmatic dimension of language and tracing patterns in language use can powerfully reveal implicit understandings that impact care. Cara is unlikely to trust that she will receive good care at that hospital moving forward, where she is "Mom" and not "Cara." It is critically important for those engaged in medicine to understand that the ways in which healthcare providers talk to and about patients can have a profound impact on how they are seen, understood, and cared for.

Little academic work has been done on this subject. As far as we are aware, we are the only authors currently publishing on the impacts of maternalism in healthcare. Until further research is done, we can only propose steps to combat maternalism at an individual level, not at a systemic level. Since maternalism is an ideology, and not something that people generally hold as conscious thoughts or beliefs, it is particularly insidious. The best way to combat maternalism and improve the quality of care for pregnancy-capable patients is for healthcare providers to exercise reflectiveness. Clinicians can improve their awareness of their own talk patterns by paying attention to how they talk with colleagues about patients, even when patients are not immediately present. Clinicians who can engage in this reflective work and recognize when they are making assumptions about the reproductive futures and desires of their patients will be better positioned to reconsider maternalist patterns of talk and revise them. Changing these language patterns can convey respect and meaningfully communicate to pregnancy-capable patients that they have the same autonomy and right to self-determination as any other patient.

Questions for Reflection and Discussion

Reflection Questions

1. The authors use the term "pregnancy-capable person." Have you come across this term before? Where? If not, what was your experience reading this term for the first time? How does this decision reflect the power of labels that the chapter focuses on?
2. What was your reaction to reading about Cara's experience? How did her story make you feel? Why do you think you responded in this way?
3. Can you think of a time when you were labeled in a particular way that called you to embody a specific role in an interaction? Why do you think this label was used? How did you react? How did you feel about it?

Looking In: Small Group Discussion Questions

1. What is maternalism? Provide a definition in your own words and identify some examples from the chapter or other contexts.
2. What is interpellation? Provide a definition in your own words and identify some examples from the chapter or other contexts.
3. The chapter includes cases in which clinicians directly call patients "mom" and also cases in which clinicians referred to patients as "mom" when talking with the researchers. Do you think these different contexts matter for how this label works? Why or why not?

Looking Out: Large Group Discussion Questions

1. Why does maternalism matter for healthcare?
2. How are gender, patriarchy, and sexism relevant to maternalism? How does maternalism relate to other understandings of gender identity?

3. How does the language that clinicians use to label patients matter for healthcare?
4. If you were a nurse, what would you take away from this chapter? How might the chapter influence your practices at work?

References

Andaya, Elise. 2019. "I'm Building a Wall around My Uterus": Abortion Politics and the Politics of Othering in Trump's America. *Cultural Anthropology* 34(1): pp. 10–17. doi:10.14506/ca34.1.03.

Davis, Dána-Ain. 2019. *Reproductive Injustice: Racism, Pregnancy, and Premature Birth.* New York: New York University Press.

Dick, Hilary Parsons. 2018. *Words of Passage: National Longing and the Imagined Lives of Mexican Migrants.* Austin: University of Texas Press.

Ginsburg, Faye D. 1989. *Contested Lives: The Abortion Debate in an American Community.* Berkeley, CA: University of California Press.

Lewin, Ellen. 1996. On the Outside Looking In: The Politics of Lesbian Motherhood. In *Conceiving the New World Order*, ed. Faye D. Ginsburg and Rayna Rapp, pp. 103–121. Berkeley, CA: University of California Press. https://doi.org/10.1525/9780520915442-007.

Mahmoud, Zaina, and Elizabeth Chloe Romanis. 2023. On Gestation and Motherhood. *Medical Law Review* 31(1): pp. 109–140. https://doi.org/10.1093/medlaw/fwac030.

Mullings, Leith. 1995. Households Headed by Women: The Politics of Race, Class, and Gender. In *Conceiving the New World Order: The Global Politics of Reproduction*, ed. Ginsberg, Faye and Rapp, Rayna, pp. 122–139. Berkeley, CA: University of California Press.

Patel, Sima. I., and Paige P. Pennell. 2016. Management of Epilepsy during Pregnancy: An Update. *Therapeutic Advances in Neurological Disorders* 9(2): pp. 118–129. https://doi.org/10.1177/1756285615623934.

Ross, Loretta, and Rickie Solinger. 2017. *Reproductive Justice: An Introduction.* Oakland: University of California Press.

Shepherd, Katie, and Frances Stead Sellers. 2022. Abortion Bans Complicate Access to Drugs for Cancer, Arthritis, Even Ulcers. *The Washington Post*, August 8. https://www.washingtonpost.com/health/2022/08/08/abortion-bans-methotrexate-mifepristone-rheumatoid-arthritis/.

Sonenberg, Andrea, and Diana J. Mason. 2023. Maternity Care Deserts in the US. *JAMA Health Forum.* https://doi:10.1001/jamahealthforum.2022.5541.

Sun, Michael, Tomasz Oliwa, Monica E. Peek, and Elizabeth L. Tung. 2022. Negative Patient Descriptors: Documenting Racial Bias in the Electronic Health Record. *Health Affairs* 41(2): pp. 203–211. https://doi.org/10.1377/hlthaff.2021.01423.

Waggoner, Miranda R. 2013. Motherhood Preconceived: The Emergence of the Preconception Health and Health Care Initiative. *Journal of Health Politics, Policy and Law* 38(2): pp. 345–371. https://doi.org/10.1215/03616878-1966333.

Wolf, Lisa, Hannah S. Noblewolf, Michael Callihan, and Michael D. Moon. 2023. What If It Were Me? A Qualitative Exploratory Study of Emergency Nurses' Clinical Decision-Making Related to Obstetric Emergencies in the Context of a Post-Roe Environment. *Journal of Emergency Nursing*. https://doi.org/10.1016/j.jen.2023.06.009.

Zimman, Lal. 2017. Transgender Language Reform: Some Challenges and Strategies for Promoting Trans-Affirming, Gender-Inclusive Language. *Journal of Language and Discrimination* 1(1): pp. 84–105. https://doi.org/10.1558/jld.33139.

2

Talking about Pain in Traditional Korean Medicine Clinics

Hyemin Lee

Introduction

One afternoon in late May 2015, I entered the doctor's office in Willow Clinic, a small traditional Korean medicine (TKM) clinic in a suburb near Seoul, South Korea. For weeks, I had been shadowing Dr Jeong, the head doctor, for my research on doctor-patient communication in TKM clinics. After a quick review of the patient forms, Dr Jeong welcomed Eunju, a female patient in her 50s who had presented with a fever. Dr Jeong examined Eunju's face, took her pulse, and asked about her symptoms. While taking notes, I sensed some subtle tension when Dr Jeong asked Eunju about her headache.

Example 2.1 Dr Jeong asks Eunju about her symptoms (for transcription conventions, see chapter appendix)

(01) EUNJU: I can't really explain what the pain is like ... I don't know (laugh)
(02) DR JEONG: You can take your time (smile)
(03) EUNJU: ... Oh, how can I put this in words ... (laugh)
(04) DR JEONG: Was it stiff, tingling, or heavy? Or ...
(05) EUNJU: It just really hurts (smile)
(06) DR JEONG: ... Okay

After the lengthy consultation with Dr Jeong, I met Eunju for a short interview at a café near Willow Clinic. I was curious about Eunju's evasive laughter, which hinted to me that some difficulties had arisen in the conversation with Dr Jeong about her headache. To my question about how she felt when asked to "explain what the pain is like," Eunju answered, "To me, when my head hurts, that's a headache. Telling the doctor what my headache is like ... is challenging. It is not a matter of my speech fluency, but talking about pain itself is difficult." She added, "I have believed that language is unlimited and infinite, but when it comes to explaining my pain ... the language doesn't really do its job. It has limitations, at least in talking about pain."

On the next observation day, I reminded Dr Jeong of the conversation with Eunju and asked what her expectations were when communicating pain with her patients. Dr Jeong answered,

Hyemin Lee, *Talking about Pain in Traditional Korean Medicine Clinics*. In: *Language and Health in Action*. Edited by: Lynnette Arnold et al., Oxford University Press. © Hyemin Lee (2026). DOI: 10.1093/9780198933953.003.0002

> I don't think there is something like a clear language for describing our pain and sensations. The goal is not to translate the pain into words. Rather, it is to make sketches based on my impressions of the patient's pain, because our body speaks about pain beyond what we could capture in words.

This chapter introduces the cultural perspectives of language and the body shared in TKM clinics in South Korea by focusing on how TKM doctors and patients talk about pain in TKM clinical settings. As Eunju and Dr Jeong implied, in TKM clinics, language is understood as less capable of clearly explaining pain. I pay close attention to how pain and bodily sensations are articulated in interactions between clinicians and patients, as well as in interviews with TKM practitioners. This chapter is based on data collected during ethnographic fieldwork in TKM clinics and hospitals from April to August 2015 and two follow-up field research trips in April 2016 and February 2017.

TKM is a traditional medical system that has developed and is popularly used on the Korean peninsula. It shares some characteristics with traditional Chinese medicine and other East Asian healing practices. Its main therapeutic methods include acupuncture, moxibustion, cupping, manual therapies, and herbal medicine, where the most popular therapeutic practice is *ch'im* (acupuncture), a technique of inserting a special needle into specific points of the body (also called acupoints). Most South Koreans are familiar with TKM and acupuncture treatment for treating musculoskeletal pain, such as aching, stiffness, twitches, and burning sensations in muscles, tendons, ligaments, joints, and bones. In 2022, approximately 74% of TKM clinic visitors sought treatment for musculoskeletal pain, and 94% of these patients received acupuncture treatment (MOHW 2023). Aligning with these statistics, many patients that I met in Willow Clinic and other TKM clinics disclosed that physical pain, for example backache or ankle sprain, motivated their visits to TKM clinics. A few of them reported that they had gone to spine and orthopedic clinics before coming to TKM clinics, where an invasive procedure (e.g., surgery) was recommended. These patients added that they decided to receive TKM treatments in order to avoid going through surgical procedures.

Today, South Korea has a dual medical system where biomedicine and TKM stand on equal terms with exclusive practice boundaries, meaning that biomedicine and TKM have separate systems for medical education, national licenses, and therapeutic practices. This also means that in South Korea, despite the term "traditional" in its name, TKM is not classified as complementary and alternative medicine (CAM) but is instead regarded as conventional medicine. As such, it has been integrated into the Korean national healthcare system since 1987 (Ryu et al. 2013). South Korea was home to 2,708 TKM hospitals and 17,159 TKM clinics. Approximately 71% of the Korean population visits TKM practitioners ten times yearly (KOSIS 2023). Although every society has some degree of medical pluralism, the everyday and legal coexistence of biomedicine and TKM clearly distinguishes South Korea as a medically pluralistic society.

Medical pluralism describes a context in which people make use of different medical systems, traditions, and practices to make sense of their pain, seek treatments, and pursue health. In contexts with medical plurality, there are different ways of talking about pain in accordance with the different ways of understanding it. For example, in an orthopedic clinic, doctors provide a numerical pain scale for patients to articulate their pain by identifying a number. Here, pain is understood as scalar, where each number is a proxy for pain intensity. In a TKM clinic, as we will see, doctors use visual and poetic expressions, rather than scales and numbers, to ask patients about their pain in detail. Pain is perceived less as scalar and more as impressions, and TKM doctors use these impressions to diagnose and prescribe treatments.

As an inherently subjective experience, pain is particularly difficult to capture in language. Different medical systems have developed strategies for dealing with this problem (see, for example, Buchbinder 2015 and Scarry 1985). Talking about pain is one such strategy and is also one of the first steps of medical examination to treat a patient's discomfort: the diagnosis. This chapter explores the ways of talking about and understanding pain from the TKM perspective. With this focus, this chapter calls attention to how talking about pain has far-reaching consequences for diagnosis, not only in TKM but also in other medical systems. It also illuminates that medical systems, whether TKM or biomedicine, rely on ideologies about how pain is expressed, ideologies that shape how medical diagnoses are made. In essence, the focus on how pain is articulated reveals that medical systems are, at their core, cultural systems.

Language Ideology and Semiotic Ideology

In this section, I turn to two important sets of beliefs that inform TKM doctors' thinking about the role of language and the body in talking about pain: language ideologies and semiotic ideologies.

Linguistic anthropologists have theorized **language ideologies** as involving people's shared attitudes, opinions, and beliefs about language, including language in general, language varieties, language use, linguistic structures, and speakers. For instance, the pain scale is based on the idea that speaking in numbers is a convenient, accurate, and effective way for patients to describe their pain intensity to doctors. Doctors expect the scale to facilitate clear communication about pain, which is important for effective pain management. This idea that numbers promise clarity is part of a language ideology widely shared in biomedical fields, where language (e.g., speaking in numbers) is believed to represent and name what is out there in the world (e.g., pain). Just as these ideas are debatable and may not be shared by all medical practitioners, scholars, and patients, language ideologies are neither true nor false. Rather, language ideologies are always partial and open to contestation (Gal and Irvine 2019; Woolard 1998). Whether the members of a social group are aware of their own language ideologies or not, those language ideologies have profound social consequences, for instance shaping how pain is diagnosed.

In addition to verbal and written forms of language, there are other means of communicating pain in clinical settings. Linguistic anthropologists have long focused on how specific words, objects, or sensations come to have meaning, an approach known as semiotics. **Semiotics** expands the scope of meaning making by incorporating other forms of expression such as gestures, sounds, colors, images, dress styles, and other aspects of the body. In semiotics, these are all understood as signs that can potentially carry meaning, depending on the beliefs people hold about what and how meanings are being invested. In other words, anything can be a sign if it stands for something else and if someone believes that it stands for something else. For example, the white coats that some doctors wear serve to indicate their professional status and distinguish them from other healthcare workers, signaling their technical competence and professional knowledge. Here, a white coat serves as a sign that can communicate such meanings even in the absence of words.

Linguistic anthropologists have introduced the concept of **semiotic ideology**, which refers to a set of beliefs about signs held by people, such as what signs are, their functions, and possible consequences (Keane 2018). Let us look at one example from the Willow Clinic.

Example 2.2 Jimin (a kindergartener) visited Willow Clinic for stomach pain

(01) DR JEONG: How much does your belly hurt? Can you tell me?
(02) MOM: Go ahead
(03) JIMIN: (making a small circle with her hands) Outside the bathroom
(04) DR JEONG: Great! How about in the bathroom?
(05) JIMIN: (making a big circle with her arms) This much!
(06) DR JEONG: Great

When Dr Jeong asked Jimin how intense her stomach pain was, Jimin answered by using her hands and arms together with spoken language. Jimin's first gesture, drawing a small circle with her hands, was similar to the famous hand motions in the children's song "The Itsy-Bitsy Spider." For the second gesture, Jimin raised her arms to make a big circle and lightly shook her hands to add action to her gesture. By using two gestures that could be compared to one in terms of their scale, Dr Jeong and Jimin communicated about the intensity of Jimin's stomach pain. While Jimin's gestures were not linguistic, they nevertheless stood as signs that conveyed important meaning in doctor-patient communication. Moreover, Jimin's hand gestures were interpreted as signs because of the semiotic ideology shared by Jimin, Jimin's mother, and the doctor. Dr Jeong recognized Jimin's hand gestures as signs that stand for the intensity of pain, where the scales of the gestures correspond to the severity of Jimin's stomach pain.

In the following sections, I introduce the language and semiotic ideologies shared by TKM doctors and patients in TKM clinics. These ideologies inform how TKM doctors and patients understand the role of language in articulating pain and provide a framework for understanding what the body is and how to perceive and interpret bodily sensations. Together, they illuminate why TKM doctors use poetic and descriptive words to describe pain.

"Blank Space of Words": Language Ideology in TKM Clinics

In TKM clinics, doctors and patients consider communication an important part of the diagnostic process. TKM doctors have told me that asking patients many questions and guiding them to tell their stories about pain are essential steps when collecting information that leads to diagnoses. Indeed, TKM doctors take pride in their reputation for talking more, touching more, and paying more attention to patients than biomedical doctors do. Dr Lim, a TKM doctor at a big TKM hospital in Seoul, South Korea, proudly stated, "We do not do the three-minute consultation." The three-minute consultation is a popular phrase that reflects the time constraints in many biomedical settings, where the average consultation time per person is less than three minutes due to the high volume of primary care patients (Sohn et al. 2019). In contrast, doctor-patient interactions in TKM settings are lengthy and more patient centered. Dr Lim told me, "Doctors invest more time in patients in TKM clinics" and added, "TKM doctors talk a lot [to patients]."

When it comes to communicating about physical pain, however, TKM doctors and patients report that there is a limitation in expressing pain transparently through words. As in the first example between Eunju and Dr Jeong, having difficulty talking about pain is not about an individual's capacity to use language. Instead, as Eunju understands it, the limitation is inherent in language itself and how it explains experiences of pain.

Similarly, TKM doctors also believe that bodily sensations like pain cannot be fully described in language. Here, it is notable that TKM doctors used the term "words" (*mal*) rather than other relevant terms like "letters" or "writings" (*kŭl*). In Korean, *mal* refers to the "human voice" or "sound" through which "thoughts or feelings are expressed or conveyed" (National Institute of Korean Language 2024). This use of "words" indicates that TKM doctors' ideas about language are bound to verbal expression, that is, talking and speaking. Hence, talking and speaking about pain is understood as inherently limited, creating difficulties and challenges for patients and doctors during their conversations in TKM clinics.

Both Eunju and TKM doctors' commentaries are informed by their shared **language ideology of inexpressibility** (Lee 2016, 2022), which emphasizes the limited capacity of verbal expression of pain. In one interview, Dr Jeong introduced a metaphor that epitomizes the TKM language ideology of inexpressibility.

Example 2.3 Blank space of words

DR JEONG: Let me give you an analogy. "Blank space of words." It means there is an empty space where one cannot express the pain and, therefore, cannot fill it. [...]

Broadly, it refers to the limitation of language. In a narrow sense, it says there are not enough words to describe pain clearly.

In this commentary, Dr Jeong explains that the "blank space of words" figuratively indicates one's inability to verbalize pain, which points to the idea that language cannot express bodily sensations clearly and thoroughly. Moreover, "blank space" also implies that there is not a sufficient number of "words" to describe pain. Because of this language ideology of inexpressibility, patients in TKM clinics use gestures (see Example 2.2) or rely on TKM doctors' descriptive expressions, as illustrated in the following list of questions that TKM doctors ask their patients about their pain experience (Table 2.1).

These examples show how TKM doctors speak about the details of their patient's pain. Dr Kim used words that imitate the sounds (onomatopoeia) and physical movement (mimetic) of *p'a-lŭ-lŭ-p'a-lŭ-lŭ* (fluttering) to ask the patient about a tic in the eyelid. In Dr Park's and Dr Lim's questions about the details of pain experiences, they gave their patients choices made up of descriptive expressions. Note that the question asked by Dr Park is the same one that Dr Jeong asked Eunju about her headache. Descriptive expressions used by Dr Park included "stiff," "tingling," and "heavy." In Korean, these adjectives denote slightly different but common sensations of muscle pain and headache. Similarly, Dr Lim used the adjectives "dry and stiff" and "sandy" to describe eye pain. In one interview, a TKM doctor explained that they borrow these descriptive expressions from classical medical texts and rephrase them as questions. These examples show that TKM doctors use lengthy, picturesque, and descriptive expressions to ask patients detailed questions about their pain.

This practice is rooted in the language ideology of inexpressibility. TKM doctors do not insist on absolute clarity when it comes to verbally expressing bodily sensations like pain. They do not expect doctors or patients to comprehend pain with such clarity, and there is no single word that can fully and concisely describe a specific bodily sensation. Instead, doctors use questions to suggest several descriptions of pain and let their patients choose the most accurate. The "blank space of words," then, points to TKM's perspectives on the communicative and interpretive limitations that arise from the difficult task of clearly, thoroughly, and transparently explaining pain.

Table 2.1 Questions asked by TKM doctors to their patients about their pain experience

A. Dr Kim: Were your eyelids twitching like *p'a-lŭ-lŭ-p'a-lŭ-lŭ*, like falling autumn leaves?

B. Dr Park: Was it [the pain] stiff, tingling, or heavy?

C. Dr Lim: Did the pain in your eyes feel dry or stiff? Or was it like sandy, like when something gets into your eyes?

"The Song of the Body": Semiotic Ideology in TKM Clinics

In addition to lengthy conversations between TKM doctors and patients in the doctors' offices, another significant part of doctor-patient interaction involved touch, which was crucial to the diagnostic process. Feeling and interpreting sensations through touch is the modality through which medical information about pain is mediated. When touched, the patient's body serves as a more expressive medium for representing pain than their verbal descriptions. To borrow Dr Jeong's phrase, the patient's body "speaks about pain beyond what we could capture in words."

Maek-chin (pulse diagnosis) is a good example (see also Farquhar 2014 and Kuriyama 1999 for Traditional Chinese Medicine perspectives on pulse diagnosis). It is one of four TKM diagnostic methods and involves palpating three positions on a patient's wrist. According to many TKM doctors, pulse diagnosis is a vital part of the TKM diagnostic process because it provides an overview of the patient's body, including medical information about pain.

Example 2.4 Pulse as TKM version of endoscopy and X-ray

DR JEONG: As soon as I positioned my fingers on the patient's wrist, I would see the different aspects of the pulse based on the patient's status. And there would be many different aspects of the pulse. In this respect, the pulse is an endoscopy that allows us to figure out the patient's body. [...] It is a TKM version of X-ray.

In this interview, Dr Jeong called taking a patient's pulse the TKM version of X-ray images or endoscopy, a procedure to examine the interior of the organ or cavity of the body. This is because the pulse gives crucial medical information about the patient's body, health, and pain. Hence, the body reveals much more comprehensive and precise information about the pain than any verbal description.

Once the pulse is taken, doctors judge its quality based on twenty-eight variables. This is called a *maek-sang* (pulse image), which is a visualized description (i.e., image) of tactile sensations (i.e., pulse). Classical medical texts, such as *Introduction to Medicine*, introduce the canonical list of twenty-eight pulse images, describing pulse images using expressions like "floating," "hollow," "sunken," and "empty." When I asked Dr Jeong about the pulse images, she pulled out her memo (see Figure 2.1). This memo included her interpretations of the pulse image (the upper right) and the original text from *Introduction to Medicine* (the lower right).

Dr Jeong's "Rough Pulse" memo illustrates that TKM doctors figuratively interpret and translate pulse sensations. Note that the original text of "Rough Pulse" from *Introduction to Medicine* already includes metaphoric and poetic expressions, such as "goes back and forth" and "scratching the bamboo skin." However, Dr Jeong's interpretations add more poetic expressions based on her own experiences of touching the rough pulse. For example, she translated her tactile experience of the rough pulse as having "empty spots" that are "scattered," and she visualized this sensation as "raindrops on the sand." Dr Jeong also described the slow and inconsistent

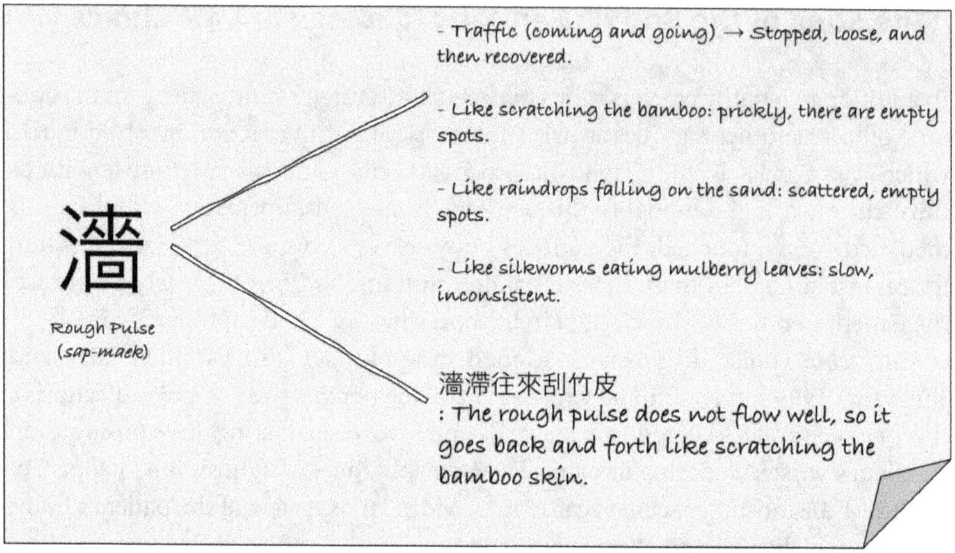

Fig. 2.1 Dr Jeong's memo on "rough pulse."
Reproduced by Hyemin Lee.

pulse speed as "silkworms eating mulberry leaves." These figurative expressions and descriptions of rough pulse, as well as the original text from *Introduction to Medicine*, illuminate that TKM doctors understand a type of pulse and its qualities through making vivid images. More importantly, the pulse image and Dr Jeong's interpretations all point to TKM's perspective on the body, where the body discloses much more information about a patient's health.

TKM's understanding of the body as expressive suggests that TKM practitioners share a particular semiotic ideology. In one interview, Dr Jeong used the metaphor of "song" to describe TKM's understanding of the body.

Example 2.5 The song of the body

DR JEONG: A song is no longer a song if it is segmented into individual musical notes. Continuity and temporality must intervene together to make up a song. This is how TKM works. TKM does not segment the body but takes continuity and temporal change seriously. We must see the continuity of the whole body. That is, the song of the body is significant in looking at the illness.

The above commentary encapsulates how a TKM doctor understands what a body is and how it works. A musical song is composed of individual notes, which are connected by following variations in tempo. Similarly, TKM's understanding of the body prioritizes incorporating the flows and changes in the patient's body. Because TKM doctors know that the body keeps expressing itself, they look for the aspects of the whole body that are constantly changing. "The song of the body," then, highlights the expressiveness of the body by emphasizing continuity, change, and flow over time.

As a semiotic ideology, "the song of the body" resonates with how pulse images are described in the classical medical text and in Dr Jeong's memo. In Figure 2.1, Dr Jeong's interpretations of rough pulse include its rhythm, speed, and motion (e.g., "traffic" and "stopped, loose, and then recovered"). Rather than a snapshot capturing a state frozen in time, Dr Jeong describes the pulse as if it is an animated image, like a GIF. TKM doctors describe this way of perceiving the body and bodily sensation as looking at the "aspects" or "impressions" of the body. It refers to "a bigger picture" of the body that includes not only the body itself but also the changes that the body has gone through. In this sense, "the song of the body" highlights its expressiveness and undergirds how TKM doctors attend to the bigger picture of the bodily state in order to detect aspects and impressions of the patient's body.

Thus, when it comes to communicating pain with patients, TKM doctors do not strive to talk about the pain as if it is something that could be captured. Although some TKM doctors agree that numbers promise absolute clarity (also a language ideology), they claim that they do not use numbers to talk about patients' pain in TKM clinics. This is not because TKM doctors lack statistical or scientific knowledge about pain measurement but rather because they prioritize seeing the aspects or impressions of pain to better understand patients' pain experiences. This is why TKM doctors like Dr Jeong refrain from asking patients to rate their pain on a scale and instead let patients speak about their pain by giving them descriptive phrases to choose from (e.g., "stiff, tingling, or heavy").

It is important to note that there is a synergy between the language ideology and semiotic ideology in TKM clinics (Lee 2022). Because practitioners and patients both think language has limitations when it comes to articulating pain, they do not expect a clear articulation of pain experiences in doctor-patient communication in TKM clinics. TKM doctors seek other ways to describe the pain experience, such as figurative expressions and descriptions. For their part, patients try their best to describe their pain experiences, for example using gestures or borrowing expressions and descriptions from TKM doctors. The use of figurative descriptions illuminates how the language ideology of inexpressibility reaffirms the notion of the body being more expressive than language, which is the TKM's semiotic ideology of the body. Moreover, TKM's way of interpreting bodily sensations reinforces the language ideology of inexpressibility. Because TKM doctors see the aspects and impressions that are created by bodily sensations like the pulse, they do not seek concise and clear articulation of pain experience. Hence, TKM doctors' explanations of pain are lengthy, picturesque, poetic, and figurative.

Conclusion

This chapter has focused on language ideology and semiotic ideology in TKM clinics, discussing what these ideologies reveal about pain talk in TKM clinical interactions. The language ideology of inexpressibility, the "blank space of words," informs TKM doctors' and patients' understanding of the limited capacity of words to describe pain. Unlike language, the body is thought to be a more comprehensive and expressive medium for representing pain, which points to the semiotic ideology called "the song of the body." Taken together, these ideologies reveal how TKM doctors privilege a holistic approach when it comes to perceiving, understanding, and interpreting the body and bodily sensations. This results in TKM doctors' tendency to use descriptive and metaphoric expressions and patients' willingness to borrow those expressions from TKM doctors. While at first glance, this poetic speech may seem inefficient and imprecise, it is through these expressions that TKM doctors and patients work toward reaching a mutual understanding of pain, despite their shared language ideology of inexpressibility.

As societies become more medically pluralistic, so do the styles and practices of medical communication. This chapter discussed this diversity of medical systems and medical communication by looking into one clinical interaction in TKM clinics. In order to increase recognition for and inclusion of diverse medical systems and practices, it is important to understand the cultural ideologies about language and the body included in each medical system. As this chapter shows, a close examination of how people articulate their pain is a good place to start. Moreover, learning that these cultural ideologies of language and the body further influence medical diagnosis demonstrates that medical systems are also cultural systems. These understandings are necessary for fruitful discussions about how to incorporate different medical systems in a single society while creating space for their unique styles and practices of clinical interaction.

Questions for Reflection and Discussion

Reflection Questions

1. What complementary or alternative medicine practices are available where you live? What is your experience with them? Have you, a family member, or a friend received care from a practitioner of a different medical tradition than biomedicine? What do you recall from the experience?
2. In your own medical care, what diagrams, models, images, and terms have clinicians used to talk about your pain? What assumptions or beliefs did these ways of representing pain rely on?

Looking In: Small Group Discussion Questions

1. What is a sign? What makes something into a sign? Give an example of a sign different from the one in the chapter.
2. What are language ideologies? Provide a definition in your own words and identify some examples from the chapter or other contexts.

3. What are semiotic ideologies? Provide a definition in your own words and identify some examples from the chapter or other contexts.
4. What do the terms "blank space of words" and "the song of the body" suggest about the approach to pain in TKM?

Looking Out: Large Group Discussion Questions

1. List examples of how TKM doctors' describe a person's pulse, pain, or other bodily phenomena. What are some common patterns you notice in these descriptions? What similar or different patterns can you think of from other medical systems?
2. Why is it important to pay attention to language ideologies and semiotic ideologies in clinical interactions? How do they matter for healthcare?

Appendix

Notes on Romanization, Translation, Transcription, and Names

I have followed the McCune-Reischauer Romanization system of Korean, except for the widely circulated words that follow the Revised Romanization System of Korean (e.g., Seoul, Jeong). In examples, tables, and figures, I only included the English translations for better clarity of transcripts. All translations from Korean to English are mine. Transcription conventions are as follows:

()	Visual and auditory information
[...]	Ellipsis
...	Pause
[]	Transcriber's note for clarifications for the reader

I have anonymized all personal names and clinic names.

References

Buchbinder, Mara. 2015. *All in Your Head: Making Sense of Pediatric Pain*. Berkeley: University of California Press.

Farquhar, Judith. 2014. Reading Hands: Pulse Qualities and the Specificity of the Clinical. *East Asian Science, Technology and Society: An International Journal* 8: pp. 9–24. DOI 10.1215/18752160-2405767.

Gal, Susan, and Judith Irvine. 2019. *Signs of Difference: Language and Ideology in Social Life*. Cambridge: Cambridge University Press.

Keane, Webb. 2018. On Semiotic Ideology. *Signs and Society* 6(1): pp. 64–87.

KOSIS (Korean Statistical Information Service). 2023. 평생 한방의료 이용 경험—일반국민 [Lifetime Experience in Using Traditional Korean Medicine—General Public]. Ministry of Health and Welfare. April 25. Accessed on June 27, 2023.

Kuriyama, Shigehisa. 1999. *The Expressiveness of the Body and the Divergence of Greek and Chinese Medicine*. Princeton, NJ: Princeton University Press.

Lee, Hyemin. 2016. "말의 여백, 몸의 노래": 한의원에서의 언어 사용과 "아픔"의 언어화 ["Inexpressibility of Words, Expressiveness of Bodies": Verbalization of "Pain" in Medical Interactions in Traditional Korean Medicine Clinics.] Master's Thesis, Seoul National University, South Korea.

Lee, Hyemin. 2022. Sounds of Healing: Qualia and Medical Efficacy in a Traditional Korean Medicine Clinic. *Journal of Linguistic Anthropology* 32(2): pp. 364–385. https://doi.org/10.1111/jola.12353.

MOHW (Ministry of Health and Welfare). 2023. 2022년 한방의료이용 실태조사 결과 발표 [Results of the 2022 Survey on the Use of Traditional Korean Medicine]. March 31. Accessed on July 21, 2024.

National Institute of Korean Language. 2024. *Korean-English Learner's Dictionary*. https://krdict.korean.go.kr/m/eng.

Ryu, Jiseon, Byunghee Choi, Byungmook Lim, Sina Kim, and Youngju Yun. 2013. Medical Practices and Attitudes of Dual-Licensed Medical Doctors in Korea. *Evidence-Based Complementary and Alternative Medicine*. doi: 10.1155/2013/183643.

Scarry, Elaine. 1985. *The Body in Pain: The Making and Unmaking of the World*. Oxford: Oxford University Press.

Sohn, Kyung-Hee, Sarah Nam, Jungmin Joo, Yong Jin Kwon, and Jae-Joon Yim. 2019. Patient-Centeredness during In-Depth Consultation in the Outpatient Clinic of a Tertiary Hospital in Korea: Paradigm Shift from Disease to Patient. *Journal of Korean Medical Science* 34(15): p. e119. doi: 10.3346/jkms.2019.34.e119.

Woolard, Kathryn. 1998. Introduction: Language Ideology as a Field of Inquiry. In *Language Ideologies: Practice and Theory*, ed. Bambi Schieffelin, Kathryn Woolard, and Paul Kroskrity, pp. 3–47. Oxford: Oxford University Press.

3

Autism Diagnostics as White Public Space in US Clinics

Stephanie Keeney Parks

Introduction

"Dell? What do you like?" asks Dr X. "I like big butts and I cannot lie!" replies Dell. On this particular afternoon, about fifty graduate students are packed into an auditorium watching a live demonstration of an Autism Diagnostic Observation Schedule or ADOS. The ADOS is a diagnostic tool commonly referred to as the "gold standard" in testing for autism. I am seated off to the left of the stage in the second row of the auditorium, watching my son, Dell, offer up a famous rap lyric as a response to a question from the clinician.

Our day started much earlier when I received a phone call from the clinical director at the local medical school requesting that I bring Dell, my 11-year-old autistic little boy, to class with me. The child initially scheduled to model the ADOS had canceled at the last minute. I requested that the clinic provide Dell with a box of Hot Tamales candy and a gift certificate to the car wash as payment for his services. After the clinical director agreed to my terms, I arranged for Dell to join me on campus to model the test that afternoon.

Later that morning, I am seated in the auditorium with my laptop, ready for the seminar to begin. The room holds an interdisciplinary group of graduate students in medicine, psychology, occupational health, speech language pathology, genetics, public health, and physical therapy. I waved at a friend, the only other Black person in the room, a graduate student in psychology. He was sitting next to the sole Latina in the room. The auditorium was buzzing with energy as the medical school had brought in a well-respected clinical expert on autism to teach us how to administer the test, Dr X, an older (55–60-year-old) white male.

Dr X began the seminar by explaining that the test includes questions and activities for the patient to complete. The activities included manipulatives such as dolls, superhero action figures, cars, books, blocks, and other items that a child might play with. I noticed that the dolls and action figures represented only white people. There was not a single item that represented a person of any other race. I made a note of this and decided that I would ask Dr X about this later during the break. At some point that morning, a medical student asked Dr X if a patient's culture should

Stephanie Keeney Parks, *Autism Diagnostics as White Public Space in US Clinics*. In: *Language and Health in Action*. Edited by: Lynnette Arnold et al., Oxford University Press. © Stephanie Keeney Parks (2026). DOI: 10.1093/9780198933953.003.0003 be considered when administering and scoring the test. The student clarified their statement by stating, "You know, what if we run into culture?" to which Dr X replied: "It is not about culture; it's about a response." Given that Dr X told an auditorium packed with graduate students that culture is different than response and not something to take into consideration during the ADOS, I started to feel deeply curious about how the test would unfold with Dell, a Black child who often speaks Black language.

The Autism Diagnostic Observation Schedule

The ADOS includes four levels based on a patient's age (18 months–adult) and verbal language capabilities. There are several tasks that the patient must perform, which change based on the level of the test, age, and verbal and intellectual abilities of the patient. In the ethnographic example in this chapter, the clinician moved between two scales in the ADOS (ADOS 2 and 3) to accommodate Dell's intellectual disability, autism diagnosis, age, and verbal language capabilities. The tasks involve imaginative play activities, collective storytelling, relationship questions, and daily life. Much of the evaluation centers on the appropriate use of verbal language, as differences in social interaction and communication are central aspects of the diagnosis. One example of such communicative difference is echolalia, the repetitious use of language where the individual echoes or parrots back words, phrases, or sounds. Many clinicians, like Dr X, treat ADOS scoring as a practice that is not impacted by culture. However, as I will argue in this chapter, ADOS scoring is, in fact, a cultural process through which systems of oppression, especially those that are based on race and culture, can be seen at work.

Race and Culture

The scoring of an ADOS is grounded in the subjective assessment of the clinician administering the test and how they understand the patient's behavior in front of them. Dr X's view of his patients and how he interacts, hears, and interprets behavior and language is not only clinical. His view is shaped by his positionality as a white male physician whose life and professional training have been framed by the cultural norms of the United States. These norms influence how he both understands and experiences identities such as race and culture. These in turn shape understandings of disability, in this case, autism.

Race is a socially constructed category that sorts humans via phenotype or physical characteristics; for example, Dr X is a white man and Dell is a Black child. White and Black are the racial identities that are being explored in this chapter. Race and culture are not the same things. Culture is a set of practices a group of people engage in. Dell, the child featured in this chapter is racially Black, but his ethnicity is that of a Black American which he expresses via his use of Black language, which is a part of his cultural practices. Neither race nor culture are stable categories. Race, for example, can be based upon how one identifies oneself or how one is identified by others. Similarly, there are no hard boundaries for culture as cultural practices are dynamic and can change over time. Misrecognition of another's race, ethnicity, or culture can lead to stereotyping and other marginalizing outcomes such as health inequities.

In the United States, race is a particularly difficult topic. It is so contentious that it is avoided in polite conversation across various social settings including medical spaces. Despite this, racial categories have a significant impact on individuals' life experiences within every social system from housing and education to access to healthy food, water, and healthcare. Culture, however, is often treated as a more acceptable topic. Culture is popularly understood as being associated with things like art, food, music, etc. Often race and culture are tied together with one category indexing—quietly referencing or silently pointing to—the other. The ways that race and culture are used or not used in conversation has very real outcomes for the people involved. We can see this entanglement in the following example of Dr X's interaction with Dell.

"Cultural" Response

Dell arrives after a short lunch break and is his usual excited, happy self. A microphone is placed on his shirt, which he loves. Dell starts joyfully hollering, "Everybody can hear me!" over and over again as he skips down the aisle toward the stage. The trouble begins when Dr X asks Dell, "What do you like?" to which Dell responds, "I like big butts, and I cannot lie—woohoo, everybody can hear me!" as he giggles infectiously and continues to tap the microphone attached to his polo shirt and wiggle in his seat on the stage. Dell, Dr X, and the graduate student audience all laugh at the response, a famous lyric from Sir Mix-A-lot's popular 1990's hit song, "Baby Got Back," which includes the famous line "I like big butts and I cannot lie." Dell continues to giggle and wiggle, delighting in his newfound fame on stage.

As the model test proceeds, the clinician asks Dell a question about school. The following conversation takes place:

Example 3.1

(01) CLINICIAN: what is your favorite class at school?
(02) DELL: Ummmmmm dancing and music
(03) CLINICIAN: Whoa, whoa, whoa, your favorite class is dancing?
(04) DELL: Yeah, my favorite class is dancing and music!
(05) CLINICIAN: Dancing?

(06) DELL: Yes! We dance in music class all the time.
(07) CLINICIAN: Dell, what kind of dance?
(08) DELL: Alabama Gal in music.
(09) CLINICIAN: What?
(10) DELL: Yeah, he (music teacher) tells us to find partners.
(11) CLINICIAN: What kind of dance is that?
(12) DELL: It's the Alabama Gal, it's what we did in music this last year.
(13) CLINICIAN: Well Dell (using a stereotyped tone of Black English Vernacular [BEV]), I'm one of the best hip-hop dancers you've ever seen (laughs and mimics dropping the mic).
(14) DELL: No. We have partners! (Dell insists)

Dell references the country western song "Alabama Gal" and the corresponding square dance in the above conversation. However, Dell's inability to clarify this for Dr X leaves Dr X guessing what Dell is referring to. Dr X's immediate response, "I'm one of the best hip-hop dancers you've ever seen," embodies a Black stereotype in two ways. First, through his use of a Black language in the form of a mock Blaccent. Here I bring together McWhorter's term "Blaccent" (2017) with Jane Hill's work on Mock Spanish (1998). Non-Black people's use of a Blaccent is akin to the ways that non-Spanish speakers use mock Spanish to make themselves sound "cool." However, as in Hill's work, the use of the mock language retains derogatory implications, especially for those who are racially/ethnically tied to the language being mocked. Second, Dr X uses stereotyped Black body movements as he mimics "dropping the mic." This gesture originated with Eddie Murphy's epic mic drop in his 1983 comedy show "Delirious." President Obama also used a famous mic drop in his final speech as president during the annual White House correspondent's dinner. This gesture indicates that the speaker has said the most powerful/funny/unbeatable statement and there is nothing left to say, they are out, the mic has been dropped. While the audience laughs at Dr X's performance, Dell demands that Dr X is incorrect, stating, "No. We have partners!"—which is ignored by Dr X.

The power dynamics of a white public space allow for Dr X to style shift into a mock Blaccent and language. The audience reinforces Dr X's behavior by laughing and clapping for his performance. Dell's behavior in the form of referencing a country song is seen as non-normative and eventually factors into his diagnosis. In white public space, the non-white person must behave in ways that make sense to white norms and expectations. Dell must meet the expectations of Dr X. But these norms are complicated, unstable, and ever changing. In this vignette, Dr X expects that Dell is referencing hip-hop music and dancing, presumably because Dell is Black. This is displayed in Dr X's racialization of Dell by using Black tropes and stereotypes such as "dropping the mic" and the use of a mock Blaccent and referencing hip-hop dancing. Dell does not meet Dr X's racialized expectations. He misses the mark by referencing a country song and a square dance. As we shall see, this is a grave mistake on Dell's part that then impacts the outcome of the test.

Color Evasiveness

Dr X's response, which draws on stereotypes about Black culture, shows us that he perceives and hears Dell as a racialized other, despite his assertion "it is not about culture; it's about a response." This incident is a manifestation of what is known as **color evasiveness** (Annamma et al. 2017). This term describes the practice of avoiding talking about race in interaction. It centers racism as linguistic and ideological processes that humans actively take part in via language choices. These linguistic choices are ones that actively try to avoid the topic of race and, at times, culture. In the case of color-evasive practices, culture can index race in a way that is socially acceptable as it allows individuals to talk about race without talking about race. When Dr X references hip-hop with Dell, he does not mention race; he evades the verbalization of a racial category by instead referring to culture. This is not as simple as it seems. Dr X is implying that hip-hop equates to Black culture and thus it is appropriate to reference it with a Black person. While race is taboo, so-called color-evasive language and ideas allow for culture to be referenced in lieu of racial categories. While statements about culture might at first sound more polite because they evade the category of race, they still point to race, thus achieving the same work.

The idea that one can "run into culture," as the student in Dr X's class inquired about, or that culture is separate from response, demonstrates an imagined way of being understood to be cultureless. In this example, whiteness is treated as if it is cultureless. That means that all other ways of being, or the "culture" that one can "run into," are measured against whiteness as the unmarked normative standard. This leads to non-white cultural norms being marked as different and outside of the norm. By approaching the autism diagnostic test from this so-called "cultureless" perspective, Dr X is engaging in color evasive behavior. Instead of treating white cultural norms as what they are, cultural norms, they are backgrounded and made invisible. Non-white cultural practices are then treated as "culture," a form of otherness that future clinicians are told they might run into.

By teaching his students that ADOS "is not about culture; it's about a response," Dr X is conflating normative responses with white cultural practices. He is erasing the possibility that there could be a neurotypical response that doesn't match his white cultural practices. Dr X is teaching these students the idea that there is one normative way of being and, set against that, there is a thing called "culture" that lives separately and outside of these normative responses. Color-evasive ideologies that appear in classroom pedagogy are central to teaching medical students to believe it is not only possible but scientifically accurate to dissociate culture from their patients' behaviors.

Color-evasive ideologies are important to understand as they are often used as a moral framework. People typically engage in color-evasive practices because they believe that it will have a better outcome: one cannot be racist if one doesn't talk about race. However good the intention, as the case with Dr X shows, racism can happen even when one does not explicitly talk about race. When it comes to the racism created and perpetuated by color evasion, the displacement of ownership allows for there to be racism without the appearance of any racist or overtly racist behavior, making it a particularly difficult problem to solve as it appears that there is nobody at fault. Any attempt to negate racist behavior is undoubtedly admirable but color-evasive strategies like these are ineffective at best, as shown in the following example.

Evaluating Cultural Responses

In the final ethnographic example, Dr X guides Dell to complete one last task. Dr X asks Dell to create a story using a book that has "no words." The interaction is as follows:

Example 3.2

(01) CLINICIAN: We got something else to do, ok?
(02) DELL: What is it? It wasn't me, it wasn't me.
(03) CLINICIAN: Ok.
(04) DELL: What is it?
(05) CLINICIAN: It's a book, we are going to read a book together.
(06) DELL: Yep
(07) CLINICIAN: You know what's special about this book?
(08) DELL: We have a last one.
(09) CLINICIAN: You know what's special about this book?
(10) DELL: Tuesday, Thursday ...
(11) CLINICIAN: It doesn't have any—whole lotta words to it, so we have to make up our own story.
(12) DELL: Good, it doesn't have any words?
(13) CLINICIAN: I'll tell you what, I will take a turn, then you can take a turn.
(14) DELL: There are no words?
(15) CLINICIAN: Well they're a couple of words, let's see ... Let's start from, let's see about the frog.
(16) DELL: (Singing indistinguishably).
(17) CLINICIAN: (indistinguishable instructions; possibly, "you hold the book") Tuesday evening, around eight o'clock the sun's going down ...
(18) DELL: (singing) it's goin' down for real
(19) AUDIENCE: laughter
(20) CLINICIAN: (laughs), are you going to sing the whole book to me?

Again, Dell uses a famous rap song lyric to engage with the clinician. Dell sings "It's Going Down for Real" from Flo Rida's 2014 hit song. The audience and clinician react to Dell's lyrical choice by laughing. As the test ended, Dr X thanked Dell, who hopped up and bowed, smiled, and waved at me from the stage. Dr X then presented

Dell with a gift card to the carwash and a king-size box of Hot Tamales, to which Dell yelled, "Ohhhhh cinnamon Hot Tamales! Mom! Car wash?" indicating that he would like me to take him to the car wash, his favorite place. Dell's therapist entered the auditorium and escorted him to an indoor playground to play while I finished class.

During the break, I asked Dr X about the racial homogeneity of the manipulatives for the test. Dr X listened to my question and took a second to consider it, then said, "Well, I never really noticed; nobody has said anything. I guess it doesn't matter; they are just dolls." I thank Dr X and return to my seat. Dr X's assertion that he "never really noticed" is in alignment with his color-evasive practices that render whiteness as an invisible, normative way of being. Whiteness is so ingrained as the unmarked norm that Dr X has to be told that his manipulatives are all white because he's never noticed. To him, they are just dolls. For a family like mine, a family of color, the lack of representation, even within the manipulatives, is a physical and visual reminder of how pervasively white the experience of a clinical encounter is.

As the class reconvenes, we go over the scoring process for the ADOS. Dr X begins the session by characterizing Dell as a delightful, charming child full of energy. He then explains that Dell's charm and giggling were helpful, making Dell's "disruptive" and "inappropriate" behaviors easier to deal with. The unwanted behaviors Dr X identified included Dell's echolalia, off-topic questions, wiggling, energy level, and giggling. As we work through the test, the question regarding repetitive language gives Dr X pause. He tells us, "Dell has echolalia; he uses phrases that are not spontaneous nor independent to answer questions; that's a problem. He sang to us the rap song he used to answer questions." Dr X says, "Dell is a charmer, but he is overactive and moves constantly. If he weren't so charming, this would have been a much harder assessment. He displays some disruptive behavior; his rap songs are inappropriate." The test resulted in a higher score for Dell from his previous assessment and the addition of a new symptom: "echolalia." A symptom that, before this, had never been identified as a part of Dell's diagnosis.

The behavior that Dr X labeled as echolalic has an alternative interpretation. Throughout the nearly ninety minutes of testing, Dell displayed two instances of Black language in the form of conversational sampling. Conversational sampling within Black language is the use of popular culture as a part of everyday speech (Roth-Gordon 2009). Dell's use of a rap lyric to answer a question and elicit a response, such as laughter, is a great example. Conversational sampling is common and even desired within Black language. Dr X, however, does not recognize this language practice. He sees Dell's use of lyrics as echolalic, disruptive, and not appropriate. This is particularly important as Dr X's original assertion had been that he was looking for a response, not culture. For Dr X, Dell's response is not contextualized by Black American cultural ways of speaking in the form of conversational sampling. Dr X's color-evasive ideologies impact the diagnostic process by attempting to frame Dell's speech as a cultureless response. But culture is always at work; it shapes responses, and it shapes Dr X's analysis of Dell's responses. Dr X's color-evasive ideology centers whiteness as the unspoken norm against which Dell's language is being judged. Dell's use of Black language does not align with Dr X's understanding of what is normative (white), and Dr X pathologizes it as evidence of disability. Dr X also uses terms such as disruptive and inappropriate to describe Dell's utterances.

The Dangers of the Clinic as White Public Space

Color evasiveness is central to the creation of clinical spaces as white public spaces (Page and Thomas 1994), spaces that are inherently dangerous for non-white people. White public space includes the following language practices;

> (1) intense monitoring of the speech of racialized populations such as Chicanos and Latinos and African Americans for signs of linguistic disorder and (2) The invisibility of almost identical signs in the speech of Whites, where language mixing, required for the expression of a highly valued type of colloquial persona, takes several forms. (Hill 1998)

For children like Dell who present as non-white, the policing of language can be both racialized and disability coded. Language is a highly monitored behavior within the autism diagnosis and verbal language is a clinical ideal. Black children within the white public space of a clinic experience the policing of language in a multiplicative way. These individuals experience racialization, an example of which is the way that Dr X resorts to stereotypes of Black people to try and understand Dell. Black patients are policed for the use of language that deviates from white cultural ideals. For Dell this took two forms: when he used rap lyrics in the form of conversational sampling and when he deviated from stereotypes of Black culture by referencing a country western song and dance. At times Dell displayed behavior that was treated as too Black and at other times he was not Black enough. Simultaneously, clinicians monitor Black patients for a set of autism diagnostic criteria that are imagined to be acultural. This process ultimately ends by pathologizing what is deemed culturally inappropriate, or non-white, uses of language.

The intense monitoring of language in this context ultimately creates an additional burden for Black patients. They must be verbal and be able to read social cues well enough to know when to code switch. Difficulties with understanding social cues are a hallmark of autism diagnostic criteria. Social skills classes run by speech pathologists are among the most common therapeutic interventions taking place in both the medical and educational spaces. If Dell had been able to read the social cues that indicate Black people need to code switch in white spaces—if, for example, he had said that he likes Hot Tamales instead of big butts—Dell's language likely would not have been coded as echolalic. Echolalia is defined as using the same language or sounds over and over as opposed to the use of "spontaneous" speech. In the white public space that Dell was navigating, clinicians like Dr X do not take Black language patterns, such as conversational sampling, into consideration. This is complicated by Dell having autism which makes reading the social cues that dictate what is expected of him in white public spaces extremely difficult, if not impossible.

The creation of white public spaces includes a second criterion, the invisibility of language mixing in the speech of white people (Hill 1998). White people are allowed to showcase similar speech patterns to non-whites as it helps them craft an identity that is seen in a positive light. A great example of this is Dr X's use of Black language and the audience's positive response. The clinician uses Black language and leans into tropes of Blackness, such as "hip-hop" dancing and "dropping the mic." What is fascinating is that the clinician and the graduate students in the audience laughed, signifying that the clinician's use of Black language was funny and acceptable. Dr X and the audience also laughed at Dell's use of Black language, signifying that Dell could engage the audience in a way they found funny. Unfortunately, for Dell, his language was interpreted differently during the test scoring, at which time the behavior was pathologized as being echolalic. White public space and color-evasive practices render Dr X unable to see Dell's use of Black linguistic norms as a culturally normative and desirable trait for Black Americans. This is not without its repercussions; it increases Dell's score and potentially changes his category from moderate to severe autism—which has further ripple effects.

The Stakes Are High

In the contemporary United States, Black students are at higher risk of being overidentified for special education, but they are also at significant risk for misdiagnosis in both the medical and education systems. According to a recent 2023 study by the Center for Disease Control (CDC), researchers have found that Black children have gone from being the least likely racial group to access an autism diagnosis to becoming the most likely group to access the diagnosis (CDC 2023). The problem of misdiagnosis is that students receive the wrong services and support. Undiagnosed students receive no services or support. Hyperdiagnosis means that those who should not meet the criteria for a diagnosis but have been diagnosed anyway end up in special education again losing out on an education that meets their needs. The wrong diagnostic label leads to an inappropriate classroom placement, the inability to access appropriate services and therapeutic options, and traumatizing experiences with adverse disciplinary measures such as restraint, seclusion, and school expulsion.

For those unfamiliar with special education, behavior management methods often include restraint and seclusion. But these methods, which amount to punishment, are disproportionately used on Black disabled children (Noguera 2003). Too many special education classrooms include a seclusion room—sometimes called a "room within a room." These are small closet-sized rooms that include padding on the walls and a door with a window. Children who display unwanted behaviors are placed into these small cells and the door is locked—an adult looks in on the child through the window—and the child is released upon displaying wanted behaviors, such as quiet, calm, etc. It is difficult to miss the fact that young children—especially Black disabled children are subjected to solitary confinement within public schools as early as preschool. Education scholars have referred to special education as the "playground for the pipeline to prison" (Powell and Keeney Parks 2021; Wald and Loosen 2003). The National Center for Learning Disabilities 2022 report on Black disabled students in special education states that these students constitute the most significant portion of students suspended annually. Of youth in juvenile detention facilities, 60–75% percent have disabilities that make them eligible for special education services. However, the majority of these students cannot access much-needed support from either the education or medical systems.

In many states, special education students with IEPs (Individual Education Plans) do not receive a diploma for high school completion but rather a certificate, sometimes referred to as a "certificate of attendance." The refusal to allow all disabled students to access a diploma further limits their ability to gain access to gainful employment. Subminimum wage remains enshrined in US federal labor laws, which means that it is legal to pay disabled people a significantly lower wage than their non-disabled peers. The average is currently around $3.40 per hour. Black disabled people are considerably more likely to experience these outcomes.

Conclusion

In this chapter, I have argued that color-evasive ideologies create white public space where clinicians police non-white bodies and conflate a Black child's use of Black language with disability. Color-evasive frames allow for the evasion of the taboo category of race and replaces references to race with culture as a proxy. However, the category of culture still creates racialized outcomes. Culture becomes a proxy for race—and normativity becomes synonymous with whiteness. Language practices and ideologies work powerfully to produce and maintain biomedicine as white public space.

Blame for racial inequities in healthcare is too often placed upon Black families and patients in the familiar refrains of "Black people mistrust medicine" or "Black people don't talk about disability." Instead of placing the blame for racism and inequities in healthcare on Black families, we should interrogate the clinicians and the color-evasive frameworks that they reinforce in the clinical classroom. Teaching is one of our most powerful tools to combat racism. What one teaches in the classroom profoundly impacts how clinicians diagnose and interact with non-white individuals when they enter into practice. The stakes for Black disabled children are incredibly high. Disability is not contained in clinical spaces; it is lived in all spaces and systems across the lifespan. A misdiagnosis of any kind has a ripple effect that has devastating consequences on the lifetime outcomes of Black disabled people.

Acknowledgments

I would like to thank the following scholars and community members who agreed to read and edit this chapter. Thank you for your support and friendship and for sharing your thoughts on this piece: Sireen Irshied, PhD, Abigail Mack, PhD, Temell Purkett, MS, MBA, and Jeffery Wilson.

Questions for Reflection and Discussion

Reflection Questions

1. What part of this chapter impacted you the most? Choose a specific quote or example and discuss how you responded to it. How did it make you feel? Why do you think you had this response?
2. Have you come across the concept of "white public space" before? Where? If not, why do you think it is a new concept for you?

Looking In: Small Group Discussion Questions

1. What is the ADOS? How does this evaluation guide the way that the clinician in this example listens to Dell's language?
2. What is color evasiveness? Define this term in your own words and provide examples from the reading or other contexts.
3. How do ideas of "culture" get mobilized in color-evasive frameworks? Discuss examples from the chapter to illustrate.
4. What is white public space? Define the term in your own words. Are there spaces you move through in your life that might be considered "white public spaces"? What have you noticed about these spaces that makes you think of them as white public spaces?

Looking Out: Large Group Discussion Questions

1. How are white public spaces enacted and perpetuated in the training of future clinicians, as in the graduate class shown here?
2. What are other examples of white public spaces in contexts related to health? What aspects of language and communication contribute to producing these as white public space?
3. In the chapter, what linguistic practices were observed as part of the ADOS? What practices were ignored? (It may be helpful to think about the use or avoidance of terms like echolalia and conversational sampling.) Given what you learned in the chapter, how might you modify the way Dr X taught the ADOS? What changes might you implement in the ADOS itself?

References

Annamma, Subini Ancy, Darell D. Jackson, and Deb Morrison. 2017. Conceptualizing Color-Evasiveness: Using Dis/Ability Critical Race Theory to Expand a Color-Blind Racial Ideology in Education and Society. *Race Ethnicity and Education* 20(2): pp. 147–162. https://doi.org/10.1080/13613324.2016.1248837.

CDC (Center for Disease Control). 2023. Spotlight on a New Pattern in Racial and Ethnic Differences Emerges in Autism Spectrum Disorder (ASD) Identification among 8-Year-Old Children, April 6. https://www.cdc.gov/ncbddd/autism/addm-community-report/spotlight-on-racial-ethnic-differences.html.

Hill, Jane H. 1998. Language, Race, and White Public Space. *American Anthropologist* 100(3): pp. 680–689.

McWhorter, John. 2017. *Talking Back, Talking Black: Truths about America's Lingua Franca.* New York: Bellevue Literary Press.

Noguera, P. A. (2003). The Trouble with Black Boys: The Role and Influence of Environmental and Cultural Factors on the Academic Performance of African American Males. *Urban Education* 38(4): pp. 431–459.

Page, Helan, and R. Brooke Thomas. 1994. White Public Space and the Construction of White Privilege in US Health Care: Fresh Concepts and a New Model of Analysis. *Medical Anthropology Quarterly* 8(1): pp. 109–116.

Powell, Tunette, and Stephanie Keeney Parks. 2021. They Never Listen to the Parent: Parent Narratives at the Intersection of Racism, Education, and Disability. In *Racism by Another Name: Black Students, Overrepresentation, and the Carceral State of Special Education*, ed. D. Hines, M. Boveda, and E. J. Lindo, pp.227–240. Charlotte, NC: Information Age Publishing.

Roth-Gordon, J. (2009). Conversational Sampling, Race Trafficking, and the Invocation of the Gueto in Brazilian Hip Hop. In *Global Linguistic Flows: Hip Hop Cultures, Youth Identities, and the Politics of Language*, ed. H. S. Alim, A. Ibrahim, and A. Pennycook, pp. 63–77. Abingdon: Taylor & Francis Group.

Wald, J., and Daniel J. Losen. 2003. Defining and Redirecting a School-to-Prison Pipeline. *New Directions for Youth Development* 99: pp. 9–15. https://doi.org/10.1002/yd.51.

SECTION 2
LANGUAGE ACCESS
Editors' Introduction

Migration has always been a central part of the human experience. Across human history, people have at times chosen to move and at other moments have been forcibly obliged to leave their homelands and live elsewhere. Communities where people have remained in place have also been transformed by the arrival of newcomers with different languages and cultural practices. These processes continue to unfold today, resulting in increasingly diverse populations the world over. As a consequence, most regions, nations, and cities are characterized by cultural diversity and multilingualism. This diversity can include highly varied combinations of signed and spoken languages, Indigenous/Native languages, colonial languages, creole languages, and immigrant languages.

In healthcare settings, patient populations reflect contemporary realities of cultural, racial, class, national, ethnic, religious, and linguistic diversity. This means that, at least sometimes, clinicians are treating patients with whom they do not share a common language. Clinicians and patients may also have widely differing understandings, expectations, and practices concerning health and illness. Though these kinds of diversity are pervasive, healthcare institutions often treat the dominant language and culture as the default or the norm for medical care, turning language into a barrier for accessing care (Martínez 2020).

In light of this reality, practitioners, community organizations, researchers, and governing bodies have developed innovative solutions (e.g., Flood et al. 2019). The design and implementation of these strategies are shaped by multiple factors, including: assumptions about the role of verbal or signed interpretation, preconceived ideas about translation, stereotypes about certain patient populations, attention to what linguistically diverse patients say they want and need, awareness of and concern for patients' material circumstances, and a willingness and ability to allocate resources (cf. Byrd and Monaghan 2019). When institutional support is unavailable, multilingual family members, including children, are often obliged to moderate clinical communication (García-Sánchez 2014; Reynolds and Orellana 2009).

The chapters in this section explore communicative challenges in healthcare across three settings and describe the interventions that have been implemented in these places to address these challenges and improve language access to healthcare. Rachel Showstack, Raúl Rangel Fernández, and Margarita Francisco lay out the complex ways that language constitutes a social determinant of health and describe an academic-community partnership that has created accessible health education materials for Mayan Guatemalan communities in Kansas in the United States. Lissie Wahl's chapter demonstrates that even when there is a legal obligation for healthcare organizations to provide interpretation, multiple factors moderate how effectively professional interpreters are able to support patients. Paula Saravia and Tibor Gutiérrez describe the important work that Mapuche intercultural facilitators do to provide support for patients receiving care in Chile's public healthcare system.

References

Byrd, Mark, and Leila Monaghan. 2019. Interpreting Deaf HIV/AIDS: A Dialogue. In *Language and Social Justice in Practice*, ed. Netta Avineri, Laura R. Graham, Eric J. Johnson, Robin Conley Riner, and Jonathan Rosa, pp. 128–135. New York: Routledge.

Flood, David, Anita Chary, Peter Rohloff, and Brent Henderson. 2019. Language as Health: Healing in Indigenous Communities in Guatemala through the Revitalization of Mayan Languages. In *Language and Social Justice in Practice*, ed. Netta Avineri, Laura R. Graham, Eric J. Johnson, Robin Conley Riner, and Jonathan Rosa, pp. 136–143. New York: Routledge.

García-Sánchez, Inmaculada Ma. 2014. *Language and Muslim Immigrant Childhoods: The Politics of Belonging*. Malden, MA: Wiley-Blackwell.

Martínez, Glenn A. 2020. *Spanish in Health Care: Policy, Practice and Pedagogy in Latino Health*. New York: Routledge.

Reynolds, Jennifer F., and Marjorie Faulstich Orellana. 2009. New Immigrant Youth Interpreting in White Public Space. *American Anthropologist* 111(2): pp. 211–223.

4

Health Care Access for Mayan Communities in Kansas

Rachel Showstack, Raúl Rangel Fernández, and Margarita Francisco

Introduction

In the rural highland community in Guatemala where Sandra (a pseudonym) grew up, everyone spoke the Mayan language Akateko. Occasionally Sandra spoke Spanish when communicating with individuals outside of her community, but she had never been to school and had not learned to read or write in either language. When she was 18 years old, Sandra, her husband, and their two children relocated to Coffeyville, Kansas, to find work and a better life. They had not lived in Coffeyville for long when Sandra began experiencing tooth pain and found a dentist who could see her even though she didn't have insurance. At the dental office, a receptionist handed her a form to fill out, but Sandra was unable to read it. She left the office and took the form to a bilingual community leader named Blanca to ask what to do with it. Since Blanca did not have experience with dental office paperwork, she suggested that Sandra go back to the receptionist to request assistance. Following Blanca's suggestion, Sandra returned to the office with the form and asked the receptionist for help. The receptionist looked at the form and then looked at Sandra and said: "This form is in Spanish!" Feeling ashamed that she did not know how to read or know enough Spanish to answer questions about her health, Sandra left the office again. Eventually, Blanca called the office to request that additional support be provided, and Sandra and her family were finally treated.

In this chapter, we describe a process of coalition building and community engagement to work toward improving institutional and community contexts in Southern Kansas, so that individuals like Sandra can receive the resources, assistance, and treatment they need to be healthy. The project we describe is an initiative we are involved in called Alce su Voz (Speak Out) at Wichita State University, an interdisciplinary center that utilizes a community-based approach to improve health equity for Latinx and Indigenous communities across the state. Our three-pronged approach to improving health equity includes community engagement and education, workforce development, and policy-maker engagement. This chapter

Rachel Showstack, Raúl Rangel Fernández, and Margarita Francisco, *Health Care Access for Mayan Communities in Kansas.* In: *Language and Health in Action.* Edited by: Lynnette Arnold et al., Oxford University Press. © Rachel Showstack, Raúl Rangel Fernández, and Margarita Francisco (2026). DOI: 10.1093/9780198933953.003.0004 focuses primarily on the first component of our work, and we describe our processes of engaging with Mayan communities in rural parts of Kansas.

Sandra's story demonstrates how a constellation of different factors related to communities and the healthcare system can interact with each other and lead to barriers to healthcare access. These include elements of an individual's experience within their communities, such as low literacy levels in families, a lack of educational opportunities, shame related to Indigenous languages and identities, and a distrust of the healthcare system. They also include conditions within the healthcare system, such as limited awareness about multilingualism and literacy, insufficient sensitivity to Indigenous perspectives on health, limited resources to support communication with Indigenous communities, and health insurance systems that do not cover all residents. Xenophobia and hostility toward immigrants also shape conditions within the healthcare system, affecting the ways that individuals are treated within the system and leading to fear of interactions with authorities, including doctors and hospitals. These experiences and conditions create barriers to **health equity**, a state in which everyone has the opportunity to achieve optimal health. The community and systemic elements that impact health equity are examples of **social determinants of health** or **SDoH**, which the United States Department of Health and Human Services (HHS) defines as "the conditions in the environments where people are born, live, work, play, worship, and age that affect a wide range of quality-of-life outcomes and risks." Officially, HHS categorizes SDoH into five domains: economic stability, education access and quality, health care access and quality, neighborhood and built environment, and social and community context (Office of Disease Prevention and Health Promotion 2030).

As Sandra's story demonstrates, language is a key SDoH (Showstack et al. 2019). However, there is no simple correlation between language skills and health outcomes; rather, health communication experiences of linguistically minoritized groups are impacted by the availability of same-language care, the willingness and abilities of healthcare workers and patients to strive for shared understanding, and other contextual factors (Martínez 2020; Santos et al. 2023). Sandra's story also suggests how language proficiency interacts with other factors, such as immigration status, socioeconomic status, access to quality education, and acceptance (or lack thereof) of linguistically diverse individuals. This is an example of how multiple interacting SDoH impact health outcomes differently than each would on its own (Singer et al. 2006).

Like many healthcare entities in rural Southeast Kansas, Sandra's dental office was not prepared to provide equitable care for Mayan patients, who often do not understand English, speak limited Spanish, and may not be able to read. The receptionists and dental clinicians were unaware of the needs of the community, and the office did not offer qualified professional interpreting services. Though one receptionist spoke Spanish, she was not trained in healthcare interpreting. Because of Sandra's undocumented immigration status and her awareness of xenophobic discourses circulating in Coffeyville, she was reluctant to ask for help. Furthermore, since Sandra had not lived in the US for long and did not have access to information about her rights, she was not aware that the dental office had a legal obligation to assist her in understanding and filling out their forms at no cost.

Sandra was also hesitant to reveal that she spoke a Mayan language because she had learned to avoid divulging this information, perhaps due to the history of oppression and violence against Mayan communities in Guatemala. Mayan people have been an "underprivileged majority" in Central America since the region was conquered by Spanish colonizers in the sixteenth century (Holocaust Museum Houston 2023). Mayan immigration to the United States began in the late 1970s and has accelerated since, driven largely by Guatemala's thirty-six-year civil war, during which a genocide inflicted by US-backed dictators killed hundreds of thousands of Mayan individuals through violence that included raids and the burning of villages and crops (Commission on Historical Clarification 1999; Holocaust Museum Houston 2023).

Like other states in the Great Plains region, Kansas has recently experienced an increase in immigration from Central America, particularly from Mayan communities in Guatemala (Hamann and Harklau 2021). This is in part due to recruitment practices in industries that rely on immigrants for their workforce. Southeast Kansas, where Coffeyville is located, is home to thousands of Guatemalans, many of whom are from the Huehuetenango region, where the mutually intelligible Mayan languages Akateko and Q'anjob'al are spoken. In Southwest Kansas, the primary Mayan languages spoken are K'iche', Aguacateco, Kaqchikel, and Mam. Many Guatemalan migrants travel to Kansas directly from Guatemala; others arrive via California or southern states such as Florida, drawn by the low cost of living, tranquil lifestyle, and employment opportunities in factories and meatpacking plants. For example, in Arkansas City (known as Ark City) in South-central Kansas, the main source of employment for Mayans is the Creekstone Farms meatpacking plant, which was established in the region in 2003. Other work opportunities include factories such as the Acme Foundry, which specializes in iron castings.

Migrants from Indigenous communities in Latin America (particularly Mexico and Guatemala), who have settled in large numbers in California, the Great Plains, and Florida, commonly experience combinations of barriers similar to Sandra's, leading to difficulties with attaining health care (Bonessi and Turner 2021). Meanwhile, the region's healthcare facilities are in the beginning phases of addressing barriers to access for linguistically diverse communities. Federal legislation provides strong protection against discrimination based on language, and failure to provide qualified language access services in just about any type of healthcare entity is against the law; yet healthcare facilities in Coffeyville and Ark City have struggled to provide these required services, perhaps in part due to the state's inefficient system for financing them (see Showstack 2022). In addition to the issues within the healthcare system, problems exist within the Mayan communities in Kansas that create additional barriers, such as low levels of literacy and distrust of the US healthcare system.

This chapter situates the barriers to health equity experienced by Mayan community members in Southeast and South-central Kansas within the SDoH framework and calls for a rethinking of the framework that considers the complexities of the relationship between language and health equity. Furthermore, we demonstrate how university faculty and students can develop community partnerships to improve access to healthcare for linguistically diverse communities by describing a partnership to address health equity for Mayan communities in Kansas that was developed between 2022 and 2023, during the COVID-19 pandemic.

Health Disparities in Mayan Communities in Kansas

The severity of the COVID-19 pandemic exacerbated existing health inequities, leading to disproportionately high infection rates and mortality rates among communities of color (especially Black, Latinx, and Indigenous communities) in the United States. The pandemic therefore serves as an illustrative example of how SDoH can lead to poor health outcomes in certain populations. The preventable differences in health outcomes that correspond with SDoH are known as **health disparities** and are often measured based on health indicators such as infant mortality, the presence of diabetes, life expectancy, and cancer mortality. In the case of COVID-19, comorbidities (i.e., having additional, often preventable, health conditions, such as uncontrolled diabetes) increase the risk of severe illness from the virus. Health disparities occur because the SDoH lead to a context in which different groups have unequal opportunities to attain the highest possible level of health. The purpose of community health work is to reduce, and ultimately do away with, health disparities, and achieve health equity. Health equity does not mean that every person has access to the same assistance, services, and resources as everybody else; rather, it means that every person has access to the assistance, services, and resources that they need to thrive. For example, not everybody needs language access services, but individuals like Sandra, who are not able to communicate about their health in the language spoken by their clinicians, do need them. For these individuals, qualified professional interpreting services are shown to reduce miscommunication and improve patient satisfaction, which ultimately leads to improved health outcomes (Diamond et al. 2019; Karliner et al. 2007).

It is difficult to collect data on health outcomes from COVID-19 in Latin American Indigenous communities in the US because individuals from these communities are often classified as Hispanic/Latinx and Spanish speaking, erasing their indigeneity in the data (CIELO et al. 2022; Foo et al. 2021). However, based on conversations with community leaders and Mayan community members in Kansas, we know that various factors placed this demographic at higher risk for poor outcomes from the virus. For example, barriers to healthcare access experienced in Kansas Mayan communities can lead to poor control of chronic conditions like diabetes, increasing the risk of severe outcomes from the COVID-19 virus.

Mayan workers were also at increased risk for contracting the virus early in the pandemic. Meatpacking plants, which have a history of actively recruiting workers from disadvantaged communities abroad, employ many Mayans. Workers at these plants, because they were essential workers, could not stay at home during the lockdown and had to continue working in close quarters with each other. The resulting outbreaks of COVID-19 in the plants primarily affected immigrant communities, including the many Mayan workers.

When Kansas vaccinated its meatpacking workers in the spring of 2021, large numbers of Mayan residents were vaccinated. However, vaccination rates remained low for Mayans who did not work in the plants, due to barriers to health care and to health information, inadequate language access services in public health programs, lack of transportation, fears resulting from vaccine misinformation, cost, a lack of prior experience with local health clinics and vaccines in rural communities in Guatemala, and a preference for natural home remedies over biomedical treatment.

Community Partnerships for Health Equity

In this section, we illustrate the role of language scholars in addressing health disparities by describing the process through which we formed a coalition with Mayan communities and health care leaders in rural Southern Kansas as part of a pandemic relief project that focused on addressing key factors that generate health disparities for Mayan immigrants. Each of the authors of this chapter has a unique role in the project: Rachel, an applied linguist and associate professor of Spanish at Wichita State University, is the director of Alce su Voz, a community-based initiative at Wichita State whose mission is to support health equity for Spanish speakers and speakers of Indigenous languages in Kansas. Raúl, a graduate student in Spanish and linguistics, was a research assistant on the project and has been engaging with Mayan community members and collecting data on the Mayan languages spoken in Kansas. Margarita, who grew up in Guatemala and speaks Akateko, Spanish, and English, is a community liaison on our project and is working on information dissemination and community engagement. We wrote this chapter together to present our diverse perspectives on SDoH within Mayan communities in Kansas and our experiences with coalition building for health equity.

Alce su Voz was formed in Wichita, a mid-sized city in Central Kansas and the largest city in the state, after a series of community meetings that Rachel and her students organized in spring 2020 to engage Spanish-speaking Kansans in conversations about language barriers and interpreting services in healthcare encounters. These meetings were organized in collaboration with faculty in the Wichita State University Department of Public Health Sciences and with support from local Latinx community leaders. We structured the meetings within the framework of community-based participatory research (CBPR), a collaborative approach that includes, from its inception, the voices and perspectives of the individuals a project is designed to serve (Minkler and Wallerstein 2012). Through the sharing of *testimonios*, personal stories about challenging experiences related to a sociopolitical context, the participants identified a need to improve: (1) the availability of Spanish-language public health information and information about how the healthcare system works, and (2) healthcare interpreting services for in-person and telemedicine health appointments. This community story sharing and identification of issues led to the formation of a community coalition that would later become Alce su Voz.

The organization's work with Mayan communities began in 2022, two years after the initial community meetings, when Rachel learned from a state-level vaccine equity official that there was a need for vaccine equity work in the state's Mayan communities. At that time, data from the Kansas State Department of Education showed that thousands of Mayan families lived in Southwest Kansas and that similar communities were growing in Southeast Kansas as well. Alce su Voz began building connections with our partners in rural Southern Kansas and simultaneously developed a proposal for a COVID-19 relief funding grant, which we attained in fall 2022. In our process of coalition building, we aimed to focus primarily on listening first, carefully planning meeting agendas to include only very basic introductions before allowing participants to share their perspectives on challenges to healthcare access in their communities. Meetings with partners included two types of groups: (1) healthcare leaders, such as directors of Federally Qualified Health Centers (FQHC) and county health departments, and (2) community health workers and others who work closely with Mayan communities.

After initiating a process of building regional coalitions, the next step was to engage with Mayan community members in each region. We did this through meetings with individuals and families organized by our community partners, a quantitative and qualitative questionnaire administered verbally, and larger community engagement workshops organized in collaboration with community partners and Mayan community members. Although the overall objective of the funded project was increasing vaccine confidence and promoting vaccination efforts in Mayan communities in Kansas, we knew that we needed to better understand the experiences and circumstances of the target communities and have time to gain community trust before engaging in vaccine messaging and education activities. Specifically, we were interested in learning who the trusted voices in the community were, where people got their information about public health issues, and what challenges they encountered when seeking care.

When meeting with community partners and Mayan families, the team leaders paid careful attention to different Mayan cultural practices so that we would be able to interact with Mayan communities appropriately, but we entered this process with a naïve assumption that all Mayans share the same cultural practices. For example, when we attended a mobile Guatemalan consulate event, a team member asked a few different women if she could take photos of them and their children, and they asked their husbands for permission. Based on this observation, we assumed that in Mayan communities the men generally made decisions for family members; however, this was an erroneous assumption because every Mayan community has its own set of cultural norms. From before the colonization of the Americas, Mayan people have never been unified under one government, and ongoing conflicts exist between some communities. Each Mayan community (e.g., Akateko people) has its own traditions and cultural practices, including interactional norms, dress, cuisine, and gender expectations; furthermore, like anywhere else, each family has its own culture. This observation is a valuable reminder of the importance of cultural sensitivity, an openness to learning about and respecting an individual's cultural practices.

We also spent time getting to know the rural regions of Kansas where Mayan communities are centered. For example, Rachel spent a period of several days in Coffeyville meeting with diverse individuals along with different team members each day. By spending time with an Akateko family that Rachel had met previously, Rachel and Raúl were able to develop a stronger relationship with that family. Shared time together is a way that team members associated with the university have been able to build rapport and trust with Mayan families and individuals, which is an important step toward engaging a larger community. We also explored the town by car and visited the different spaces where Mayan community members spend time, including the Mexican store, the Guatemalan store, the Boys & Girls Club, local churches, and the local FQHC. Spending time in Coffeyville also allowed the team to meet healthcare leaders, gain a better understanding of the resources available and the challenges the community was facing, and become familiar faces in the process of developing community trust.

In this section, we narrated the formation of partnerships for health equity in Kansas Latinx and Mayan communities. In the next section, we describe what we learned from Kansas Mayan communities about barriers to health equity during the COVID-19 pandemic.

Health Equity for Mayan Communities during the COVID-19 Pandemic

We learned from Mayan community members in Southwest, South-central, and Southeast Kansas that church leaders were some of the most trusted and respected voices, and that many community members obtained health information from Facebook and other forms of social media. Blanca, a resident of Coffeyville, explained that the pastors of one of the churches had told their congregation that God would punish them if they got vaccinated against the COVID-19 virus. However, this was the only case of blatant anti-vaccination discourse that we heard of at a religious institution. In many other cases, churches were an important source of information on COVID-19 safety protocols and vaccination opportunities for Mayan communities. Common barriers to healthcare access included: difficulties obtaining accessible sources of reliable information, the spread of misinformation on social media and within families and communities, differences between healthcare practices and requirements in Guatemala and those that exist in the United States, fear of US Immigration and Customs Enforcement (ICE), being uninsured, a lack of information about healthcare payment plans and where to receive the most affordable healthcare, and lack of knowledge within the healthcare system about Indigenous peoples.

Additionally, many people experienced the same challenges as Sandra related to language and literacy. Most of the Mayan community members whom we have met speak Spanish as a second language; they explain that Spanish is the language they used to communicate with people from different communities back home in Guatemala. However, levels of proficiency in Spanish vary greatly, and additional scaffolding may be needed in Spanish-language conversations, especially in high-stakes situations like medical encounters. Men in Mayan families are more likely to be proficient in Spanish because they tend to have more schooling and are usually the ones engaged in communication outside of their own neighborhood. Furthermore, people from isolated rural communities were less likely to have access to education and are therefore less likely to be literate and proficient in Spanish. We also found that some Mayan community members were hesitant to share with us that they spoke a Mayan language. Some may be accustomed to hiding their Indigenous identity because of the recent genocide and long legacy of colonialism in Guatemala. Another reason people may not mention that they speak a Mayan language is the prevailing ideology that Mayan languages are not real languages; in Kansas, most people from within and outside of the Mayan communities refer to Mayan languages as *dialectos* (dialects).

We have also observed that Mayan individuals living in Kansas tend to have very limited literacy, reflecting low levels of literacy in Guatemala (Hallman et al. 2006). When healthcare entities do not have trained interpreters and clinicians are not accustomed to the communication needs of Mayan patients, a Mayan individual with limited Spanish language and literacy skills is unlikely to receive quality care. This scenario created a significant hurdle for our project because, although we aimed to connect Mayan communities with health care in their own town, or at least in their county, many individuals reported facing inadequate language access services; it is common for people to travel three hours from Coffeyville to Wichita for care to visit a clinic with Spanish-speaking staff. This situation demonstrates why it is important to work with both communities and health care facilities to address SDoH. We can learn from communities about barriers to healthcare and share information about rights and resources, but those individuals will not be able to attain adequate care unless facilities are able to provide the services that people need.

Improving Health Equity for Mayan Communities in Kansas

Our initiative to improve health equity in Kansas Mayan communities includes different forms of information dissemination within Mayan communities and collaboration with local healthcare entities to address problems within the healthcare system. In this section, we describe the approaches we utilized for these activities and how we implemented them.

Our methods of information dissemination are community workshop presentations, tabling at community events, and creating and disseminating informational videos and testimonials that target Kansas Mayan communities. The first community engagement workshops in Ark City and Coffeyville took place in fall 2023, after we had spent a year building rapport in the communities. The purpose of these meetings was to continue learning about barriers to health equity for Mayan communities and to provide information about patients' rights and local health resources. Our Ark City event was attended by speakers of the Mayan languages Akateko, Q'anjob'al, K'iche', and Aguacateko, and Margarita arranged for interpreters for each of these languages. We facilitated the event in Spanish, and participants were grouped according to language, so that they could have access to interpretation and converse with each other easily. At our Coffeyville event, the participants spoke either Akateko or Q'anjob'al, and Spanish-Akateko and Spanish-Q'anjob'al interpreting was provided. Concerns about lack of access to information and services due to limited literacy skills emerged as a salient theme in our conversations in both workshops, and participants shared information with each other about accessing and paying for certain health services.

The initial set of videos that we created in Spanish and Akateko for Mayan community members in Kansas aimed to dispel common myths about the COVID-19 vaccine (e.g., that it was created by the US government to place a chip inside people's arms for surveillance purposes), assuage fears (e.g., of getting sick from the vaccine, having to pay for it, or being forced to share personal data); and to disseminate information on boosters. The videos featured both healthcare providers offering vaccine information and Mayan community members sharing their personal stories of why they chose to get vaccinated and what their vaccination experience was like. We utilized information obtained through our community engagement activities to inform our dissemination plan; since Facebook was a common source of information and interpersonal communication often occurred through WhatsApp, we designed our campaign to be compatible with both modalities. The use of video allowed us to provide information in a way that could reach individuals with low levels of literacy, and the use of community members' personal narratives aimed to be reflective of beliefs and experiences within the community.

In addition to disseminating information to address barriers within the communities, we also worked with healthcare leaders to address barriers within the healthcare system. When meeting with healthcare leaders, we found that a lack of information and resources and a limited multilingual workforce in rural Southeast Kansas created barriers to providing care for newcomer families. At the time of writing, we are building partnerships with healthcare leaders in Southeast and South-central Kansas and working toward supporting local health clinics in their efforts to disseminate information about available services, provide equitable language access services, and create a welcoming environment. We have also initiated conversations with *promotores de salud* (community health workers) who want to help connect Mayan communities with local resources, a key strategy for improving health equity for Mayan communities in the United States (Zhen-Duan et al. 2017).

Conclusions and Implications

In this chapter, we have demonstrated that language is one of the many SDoH affecting Mayan communities in Kansas, and that language interacts with other social determinants. We have argued that community partnerships are important for health equity and that these partnerships should start with coalition building and listening to community members. Finally, we have identified some of the challenges of addressing SDoH in Mayan communities and shared our approaches to addressing those challenges. We focused on improving healthcare language access through both supporting improvements to systems and policies, and through community education about language access rights and protocols. Our community-based participatory approach has allowed us to begin to gain community trust and buy-in through engaging community members in conversations about what issues need to be addressed and collaborating with community members in the development of community and systemic interventions. We hope that our description of the coalition-building and information dissemination process led by Alce su Voz in rural Mayan communities in Kansas can help readers consider their own roles in addressing health disparities in linguistically marginalized communities.

Questions for Reflection and Discussion

Reflection Questions

1. Map out the steps that the authors took to develop Alce su Voz. If you were to engage in an initiative similar to Alce su Voz, what steps would you include in your process? What types of skills and knowledge would you bring to the table and what other types of skills and expertise would be needed to complement yours?

Looking In: Small Group Discussion Questions

1. What does health equity mean? Provide a definition in your own words and identify some examples from the chapter or other contexts.
2. What are SDoH? How does language function as an SDoH? Consider factors related to patients' language skills as well as factors in the healthcare system.
3. What factors in Guatemala and the United States have led many Mayan people and families to leave Guatemala and settle in Kansas? How do these factors complicate healthcare access for Mayan communities in Kansas?
4. In Kansas, what factors put Mayans at higher risk of contracting COVID-19 and of having more serious complications from the virus if they contracted it? What factors shaped Mayan residents' access to COVID vaccination and their attitudes toward vaccination?

Looking Out: Large Group Discussion Questions

1. Based on the community work outlined in this chapter, what measures are necessary to ensure access to care for multilingual communities? Be sure to consider examples that go beyond simply providing multilingual resources.
2. What distinguishes CBPR from ethnographic research? How is language important in this research? What makes CBPR a particularly good approach for projects focused on community health?
3. In what ways does Alce Su Voz seek to improve health equity for Mayan communities in Kansas? How did the conversations with stakeholders influence the approach they took to community education? How did the conversations shape the health-related resources they developed? What elements of their approach do you think could be usefully applied in other communities or in relation to different health issues?

References

Bonessi, Dominique Maria, and Tyrone Turner. 2021. Local Maya Immigrants Seek Services—and Visibility—in Their Indigenous Languages. *The DCist*, November 23. https://dcist.com/story/21/11/23/maya-immigrants-dc-md-va/.

CIELO (Comunidades Indígenas en Liderazgo), UCLA AISC, UCLA Promise Institute for Human Rights, and UCLA Bunche Center. 2022. We Are Here: Indigenous Diaspora in Los Angeles. Comunidades Indígenas en Liderazgo, January 31. https://storymaps.arcgis.com/stories/618560a29f2a402faa2f5dd9ded0cc65

Commission for Historical Clarification. 1999. Guatemala Memory of Silence Tz'inil Na'tab'al: Report of the Commission for Historical Clarification Conclusions and Recommendations.

Diamond, Lisa, Karen Izquierdo, Dana Canfield, Konstantina Matsoukas, and Francesca Gany. 2019. A Systematic Review of the Impact of Patient-Physician Non-English Language Concordance on Quality of Care and Outcomes. *Journal of General Internal Medicine* 34(8): pp. 1591–1606. https://doi.org/10.1007/s11606-019-04847-5.

Foo, P. K., Berenice Perez, Neha Gupta, Gerardo Jeronimo Lorenzo, Nana-Yaa Misa, Brissa Santacruz Gutierrez, Olivia Madison, U. Mini B. Swift, and Erik S. Anderson. 2021. High Rates of COVID-19 Infection among Indigenous Maya at a US Safety-Net Health System in California. *Public Health Reports* 136(3): pp. 295–300. https://doi.org/10.1177/0033354921990370.

Hallman, Kelly, Sara Peracca, Jennifer Catino, and Marta Julia Ruiz. 2006. Multiple Disadvantages of Mayan Females: The Effects of Gender, Ethnicity, Poverty, and Residence on Education in Guatemala. Population Council. https://knowledgecommons.popcouncil.org/departments_sbsr-pgy/58/.

Hamann, Edmund T., and Lisa Harklau. 2021. Changing Faces and Persistent Patterns for Education in the New Latino/a/x Diaspora. In *Handbook of Latinos and Education: Theory, Research, and Practice*, Second Edition, ed. Enrique G. Murillo, Jr., Dolores Delgado Bernal, Socorro Morales, Luis Urrieta, Jr, Eric Ruiz Bybee, Juan Sánchez Muñoz, Victor B. Saenz, Daniel Villanueva, Margarita Machado-Casas, and Katherine Espinoza, pp. 81–92. New York: Routledge.

Holocaust Museum Houston. 2023. Genocide in Guatemala. https://hmh.org/library/research/genocide-in-guatemala-guide/.

Karliner, Leah S., Elizabeth A. Jacobs, Alice Hm Chen, and Sunita Mutha. 2007. Do Professional Interpreters Improve Clinical Care for Patients with Limited English Proficiency? A Systematic Review of the Literature. *Health Services Research* 42(2): pp. 727–754. https://doi.org/10.1111%2Fj.1475-6773.2006.00629.x.

Martínez, Glenn A. 2020. *Spanish in Health Care: Policy, Practice and Pedagogy in Latino Health*. New York: Routledge.

Minkler, Meredith, and Nina Wallerstein. 2012. Improving Health through Community Organizing and Community Building: Perspectives from Health Education and Social Work. In *Community Organizing and Community Building for Health and Welfare*, ed. M. Minkler, pp. 26–50. New Brunswick, NJ: Rutgers University Press.

Office of Disease Prevention and Health Promotion. 2030. Healthy People. U.S. Department of Health and Human Services. https://health.gov/healthypeople/priority-areas/social-determinants-health.

Santos, Maricel G., Rachel Showstack, Glenn Martínez, Drew Colcher, and Dalia Magaña. 2023. *Health Disparities and the Applied Linguist*. New York: Routledge.

Showstack, Rachel. 2022. Kansas Hasn't Paid for Medically Necessary Interpreting Services: You Can Help Change the System. *The Kansas Reflector*, October 17. https://kansasreflector.com/2022/10/17/kansas-hasnt-paid-for-medically-necessary-interpreting-services-you-can-help-change-the-system/.

Showstack, Rachel, Maricel G. Santos, Emily Feuerherm, Holly Jacobson, and Glenn Martínez. 2019. Language as a Social Determinant of Health: An Applied Linguistics Perspective on Health Equity. https://www.aaal.org/news/language-as-a-social-determinant-of-health-an-applied-linguistics-perspective-on-health-equity.

Singer, Merrill C., Pamela I. Erickson, Louise Badiane, Rosemary Diaz, Dugeidy Ortiz, Traci Abraham, and Anna Marie Nicolaysen. 2006. Syndemics, Sex and the City: Understanding Sexually Transmitted Diseases in Social and Cultural Context. *Social Science and Medicine* 63(8): pp. 2010–2021. https://doi.org/10.1016%2Fj.socscimed.2006.05.012.

Zhen-Duan, Jenny, Farrah Jacquez, and Lisa Vaughn. 2017. Demographic Characteristics Associated with Barriers to Healthcare among Mexican and Guatemalan Immigrants in a Nontraditional Destination Area. *Family and Community Health* 40(2): pp. 101–111. https://doi.org/10.1097/fch.0000000000000141.

5

Of Worlds and Words

Medical Interpretation in a US Primary Care Clinic

Lissie Wahl

Introduction

This chapter explores what is at stake in interlinguistic medical encounters in which patients seeking care do not share a language with their medical providers and must rely on professional interpreters to communicate about symptoms, diagnoses, treatment plans, and more. How interpretation is handled in these contexts matters because communication in medical care can have life or death consequences. Effective communication, however, involves much more than word-to-word translation, as the following observations from a Khmer-English interpreter illustrate. Here the interpreter explains to me how a diabetic Cambodian immigrant patient, after being advised to increase intake of fruits and vegetables and avoid or reduce that of rice, oils, and carbohydrates, tells her outside the exam room that she will not comply with her US American physician's recommendation to cut down on eating rice:

> You have to understand, they were surviving through [civil] war, [with] lots of family member[s], where they have nothing ... For you to say, "Don't eat rice," it's almost like telling them, "Hey, I'm going to cut one of your arms off." ... [They respond], "Wow, I lived off of nothing for me to be here to have food! food! food! And now you want to tell me I can't eat this? ... No, I'm going to eat, before I'm going to die!"

Here, "rice" is clearly not just a word for a type of food, but a historically situated concept with strong emotional associations. The single word "rice" implicates an entire social world that is not shared among all participants in the medical encounter.

In the United States, medical interpreters are often asked to translate for immigrants who speak languages other than English. The professional practice of medical interpretation is tied to the social political history of civil rights. In 1964, Title VI of the Civil Rights Act was enacted to prevent discrimination against persons of different national origin, including those with "limited English proficiency." LEP Title III of the American with Disabilities Act (U.S. Department of Justice Civil Rights Division 2020) and Section 1557 of the Affordable Care Act (U.S. Department of Health

Lissie Wahl, *Of Worlds and Words*. In: *Language and Health in Action*. Edited by: Lynnette Arnold et al., Oxford University Press.
 DOI: 10.1093/9780198933953.003.0005

and Human Services 2010 and U.S. Department of Health and Human Services Office for Civil Rights 2023) reinforced these protections. From 2019 to the time of this writing, all medical institutions that receive federal funds have had to provide qualified and certified language access to all patients. Unfortunately, incorporating licensed medical interpreters into US medical institutions is an uphill battle. Even where interpreters are included, their ability to engage patients and medical providers in meaningful communication can be quite limited—for reasons having little to do with the words themselves and more to do with the biomedical world within which interpreted encounters are embedded.

This chapter examines structural forces outside the exam room that shape who and what is listened to in the exam room. Following an explanation about the research on which this chapter is based, the chapter is organized into sections that outline medical interpretation work, describe some of the key challenges to effective communication in medicine, explain constraints on medical interpreters and healthcare, and identify the ways these problems can undermine the quality of healthcare that immigrants receive. Across these sections I argue that monologic modes of medical communication can force medical interpreters to sacrifice potentially critical communication related to patients' worlds and life circumstances affecting their health. This has negative consequences for everyone involved in the medical encounter and contributes to health inequities in the United States. I conclude the chapter by identifying policy changes that can enhance medical interpreters' ability to contribute meaningfully in the healthcare of immigrant patients.

Research Background

Throughout the chapter, I draw on interviews I conducted with staff at a community healthcare clinic I call DePaul. The clinic is centered on primary care and is affiliated to a large university teaching hospital in the northeastern United States. I am an interpreter, medical anthropologist, and independent researcher, and I worked at this center as a medical interpreter between 2005 and 2017. During this time, it became clear to me that individuals who did not speak the dominant language (English) had little voice or space to express their own realities, needs, and thoughts regarding their health. Protocols at the clinic seemed to make it structurally impossible. To explore this, I asked two people to join me in a formal research project: Michael T. Nathan, a primary care physician and medical anthropologist practicing at the same clinic and Seth D. Hannah, a medical sociologist. Between 2012 and 2017 we interviewed eleven interpreters, fifteen medical providers (doctors, nurses, and therapists), and three clinic administrators. At least two of the three researchers were present in each interview to avoid bias. The interview quotes in this chapter were borrowed from my book manuscript, *Worlds in Words* (in progress).

The community at the time of our study had an approximate population of 54,000 people (American Community Survey 5-Year Estimates 2014–2018), predominantly working class and diverse in both countries of origin and languages spoken. Predominant languages were Spanish, Portuguese, Khmer, numerous Arabic languages, and a dwindling number of Albanian speakers. The area around DePaul was undergoing gentrification at the same time that local demographics were shifting. Between 2015 and 2019, 39% of the population in DePaul was foreign born and 51.7% of people over the age of 5 spoke a language other than English at home. By 2022 these percentages had grown to 43.9% and 57.6%, respectively (American Community Survey 5-Year Estimates 2022).

Medical Interpretation

While medical interpretation is often understood as a tool for exchanging information in which words are translated from one language to another, effective medical interpretation in fact calls for much more. Individual words, like isolated symptoms, have little meaning on their own. Talk is inevitably embedded in a context that shapes its meaning. An exchange of medical information is no different.

If medical interpreters are to facilitate meaningful communication between doctors and patients, they must be permitted to focus not just on the words being exchanged, but on the worlds that make up the context or meaning of those words, which include both the patients' worlds and the biomedical world in which the exchange is taking place. For this to happen, interpreters must be understood as active participants in a **dialogic model** of communication wherein all interlocutors engage in co-constructing meaning to facilitate mutual understanding (Bakhtin 1981; Li 2013).

Interpretation involves historical and cultural meanings that shape how people use language. All words and texts are prone to **heteroglossia**, or different possible meanings or interpretations tied to cultural and historical contexts (Bakhtin 1981). Based on Bakhtin's insights, Cecilia Wadensjö (1998) transformed the study of language interpretation by explaining that, regardless of the number of people involved, the interaction at play among patient, doctor, and interpreter is as important for medical communication—if not more important—than words alone.

Dialogic language interpretation recognizes that meaning can be co-constructed by everyone involved in the interpreted encounter. Sociolinguists have argued that medical communication and interaction should take into account patients' experiences, knowledge, and thinking for an interlanguage encounter to prove meaningful. In this model, everyone involved in the interpreted medical encounter is authorized to meaningfully participate. This requires that the interpreter—the only person who understands both languages in an interpreted medical context—actively coordinate and engage everyone to reach beyond the limits of the words, signs, and silences in order to co-construct or arrive at a meaningful exchange (Baraldi 2012; Li 2013; Sard 2006).

The training that medical interpreters receive prepares them to recognize and potentially enact a number of overlapping roles including conduit, clarifier, cultural broker, and patient advocate. The first and most recognized role is that of the conduit, which can be visualized as the process of transmitting specifically what is being said between two or more people. A second role is that of clarifier. In this role, the interpreter's goal is to make messages comprehensible and, in particular, to clarify messages from the medical provider to the patient. Medical interpreters can also play the role of cultural broker, in which the interpreter is responsible for conveying cultural context that might aid mutual understanding. A fourth role is that of patient advocate, in which the interpreter can speak up for the patient when in imminent danger.

Unfortunately, despite this training and broader orientation to dialogic communication in interpretation, medical communication in clinical settings in the US is most often **monologic**, meaning that only one voice—that of biomedicine—dominates communication and interaction. The prevalence of monologic communication in medical encounters is tied to historical and structural trajectories in clinical medicine, as well as to a larger field of economic and political forces and structures (Bruss and Titunik 2012; Volosinov [1929]1973). It is important to note that we are all embedded in a historical and cultural context, yet in biomedicine it is generally assumed that the culture of the clinic and biomedicine are not, thereby, ignoring the value of what a patient or interpreter may want to communicate.

Biomedical Authority and Monologic Communication

Biomedical practice and the protocols for interpreting medical information and narratives are embedded within a historical epistemological hierarchy that obstructs meaningful dialogic communication in the exam room. In this hierarchy, biomedical forms of knowledge, and ways of making sense of the world are construed as superior to other sources of knowledge and perspectives, as if in a zero-sum game (a competition in which one party must necessarily be wrong for the other to be right). The biomedical industry maintains this authority by counterposing science to culture and claiming that biomedical science is pure and untouched by social, historical, or structural considerations (Taylor 2003; see also Chapter 3). Biomedical institutions hold that their practices are based upon evidence-based scientific facts and thus offer a uniquely objective perspective in matters pertaining to health and wellbeing (Briggs 2024; Lock and Nguyen 2010).

The privileging of biomedical perspectives over other ways of understanding illness is tied to the political economy of health. The economic transformation of medical care into an industry has turned health into a commodity that continues to grow and amass power based on market principles (Good 1998; Rylko-Bauer and Farmer 2002). This in turn privileges the "medical gaze" as the dominant knowledge frame from medical school onward (Briggs 2024; Eisenberg 1981; Good 1994; Kleinman and Benson 2006).

Under this model, diagnosis and treatment options are arrived at through algorithms based on results that are averaged out and then termed the "gold standards" of biomedicine. In this model of evidence-based medicine, payment for medical treatment can be denied with the rationale that there is not enough research demonstrating its utility for the statistically average patient, who is a mathematical construct that in fact does not anywhere exist.

One consequence of relying on statistical abstractions is that many perspectives are silenced. The situated knowledge and experiences of interpreters, patients, and even medical professionals are excluded from consideration in order to comply with the mathematical formulas of evidence-based treatments and modes of communication dictated from afar and in which insurance and pharmaceutical companies have an inordinate interest and say. These mandates include the current reliance on standardized electronic health records (EHRs) (Hunt 2017; Lozar 2019). EHRs and various iterations of artificial intelligence (AI) facilitate the sharing of patient information across different medical systems, provide memory aides to medical personnel about what needs to be kept track of during an exam or course of treatment, and help medical providers and interpreters quickly access and compare vast amounts of curated data and research, translations, and vocabularies.

This biomedical system, however, can be problematic when it delimits who says what, when, and how. Neither EHRs nor AI can provide definitive answers out of context about how to appropriately treat a given individual patient. EHRs and AI-generated reports are the end products of human input and therefore subject to human bias (Panch et al. 2019). Sustaining the health of any human being requires considering more than the numeric biomedical and physiological markers captured in digital records.

Reliance on EHRs and the traditional focus on words in the process of interpretation omit consideration of the social, structural, and epistemological worlds inhabited by each person interacting in the exam room (Raymond 2014). Global patterns and processes of migration, structural violence, the histories of patients who do not speak the dominant language, and local living and working conditions in the US all have a serious impact upon patients' health, wellbeing, and the viability of following given medical orders or not (Keller et al. 2017; Rylko-Bauer et al. 2009; see also Chapter 10).

Training in these areas has largely been left out of the formal education that both medical interpreters and doctors receive (Knipper 2013). To be hired by a medical institution, interpreters must have a high school diploma, command medical terminology in two languages, and receive a medical interpretation certificate. Interpreters nonetheless, may often have higher degrees of education than that (Souza 2016:216). Medical interpreters must periodically recertify by taking online courses or attending conferences focused on medical terminologies, bodily systems, and the behaviors expected from them by biomedical institutions and bureaucracies.

Sharing a language also does not unify populations. The life worlds of patients who speak languages other than English vary widely, and an interpreter and a patient who share a common language may otherwise have little in common, including country of origin, class, education, values, ethnicity, biases and epistemologies. Neither medical institutions nor interpreting associations recognize officially the ways in which monologic forces and communication structures can deepen patient suffering and exacerbate health inequities (Keller et al. 2017; Leanza 2008). I elaborate summarily on these structures and the problems that result from them in the following sections.

Constraints on Medical Interpreters and Healthcare Providers

Expectations for interpretation in biomedical settings pose challenges to effective dialogic communication. Professional standards stipulate that medical interpreters enter the exam room with a provider, introduce themselves by name, state that everything said will be interpreted using first person language, and kept confidential. The interpreter is not to add, edit, or omit anything in the process and must remain "neutral." National medical interpreting certification standards and codes of ethics commit the interpreter to follow this behavior as well as require that interpreters have full command of medical terminology in both English and the language of interpretation (Certification Commission for Healthcare Interpreters).

Medical interpreters may feel hampered by these biomedical expectations that, in everyday practice, require them to execute an accurate, literal, and neutral translation in as short a time as possible. They are expected to restrain themselves from communicating anything other than the direct translation of what is said by the medical provider, regardless of what the patient has or has not understood and viceversa.

Biomedical providers and institutional administrators largely perceive interpreters' attempts to more extensively manage communications as a confrontation to medical authority and a legal liability and seek to limit how much interpreters talk, listen, and interact with patients. As one administrator we interviewed stressed, the interpreter's job is solely "to communicate what the doctor, the provider, says to the patient," not the other way around. This expectation is often unrealistic. As one interpreter pointed out to us: "interpreters and the medical professionals for whom they are translating may understand each other clearly, but it takes more time to explain to the patient." Another interpreter described the tension that arises in the exam room as a result of restrictive protocols: "Some doctors say, 'Just translate word-for-word,' and I say, 'No, I can't translate word for word.' ... They tell me, 'I say one word and you say too much.' ... [The doctors don't realize that] sometimes we [have to find the ways] ... to get ... concepts ... through."

In addition, patients are expected to submit to the authority of biomedicine. When the technical advice, lifestyle changes, or treatments recommended by primary care physicians are not followed as expected, patients are generally considered non-compliant or even delinquent (Zola 1972). Patients are rarely asked if they have a reason for not following medical orders, as in the case of the diabetic Cambodian patient at the beginning of the chapter who was reluctant to give up rice

(Donovan and Blake 1992; Farmer 2013). Not daring to speak up to her doctor, this Khmer patient was not offered alternative dietary options.

The reluctance of medical providers to engage in dialogic communication in the exam room can be attributed in large part to the relentless pressure put on them by the biomedical industry, specially within a financially strapped community healthcare center (Young et al. 2018). Physician and primary care physician burn-out is at an all-time high because of the high numbers of patients and bureaucratic paperwork they are expected to handle every day (Physicians Foundation 2024). One primary care physician doctor told us, "We're compensated purely on our ability to see patients, which I think is a very poor model." Interpreters recognize that this model puts doctors under enormous pressure:

> The [primary care physician] doctor is working under crunch time . . . They're scheduled to see a patient every 15 minutes. Fifteen minutes go by so fast, all the doctor has time for is, "How's your blood sugar today? How are you feeling? Anything bother you? You need any more medication? . . . I'll see you in three, six months."

Within that quarter hour, a patient's narrative might take up only twenty-four seconds from problem presentation to confirmation of symptoms (Heritage and Clayman 2010:106). One provider told us she wanted to know and better understand her patients, but she was afraid it would make her workload unbearable. She eventually left her job. Another provider we interviewed pointed out: "Just adding two to ten minutes of text per 12–15 minute encounter, when four or five patients will be seen per hour for a period of three and half hours can become overwhelming." He too left the job. A third provider was so upset by the dilemma between meeting her institution's productivity goals and realistic care for her patients she simply broke down during our interview. She quit her job as well.

Biomedical protocols constrain interactions in the exam room to rapid monologic communication, with negative consequences for patients, medical providers, and interpreters alike, particularly in the context of primary care. This dynamic helps explain the current situation in the US, whereby people can often not find an available primary care physician and treatments are focused on symptoms and the medications required to control these, as opposed to causes and cures.

What Monologic Biomedical Interpretation Neglects

Being constrained to structured monologic communication protocols, including having to ask patients closed (yes/no) questions from a predetermined list of health factors (Jenks 2011), prevents medical providers from learning about crucial aspects in their patients' lives and how these are affecting their health. There are numerous situations in which a yes/no model of communication may suffice, as in the case of emergencies, lab work, given exams, and follow-ups where what is crucial is not necessary for instant interaction or has already been identified and is being taken into account. Yet for effective communication to occur in the course of primary care or preventive medicine, chronic disease management, or mental health consultations, the voices and thoughts of patients, providers, and interpreters may all be necessary (Young et al. 2018). These are all areas affecting patient's lifestyles, for which a treatment plan grounded in reality proves essential and must be co-constructed.

One interpreter described key factors in patients' lives that get left out of discussion during primary care medical visits:

> Their social life, their family's statuses, ... financially, some patients may not have enough money to pay for the medication if they don't have insurance, and things like that. And then if they don't have income because they're not working ... They used to work, but now all of a sudden ... no more job because [of] the chronic disease ... And the family ... maybe they [were] kicked [out of their home], went to jail, or the kid ran away from home, they drop out of school, the kid got pregnant, got involved in a wrong crowd ... or the kid may be going through a divorce, or the [patient] may have lost a grandkid or things like that ... If they have all ... these family issues we don't know about, then it has an effect ... where [the patient says], "I'm having so much issue, I don't even think about my health ... All I think about is my family." I always say there is a reason why a patient's medical condition is under poor control.

As this interpreter's observations illustrate, the lifestyle changes prescribed by the medical system for the statistically average patient are not feasible for every individual. Some immigrant patients, for example, might not have access to green spaces for walking, unpolluted air for exercising outside, safe neighborhoods, affordable grocery stores selling healthy food, the financial means to break out of a domestically violent relationship or stay home when they are ill without worrying about losing their jobs or being unable to feed their families or pay rent. It is why Covid in the Greater Boston area hit particularly hard in its most impoverished areas.

Some doctors recognize that knowing about patients' circumstances can make a difference in whether or not a course of treatment is realistic for that patient. One psychiatrist who appreciated dialogic communication and interaction pointed out that: "Any doctor who's forced to see 25 to 30 patients a day and has no time to listen and misses key information should realize that they only stand to benefit from working with interpreters who tell them what is going on with their patients." As this provider acknowledged, medical interpreters may be better positioned than primary care doctors to learn about, discuss, and understand a patient's non-medical lived conditions of health, work, and wellbeing, particularly when they are part of an interpreter team that provides continuity of care for patients over long periods of time (Leanza et al. 2015). The DePaul community healthcare center often received new residents who, albeit supervised, could not quite make out their patients' health behaviors. In contrast, interpreters in the clinic worked with the same patients and their families over long periods of time in primary care and specialty appointments, something that provided them with significant depth of insight into the poorer and more marginalized immigrants' exposure to the structural violence affecting their patients' health.

Helping inform medical providers was not all that interpreters did at the DePaul primary care clinic. They often felt a moral duty to extend their services to patients outside the exam room. For example, because the clinic did not have the same financial or personnel resources as the hospital with which it was affiliated, some of the interpreters we interviewed helped illiterate, elderly, or otherwise compromised patients understand documents, fill out health insurance and food stamp applications, find transportation, seek follow-up care, and access medications. Research suggests that such functions can be just as important—if not more so—than language interpretation *per se* (Kirmayer et al. 2015), especially where fully caring for patients is no longer the highest priority in for-profit biomedical practice (Kleinman 2019).

Administrators in our study knew that interpreters had taken on expanded roles and realized that their actions were promoting the health and wellbeing of the clinic's immigrant patient population, thereby keeping the flow of federal funding at that time from coming in. The interpreters were nevertheless formally told to comply with institutional protocols, including the prohibition on engaging in any sort of communication with a patient except in the presence of a medical provider and in response to the latter's needs. Interpreters were disciplined and their jobs threatened for trespassing official protocols should a medical provider or administrator not want dialogic communication and interaction to take place.

Given these circumstances, I argue that silencing patients and the interpreters who stand up for and with them impedes communicative equity. Even when dialogic communication is permitted during medical visits, without broader policy change, the normative monologic model will live on. Patients who speak languages other than English, are poor, and are marginal with regard to mainstream America may have no bargaining power if they cannot count on the active support of interpreters, which is compromised when interpreters are restrained. The worlds that patients inhabit and the particular needs they have thus remain invisible to most administrators and healthcare professionals, illustrating how communicative injustice is health injustice (Briggs 2017).

Moving Forward

Economic inequities instilled by the US labor market's reliance upon bureaucrats and protocols to generate profits have had an inordinate impact upon medical communication and interaction in interpreted encounters (Applbaum and Oldani 2010; Gordon 1972; Houston 2016). The notion that there is only one best way of accomplishing clinical communication, and it is under the purview of uninformed and uncaring administrative personnel from afar, gives more weight to the medical system than to the human beings it is supposed to help or those who work within the system as healthcare providers (Hartzband and Groopman 2016). Hospitals, health insurance, and pharmaceutical companies impart standardized biomedical knowledge in ways that make monologic patterns of communication and interpretation compulsory.

With this backdrop, the challenges of interlinguistic medical encounters have yet to be tackled adequately. Interpreters and medical providers alike can and should take a moral stance to confront impediments to communicative and health justice, but they risk their jobs in doing so.

Communicative and health justice will not be achieved until (1) interpreters are validated and valued fully for their complex and multifaceted work, and (2) medical schools and biomedical institutions recognize that history, structural violence, and environmental factors are implicated in the linguistic and cultural barriers that interpreters can engaged to address.

Discussion of models for change are emerging among sociolinguists and institutions in Canada and Europe, where interpreters may be given an expanded role as mediators and recognized for their contributions to the medical team (Baraldi 2012; Leanza et al. 2015; see also Chapter 6 for an example from the Global South). Looking to these models, interpreted medical encounters will improve when: (1) communication protocols in healthcare institutions and policy acknowledge that words—like symptoms—must be set in a wide historical and structural context to determine their meaning; (2) interpreters are allowed to encourage immigrant patients to talk about non-medical factors impinging upon their health and are able to share this information with providers; and (3) medical education teaches clinicians and interpreters to advance dialogic communication as a means for supporting patient health.

Communicative and health equity for immigrant communities will improve when medical interpretation training, protocols, and discussions center not only on education about language, the body, and medical terminology but, just as importantly, on awareness and curiosity about world migration and emigration patterns; the countries, regions, and situations immigrants emerge from; and, in the receiving country, housing conditions; cultural stigma and violence; labor conditions; and other structural challenges that affect immigrants' health. Training related to cultural challenges in medical interpreting must come to address the history, structural violence, and environmental factors that underlie cultural barriers, rather than construing culture as mere ideas sitting in people's heads alone.

Questions for Reflection and Discussion

Reflection Questions

1. Think of a time when you were misunderstood as you tried to ask someone for help with a specific problem. What strategies did you employ to convey

your intended meaning? Did you rephrase your request? Did you add a bit of background history to contextualize your position? What was the result? Why do you think that was?

Looking In: Small Group Discussion Questions

1. What is monologic communication? Define in your own words and come up with a specific scenario where this happens in medical contexts.
2. What expectations for medical interpreters emerge from the monologic model of communication?
3. What are some problems with biomedical models of monologic interpretation? What gets left out of these models?
4. What is the dialogic model of communication? Define in your own words and come up with a specific scenario that demonstrates dialogic communication in action.

Looking Out: Large Group Discussion Questions

1. How is monologic communication tied to biomedical authority? How is it tied to language ideologies and structures of power?
2. The author proposes that medical interpreters be given an expanded role as mediators. Discuss the pros and cons of implementing that role in primary care clinical settings from various points of view (e.g., patients, healthcare professionals, administrators, interpreters).

References

Applbaum, Kalman, and Michael Oldani. 2010. Introduction to Special Issue: Towards an Era of Bureaucratically Controlled Medical Compliance. *Anthropology and Medicine* 17(2): pp. 113–127.

Bakhtin, Mikhail. 1981. *The Dialogic Imagination*. Austin: University of Texas Press.

Baraldi, Claudio. 2012. Interpreting as Dialogic Mediation: The Relevance of Expansions. In *Coordinating Participation in Dialogue Interpreting*, ed. Claudio Baraldi and Laura Gavioli, pp. 297–326. Amsterdam: John Benjamins.

Briggs, Charles L. 2017. Towards Communicative Justice in Health. *Medical Anthropology* 336(4): pp. 287–304.

Briggs, Charles L. 2024. *Incommunicable: Toward Communicative Justice in Health and Medicine*. Durham, NC: Duke University Press.

Bruss, Neal H., and I. R. Titunik. 2012. Preface. In *Freudianism: A Marxist Critique*, ed. V. N. Volosinov, pp. vii–xxi. London: Verso.

Donovan, Jenny L., and David R. Blake. 1992. Patient Non-Compliance: Deviance or Reasoned Decision-Making? *Social Science, and Medicine* 34(5): pp. 507–513.

Eisenberg, Leon. 1981. The Physician as "Interpreter": Ascribing Meaning to the Illness Experience. *Comprehensive Psychiatry* 22(3): pp. 239–248.

Good, Byron J. 1994. *Medicine, Rationality, and Experience: An Anthropological Perspective.* Cambridge: Cambridge University Press.

Good, Mary-Jo DelVecchio. 1998. *American Medicine: The Quest for Competence.* Berkeley, CA: University of California Press.

Gordon, David M. 1972. *Theories of Poverty and Underdevelopment: Orthodox, Radical, and Dual Labor Market Perspectives.* Lexington, MA: Lexington Books.

Griffin, Michael and Jennie Weiss Block, eds. 2013. In the Company of the Poor: Conversations with Dr. Paul Farmer and Fr. Gustavo Gutiérrez. Maryknoll, NY: Orbis Books.

Hartzband, Pamela, and Jerome Groopman, 2016. Medical Taylorism. *New England Journal of Medicine* 374(2): pp. 106–108.

Heritage, John, and Steven Clayman, 2010. *Talk in Action: Interactions, Identities and Institutions.* Malden, MA: Wiley-Blackwell.

Houston, Muiris. 2016. Has Medical Taylorism Gone Too Far? *Irish Medical Times* 50(14): p. 21.

Hunt, Linda M., Hannah S. Bell, Allison M. Baker, and Heather A. Howard. 2017. Electronic Health Records and the Disappearing Patient. *Medical Anthropology Quarterly* 31(3): pp. 403–421.

Jenks, Angela C. 2011. From "Lists of Traits" to "Open-Mindedness": Emergent Issues in Cultural Competence Training. *Culture, Medicine, and Psychiatry* 35: pp. 209–235.

Keller, Allen, Amy Joscelyne, Megan Granski, and Barry Rosenfeld. 2017. Pre-Migration Trauma Exposure and Mental Health Functioning Among Central American Migrants Arriving at the US Border. *PLOS ONE* 12(1): p. e0168692.

Kirmayer, Laurence J., Jaswant Guzder, and Cécile Rousseau, eds. 2015. *Cultural Consultation: Encountering the Other in Mental Health Care.* New York: Springer.

Kleinman, Arthur. 2019. *The Soul of Care: The Moral Education of a Husband and a Doctor.* New York: Penguin Random House.

Kleinman, Arthur, and Peter Benson. 2006. Anthropology in the Clinic: The Problem of Cultural Competency and How to Fix It. *PLoS Medicine* 3(10): p. e294.

Knipper, Michael. 2013. Joining Ethnography and History in Cultural Competence Training. *Culture, Medicine and Psychiatry* 37: pp. 373–384.

Leanza, Yvan. 2008. Community Interpreter's Power: The Hazards of a Disturbing Attribute. *Curare* 31(2–3): pp. 211–220.

Leanza, Yvan, ALessandra Miklavcic, Isabelle Boivin, and Ellen Rosenberg. 2015. Working with Interpreters. In *Cultural Consultation: Encountering the Other in Mental Health Care,* ed. L. Kirmayer Jaswant Guzder, and Cécile Rousseau, pp. 89–114. New York: Springer.

Li, Shuangyu. 2013. Co-Construction of Interpreted Conversation in Medical Consultations. *Applied Linguistic Review* 4(1): pp. 127–149.

Lock, Margaret, and Vinh-Kim Nguyen. 2010. *An Anthropology of Biomedicine*. Hoboken, NJ: John Wiley and Sons.

Lozar, D. C. 2019. *Technology and the Doctor-Patient Relationship*. Jefferson, NC: McFarland & Company.

Panch, Trishan, Heather Mattie, and Rifat Atun. 2019. Artificial Intelligence and Algorithmic Bias: Implications for Health Systems. *Journal of Global Health* 9(2): p. 020318.

Physicians Foundation. 2024. Physician Surveys. https://physiciansfoundation.org/research/the-physicians-foundation-physician-surveys.

Raymond, Chase Wesley. 2014. Conveying Information in the Interpreted-mediated Medical Visit: The Case of Epistemic Brokering. *Patient Education and Counseling* 87: pp. 38–46.

Rylko-Bauer, Barbara, and Paul Farmer. 2002. Managed Care or Managed Inequality? A Call for Critiques of Market-Based Medicine. *Medical Anthropology Quarterly* 16(4): pp. 476–502.

Rylko-Bauer, Barbara, Linda Whiteford, and Paul Farmer, eds. 2009. *Global Health in Times of Violence*. Santa Fe: School for Advanced Research Press.

Sard, Melanie. 2006. Reflected Words: Meaning and Silence in Language and Translation. *Macalester Journal of Philosophy* 15(1): pp. 15–33.

Souza, Izabel E. T. de V. 2016. *Intercultural Mediation in Healthcare: From the Professional Medical Interpreters' Perspective*. Bloomington, IN: Xlibris.

Taylor, Janelle S. 2003. Confronting "Culture" in Medicine's 'Culture of No Culture'. *Academic Medicine* 78(6): pp. 555–559.

U.S. Department of Justice Civil Rights Division. 2020. Americans with Disabilities Act Title III Regulations. https://www.ada.gov/law-and-regs/regulations/title-ii-2010-regulations/.

U.S. Department of Health and Human Services. 2010. Section 1557 of the Patient Protection and Affordable Care Act. https://www.hhs.gov/guidance/document/section-1557-patient-protection-and-affordable-care-act.

U.S. Department of Health and Human Services Office for Civil Rights. 2023. Health and Human Services Language Access Report. https://www.hhs.gov/sites/default/files/language-access-report-2023.pdf.

Valero-Garcés, Barbara Nazawa, Lissie Wahl-Kleiser, eds. 2014. Intercultural Communication in the Medical Field. *Panacea@ Revista de Medicina, Lenguaje y Traducción* 15(40): pp. 1–188.

Volosinov, Valentino N. [1929]1973. *Marxism and the Philosophy of Language*. Cambridge, MA: Harvard University Press.

Wadensjö, Cecilia. 1998. *Interpreting as Interaction*. London: Longman.

Young, Richard A., Sandra K. Burge, Kaparaboyna A. Kumar, Jocelyn M. Wilson, and Daniela F. Ortiz. 2018. A Time-Motion Study of Primary Care Physicians' Work in the Electronic Health Record Era. *Family Medicine* 50(2): pp. 91–99.

Zola, Irving Kenneth. 1972. Medicine as an Institution of Social Control. *Sociological Review* 20(4): pp. 487–504.

6

Translating the Invisible

Intercultural Health Facilitators in Indigenous Chile

Paula F. Saravia and Jorge Tibor Gutiérrez

Introduction

In Chile, contemporary Mapuche people's perspectives on and experiences with sickness, healing, and death have a problematic coexistence with the biomedical model sanctioned by the Chilean state. It is amid these challenges that we find Indigenous intercultural health facilitators navigating arduous healthcare pathways alongside Mapuche and other Indigenous patients. In this chapter, we examine how the important work of intercultural health facilitators is challenged by precarious labor conditions as well as the at times unattainable goal of translating Indigenous illness experiences for non-Indigenous providers. In our discussion about language and health, we emphasize the role of intercultural facilitators in translating the elusive and unique ways that their Mapuche patients understand and interact with the world around them.

Marcela, one of our collaborators, is a Mapuche woman who lives in a rural area near the city of Temuco in Southern Chile. She lost her husband to an illness that has strong connections to Mapuche spirituality and framing of wellbeing. When speaking about her husband's illness, she clarified to us how language, emotions, and the very notions of life and death are delicately intertwined:

> My husband always talked about death. We always talked about death … One day, after the pandemic, he says, "You know, I am feeling scared. I don't know what is happening, but I feel empty," … He didn't want to be alone. I had to be by his side all the time while eating and drinking yerba mate tea … he would say, "Don't go anywhere, stay by my side," … And in the end, he had a thrombosis. We had agreed that I was not going to let him die at the hospital like his parents, but the rest of the family took him there. He spent nine months there, and then we brought him back home for another nine months. So, I took him to a machi [Mapuche shaman] near here, and he said, "This man has been gone for many months now; his soul is not in his body." … I think what I experienced teaches us that we need to listen. We need to listen to the feeling of emptiness. That I know now.

Paula F. Saravia and Jorge Tibor Gutiérrez, *Translating the Invisible*. In: *Language and Health in Action*. Edited by: Lynnette Arnold et al., Oxford University Press. DOI: 10.1093/9780198933953.003.0006

In this testimony, Marcela tells the story of her husband's long illness and her experience as his companion and caregiver. In Mapuzungun, the Mapuche language, this role is known as ***ngen kutran*** (keeper of the sick). A *ngen kutran* is a caregiver whose responsibilities include accompaniment, ensuring that a sick person consults a healer and follows treatment, and managing communication on behalf of the individual. In her account, Marcela also highlights her husband's discomfort with the biomedical setting of the hospital and the importance of Mapuche healers and their assistants in helping the family make sense of his illness and death.

In this chapter, we examine the complexities of care as described by Marcela, in a context of **medical pluralism**, where Indigenous and non-Indigenous healing systems coexist, by bringing the perspectives of Indigenous intercultural health facilitators to the forefront. In doing so, we focus on the challenging work of Mapuche intercultural facilitators, who have become a cornerstone of Chile's national intercultural health system. Our argument centers on the asymmetric realities shaping the care work of intercultural facilitators and their strategies to empower themselves and the people they serve by speaking Mapuzungun and enacting multiple forms of communicative labor while assisting Indigenous patients seeking care in biomedical spaces. An important part of intercultural facilitators' communicative labor involves the struggle to translate experiences like "emptiness," which are deeply spiritual but also have tangible effects on the patient's wellbeing. These experiences are invisible to conventional medical providers, thus making them hard to explain from a biomedical perspective.

We discuss the role of language in healing and the contribution of intercultural health facilitators to meaningful healing processes and worldmaking that exceed mere language translation. Like other cultural brokers or cultural mediators (Kirmayer et al. 2014:90–91, 116–117), Mapuche intercultural facilitators are critically important agents who help facilitate communication across the boundaries of the hegemonic biomedical system, the scientific view of health, the Mapuche medical system, and Mapuche ways of experiencing illness and wellbeing.

For example, Doraliza Millalen, who served as an intercultural facilitator (1996–2001), told us that an essential part of her role at the medical center in the city of Nueva Imperial involved meeting with patients from rural areas and ensuring they were given medical appointments at times that accounted for the rural bus schedule. This kind of care in scheduling was crucial for achieving equity in access to care: "in the rural areas, people don't have a monthly wage. So, if you don't have money from selling produce at the market, you can't buy bus tickets to visit the clinic. So, our work scheduling medical visits helps our most vulnerable patients."

Another aspect of her work with patients involved providing a buffer of time and space for rural Indigenous patients at the clinic, before they had to contend with the rigidity of medical language and clinic protocols. Her strategy involved drinking black or yerba mate tea with patients and talking with them about their families and children. As they conversed, Doraliza would prepare a list of culturally relevant symptoms to communicate to the patient's medical provider. In developing this approach, Doraliza drew on her training as a *técnica en bienestar social* (social work assistant) and her lived experience as part of a family of Mapuche healers "I grew up with Mapuche medicine," she told us. Her grandmother was a *püñeñelchefe* (midwife), her father was a *ngütamchefe* (bonesetter), and she also had kin who performed as *llantal* assisting the *machi* (shamans). According to Doraliza, her experiences and knowledge about healing inform her more holistic approach to health, allowing her to be a good facilitator. Over and above the formal job description, Doraliza told us: "The role of the intercultural facilitator is to be sensitive to the pain and sadness of the patients. Facilitators need to be formed with a Mapuche social and religious character."

We argue that the Mapuche facilitators' communicative labor helps to create interactional spaces where patients can more safely communicate about their condition to providers at the clinic. Through their practice, facilitators educate and help providers recognize Indigenous ways of knowing and healing that are tightly connected to broader community processes, opening spaces and processes of world building that extend beyond clinical encounters. Doraliza, for example, also describes how intercultural facilitators like herself can assist patients:

> The problem is that sometimes the person, if he or she is sick, will not have the strength to ask for help and explain to his or her family that he or she needs help, that it is not enough to just take *lawen* [medicinal plants], but that he or she perhaps needs a break, needs to leave his or her house, take *lawen* with a friend, or take *lawen* with the machi, or that he or she needs to have a *machitun* [ceremony] done, and the sick person, because he or she is so sick, is not in a condition to ask for help. Or the family does not understand what is happening to the person.

We take inspiration from Lawerence Kirmayer's research, his critique of cultural competence frameworks (2012), and his analysis of the processes of knowledge differences and power imbalances that patients and providers inhabit during clinical encounters (2014) to suggest that through their daily practice, intercultural facilitators are part of the process of unsettling the established praxis of clinical care. By actively reclaiming their indigeneity and the legitimacy of Indigenous knowledge, facilitators position themselves as active agents of education and social change that can "walk alongside" their patients.

Our chapter is based on our long-standing work in different capacities in Indigenous communities in Chile. Jorge Tibor Gutiérrez identifies as Mapuche and speaks Mapuzungun fluently. He began his collaboration with Mapuche healers in Southern Chile in the early 1980s while completing his undergraduate studies. Today, he belongs to the Mapuche association of Adkin Tulen in Lampa, near Santiago. Paula F. Saravia is a non-Indigenous Chilean anthropologist who started working as an advocate and researcher with Adkin Tulen in 2015. During August and September of 2016, Jorge and Paula collaborated as part of the Chile Global Health Field School, an alliance between the Pontifical Catholic University of Chile and the University of California San Diego. Most of what we discuss in these pages comes from our conversations, in-depth interviews with intercultural facilitators, and participant observation of healing encounters in Lampa (Metropolitan Region) and Nueva Imperial (Araucanía Region) in Chile.

To write this chapter, we designed a new research protocol inspired by the work of Silvia Rivera-Cusicanqui (2018) and Shawn Wilson (2008), which made explicit our methodological strategies centered around Mapuche relationality. Our protocol on ethics to protect Indigenous collaborators was approved by the University of Washington and the Network of Indigenous Peoples Responding to HIV (human immunodeficiency virus) and AIDS (acquired immunodeficiency syndrome) (RENPO). We conducted ten additional in-depth interviews with Mapuche intercultural health facilitators and healers, including *machi* (shamans) and *lawentuchefe* (herbal healers), between April and December 2023. We conducted some interviews remotely via Zoom with follow-up in-person visits. Our interviews focused on: a) describing the role of an intercultural health facilitator within the therapeutic space (clinic or Indigenous healing center); b) individual trajectories of intercultural facilitators and their life histories; c) characterizing the perceptions of Mapuche intercultural facilitators regarding their position within the intercultural health program; d) learning about the difficulties that intercultural facilitators face as they complete their work. All collaborators preferred using their real names, so we are not using pseudonyms.

We begin the chapter by presenting the Intercultural Health Program in Chile to contextualize our research findings. Here, we highlight the care work that intercultural facilitators enact and the challenges they face doing this work in a political system characterized by coloniality and the racialization of Indigenous people.

The Intercultural Health Program in Chile

The role of the intercultural facilitator was first sketched in the 1990s by the Chilean Ministry of Health as part of the new Programa Especial de Salud y Pueblos Indígenas (PESPI; Special Program of Health and Indigenous Peoples) (Intercultural Health Program). At the time, the role was loosely defined by national legislation and health protocols. The first intercultural facilitators were hired as translators as part of the healthcare staff at specific family health centers and hospitals in regions with higher proportions of Indigenous residents. For the most part, intercultural facilitators were needed in more rural—usually remote—localities where Indigenous patients spoke one of the several Indigenous languages spoken in contemporary Chile (including Mapuzungun, Quechua, and Aymara). Doraliza Millalen was one of the facilitators hired at this early stage of the program, and this is how she describes her role within the Nueva Imperial Hospital:

> My role in the early morning depended on the distribution made by the hospital because, at the beginning, I was in the office and depending on the requirements that came to the office, I went out to other departments, be it SOME (reception), laboratory, or hospitalization, so that was how it was at the beginning. Later, they asked me to divide my time by department. And the truth is that all the departments wanted me to be there because they said that the communication I achieved with people was greater than what they achieved.

The lack of clarity of the role of intercultural facilitators within the clinics is something that we also observed in our ethnographic participant observation. Updated health protocols signed in July 2023 expanded and strengthened the role of intercultural facilitators, who are Indigenous persons hired by public clinics, to act as a nexus between the respective clinic and Indigenous persons, families, communities, associations, and organizations in the local area. Intercultural facilitators nowadays are responsible for coordinating, mediating, and managing Indigenous patients' access and utilization of the range of services offered at the public health centers where facilitators work.

One of the skills required for this position is proficiency in the respective Indigenous language and basic knowledge pertinent to the community. Indigenous facilitators today work out of intercultural health offices in family clinics and hospitals. They are responsible for helping patients to navigate medical resources, including by talking to them about the circumstances that may have produced their illness and communicating information to providers, assisting patients in accessing care, and following up with them throughout the process of receiving care with biomedical and/or Indigenous medical practitioners. Doraliza referred to this holistic aspect of her work with patients and how their communicative labor contributed to relieving the congestion of waiting rooms at urgent care and access to care, especially for Indigenous peoples who lived in the rural areas: "I remember that there were up to 300 people on the list for emergency care, and most of them were people from the countryside ... I registered their information in the system and secured an appointment for them." In addition, facilitators advocate for policies and practices that will support Indigenous patients' legal right to be offered culturally appropriate care under two pieces of legislation: the Indigenous Act of 1993 and the ILO 169 International Convention on the Rights of Indigenous Peoples, which was ratified by the Chilean Congress in 2008.

The intercultural program in Chile has been widely studied. For decades, scholars have accounted for its many faults, mainly focusing on the experiences and perspectives of providers and patients (Bonelli 2012; Gavilan et al. 2017; Guzmán 2024; Saravia 2015; see Jelves and Ñanco 2004 for one of the few studies focused on intercultural facilitators). While we agree with the observed limitations and criticisms of the program, we also acknowledge the significance of opening a space of potentialities where Indigenous facilitators can work and collaborate to better their communities. The following section expands our discussion of this work and its challenges.

Intercultural Health Facilitators' Care Work and Challenges

Mapuche intercultural health facilitators understand and engage with the asymmetrical realities they face through everyday language use at the clinic and beyond. In our research, we observed three primary forms of asymmetric realities stemming from facilitators' positionality: maintaining balance while navigating two ways of knowing, bringing to life Indigenous praxis, and rendering their holistic perspective on community and political engagement visible. We show these three patterns by drawing on quotes from our interviews with intercultural facilitators Doraliza Millalen, Ximena Lienqueo, and Florencia Melillan.

Intercultural facilitators participating in this research assist in the care of patients across settings where there are radically different assumptions about health and illness. Much of their work involves accurately interpreting Indigenous framings of health and illness in biomedical clinical settings. This requires extensive familiarity with biomedical conceptualizations of health and clinic protocols and with Mapuche medical knowledge, including conceptual knowledge and vocabulary for symptoms and signs of illness in Mapuzungun, which facilitators translate during therapeutic encounters so that biomedical providers can better understand patients' experiences.

Because of their familiarity with Indigenous medicine and community embeddedness, facilitators are also often involved in the diagnostic process and treatment carried out by *machi*s and *lawentuchefes* in the specific territories where they work. Their expertise stemming from this involvement is usually quite specialized in botanical knowledge and health-related ideas, which vary across Mapuche coastal, inland valley, and mountainous regions.

In addition to their technomedical knowledge, intercultural facilitators also must develop good rapport and interpersonal relationships with leaders and members of Indigenous communities (in rural areas), Indigenous associations (in urban areas), and physicians, nurses, dentists, and other health professionals with whom they work at the clinic. Facilitators told us that in order to foster community relationships, they sometimes propose to fund activities and community events at the local level and make a point of meeting local politicians. As an intermediary between Indigenous medicine and the biomedical system, the facilitator acts as a hinge system, receiving a message from the Mapuche patient and translating it or conveying the meaning of the Indigenous diagnosis to the treating provider (usually a physician). In this process of interpretation, the facilitator works alongside the provider in the clinical case for each Indigenous patient and registers the Indigenous symptomatology and the overall medical history.

Despite Indigenous facilitators' crucial role in patient care, their positions within the national healthcare system are precarious and undervalued by clinicians. Most facilitators do not have a physical space where they can talk to patients confidentially, they do not always have access to computers, and they often depend on the goodwill of individual clinic administrators to sort out the material conditions of their labor, including shift scheduling and compensation.

Facilitators' positionality as public employees and their role as mediators between the state and the Indigenous communities and associations they work with is also challenging due to the fraught history of state-Indigenous relations in Chile. Indigenous peoples have gone through long-standing processes of forced assimilation by the Chilean state, producing and reproducing asymmetric colonial relationships that suppress Indigenous epistemologies.

Doraliza, Florencia, Marcela, and Ximena, our collaborators in this research, live in a rural area in Wall Mapu, the traditional Mapuche territory shared by Indigenous peoples who identify ethnically as Mapuche across Chile and Argentina. While most Mapuche people live in cities, including Temuco and the Chilean capital, Santiago, they maintain tight connections to their home territories. For centuries, Mapuche communities have resisted colonial occupation, and contemporary struggles center on land and political autonomy. Over the past three decades, confrontations between branches of the Mapuche social movement and the Chilean State have escalated (see Cayuqueo 2018; Richards 2013). As we write this chapter, several Mapuche activists resist imprisonment through hunger strikes. For Mapuche communities, structural racism has consequences in shaping health outcomes because of maximized environmental vulnerabilities (Atallah et al. 2018), occupational hazards, and overcrowded housing, which results in a higher risk of tuberculosis, for example (Paluzzi 2004; Saravia 2015). Indigenous activists also mobilize to secure inclusive health policies and opportunities to engage in HIV-AIDS prevention campaigns and education (Morales 2024; Regnum 2019).

Through the "Chileanization" process, Indigenous ways of being in the world have been stifled and framed as backward and problematic. Mapuche people have been forcibly displaced from their land, compelled to learn and speak in Spanish, and pressured to ascribe to a creole-*mestizo* national identity. According to our collaborators, the result of these pressures is *awingkamiento* (becoming *winka* or white). This harmful transformation generates deep loneliness and rootlessness that can provoke illness (also see Bacigalupo 2016). In these ways, dispossession and assimilation are directly productive of culturally specific forms of suffering, such as *awingkamiento*. Our collaborators explained this affliction as an existential struggle that can only be overcome through ancestral knowledge and a sense of self-connectedness to the land. According to them, coping with illness and making sense of it is only possible if "we listen to the land that speaks."

Mapuzungun (also known as Chezungun), the name of the language of the people also means "the land that speaks." Our Mapuche collaborators explain that the land communicates through the positive and negative energies of the earth's *newen* (vital energy). Language—and Mapuzungun specifically—is, thus, crucial for bringing health and social life together as part of relationships that transcend the human. Indeed, the balance of *newen* is vital to *küme mongen*, the Mapuche framing of wellbeing that encompasses natural life, spiritual worlds, and community. The possibility of healing is contingent on *newen*, expressed through language and connected to ancestral *ngen* (keeper spirits). Therefore, we argue that health in its integrity is, in part, a linguistic phenomenon.

The official language (and perspective) of state-funded public clinics is Castilian Spanish, a language grounded in colonization and the historical dispossession of Indigenous people. Indigenous health facilitators play a role in unsettling these terms of coloniality by using Indigenous languages in biomedical contexts. As Bernard Perley argues, **linguistic dispossession** worked alongside other mechanisms of erasure that forced Indigenous peoples away from their lands and left them vulnerable to violence and coercion (Perley 2024). By speaking historically stigmatized Indigenous languages and by validating Indigenous knowledge in public clinics and hospitals, intercultural facilitators are actively creating spaces of resistance against the processes of racialization and discrimination that Indigenous peoples in Chile face every day.

Rather than translating directly, facilitators told us that they usually leave the complexities of Mapuzungun aside in favor of providing a synthesized list of symptoms that a provider can "easily read." In this sense, besides the symptomatology, the intercultural facilitator translates the state of mind and the state of health of the person consulting, establishing an interpersonal connection through these previous conversations. In many ways, facilitators are mediators between the biomedical doctor and the Indigenous patient, but their role goes beyond that.

The experience of most facilitators is that after applying for the position, they received little information about the expectations of their duties at the clinics. Our collaborators mentioned repeatedly that at the beginning, they felt "como un bicho raro" (out of place, literally "like a weird bug") because their colleagues at the clinic were either ignorant or dismissive of Indigenous medicines and did not know what the contribution of the facilitators would be. However, despite the initial resistance to their integration into the clinical settings, the facilitators gained spaces of participation and action through their persistent community engagement and communication efforts. Ximena Lienqueo reflected on her initial days leading the Amulzugun intercultural office at the Family Health Center in Nueva Imperial:

> The office was created in 2006 when the new family health center was opened in Nueva Imperial, right where the hospital used to be. It was a very thankless job. In fact, no one knew anything, and neither did I! It was a job that was created little by little, and they [the Ministry of Health] didn't give you the guidelines to be able to do it … So, it was very difficult to work, especially with colleagues, because my colleagues are trained in a different way. They are trained at the university, in other ways of knowing. The doctors themselves did not understand or know what it was like to be the *ngen kutran*, for example, "the keeper of the sick." That is where one plays an important role.

Ximena's long experience as a facilitator has not been easy. As she described in the quote above, not having a clear job description or agreed expectations generated resistance from medical providers and administrators and, worst of all, left the facilitator alone to create a path for integration. As the years went by, Ximena was able to find allies and took advantage of the lack of guidelines to benefit the office. To do so, she created new forms of advocacy that included health education and promotion.

Ximena also alludes to the way that intercultural facilitators sometimes enact the role of *ngen kutran* (keeper of the sick.) This role is profoundly linked to Mapuche ways of conceptualizing the person as fundamentally relational and interdependent. As our collaborators explained, "one never walks alone." There is always an invisible double or *Am*. A person is not just a body and spirit. Instead, a person's completeness depends on spiritual connection, and their presence remains in the space they inhabit, even when their body is no longer there. The *ngen* (keeper) is an invisible double who is found even in the more-than-human environment: for example, trees, animals, and even medicinal plants have a "keeper." In his ethnography of the Pehuenche people (Mapuche who live in the mountains), Chilean anthropologist Cristóbal Bonelli found that the *Am* and the *ngen* work as a dual ontological framework (2012). In this system, *kutran* (illness) is produced by an imbalance of positive and negative forces. Hence, when sick, a person needs a *ngen kutran*, a keeper, to take charge. This is precisely the role that Marcela took when her husband felt "empty" as his spirit was leaving his body.

Florencia Melillan, intercultural facilitator in one of the rural family health centers in Nueva Imperial, explained:

> Ngen kutran is the keeper of the sick; for example, if there is a couple, and she gets sick, then the husband takes the role of ngen kutran. He needs to care for his wife and make decisions concerning treatment. It can also be a brother, a sister, any family member. Because the sick don't know what to do, they are disoriented and might be depressed. Then, there is a need for a person to be with them: ngen kutran.

Our collaborators described their work as heavily reliant on language: conversing with patients, speaking in Mapuzungun, learning, and facilitating communication related to the coordination of care. In these ways, their work involves much more than language interpretation. And it is the Mapuche conceptualization of *ngen kutran* that differentiates Mapuche intercultural facilitators from medical translators or patient advocates. As Ximena told us:

> This is a really fundamental part of our people's culture, and it is also in the law of rights and duties of the sick (article 7 of the law number 20,584), and it is a space we gained. It is a very important issue because the *ngen kutran* is the person who knows what's happening. When one is disconsolate, sick, especially when one is sick in spirit, so to speak, the ill person does not say anything. The patient does not - they just sit there. If someone asks them

> where it hurts, they don't say anything. They stay silent, and then the *ngen kutran* plays an important role.

In this quote, Ximena explains their intermediary role as *ngen kutran* when a family member is not available: interpreting, consulting with the patient, translating to the doctor the patient's symptoms and state of mind, and often accompanying the sick, including coordinating their care so that they can recover. Because many young people have migrated away from rural areas to access employment possibilities elsewhere, it is common for older adults to remain alone in rural areas. In these cases, facilitators take on the role of *ngen kutran*, even as they reach out to patients' family members, urging them to take responsibility:

> Unfortunately, we have had to be part of it because sometimes the man or woman is very alone, they are older adults, they don't know where [to go] ... so what do they do? They come here [to ask us], "Can you come with us, ma'am, because I don't hear well, I don't understand, why don't you come with me?" Then we talk to the person, his daughter or son. We call and tell them, "You know, your mother was told this, she has to take that, she has to complete lab work, you have to ...now you have to accompany her." Because sometimes we have to tell them, "You have to accompany her because she can't walk alone. You can't care so little about her." So that is where the patient's keeper, *ngen kutran*, plays an important role.

Intercultural facilitators have a daunting task as intermediaries between patients, patient families, and a range of healthcare providers. They are expected to facilitate communication, often interpreting between Mapuzungun and Spanish, about patients' feelings of pain and illness, patients' hopes about treatment, and medical providers' diagnoses and instructions for treatment. In some cases, facilitators translate not words but an overview of symptoms and signs of pain and suffering, helping Indigenous patients present their medical narrative to clinicians.

Conclusions

In this chapter, we discussed the close connection between language and health for Mapuche Indigenous peoples in Southern Chile. We shared narratives and testimonies of Mapuche intercultural facilitators who engage in care work to validate Indigenous epistemologies and bridge the gap between two very different medical systems and worldviews within clinical spaces.

We emphasized the crucial role of language in healing, highlighting Mapuzungun as a means of communication and a way to connect with the land's vital energy (*newen*) and ancestral spirits (*ngen*). This linguistic connection is essential for achieving a culturally accepted sense of wellbeing (*küme mongen*) among Mapuche people. Additionally, we underscored the significant role of intercultural health facilitators who help translate both language and cultural and spiritual experiences, which are often invisible to conventional medical providers. Intercultural facilitators act as *ngen kutran* when needed and offer safe spaces for patient interaction, facilitating communication between patients and healthcare providers at the clinic.

The care work of intercultural facilitators is rooted in Mapuche concepts and ideals, representing a crucial form of communicative care labor (Arnold 2024). By using Mapuzungun and advocating for the legitimacy of Mapuche medical models, facilitators actively prevent the erasure of linguistic dispossession, resist colonial influences in Chilean clinical settings, and promote culturally sensitive and inclusive healthcare. Rather than merely translating medical terms or lists of symptoms, intercultural health facilitators make Indigenous ways of being-in-the-world possible by connecting patients with the vital energy and essential spirits, thus bringing balance to patients and communities while reproducing ancestral knowledge. In their daily labor of care, intercultural facilitators defy the entrenched biomedical space of the clinic and empower themselves and their communities by making visible what cannot be seen. Bringing these invisible possibilities to life through Mapuzungun makes all the difference for Indigenous patients.

Questions for Reflection and Discussion

Reflection Questions

1. Reflect on a time when you were injured or sick. Who assisted you? Did you need help with physical care? Comfort and encouragement? Did someone help with keeping track of information, getting medications, scheduling appointments, or communicating with your provider (in person, over the phone, or through email)? What other forms of support did you need until you recuperated?
2. Have you ever assisted someone during an illness, a doctor visit, or a hospitalization? What support did you provide? What communication tasks were involved? What was challenging and what was rewarding about this caregiving experience?

Looking In: Small Group Discussion Questions

1. According to Mapuche perspectives and knowledge, how are health, language, and land related?
2. Describe the role that intercultural facilitators play in healthcare in Chile. How is their role similar to and different from the work of medical interpretation described by Wahl (Chapter 5)?

3. In Mapuche understandings of health, what does *ngen kutran* mean? Who generally occupies this role, and what does the role entail? How is the role of intercultural facilitator related to that of *ngen kutran*?
4. What are some of the challenges that intercultural facilitators have faced in their work within the public healthcare system? How have they responded to these challenges?

Looking Out: Large Group Discussion Questions

1. Given what you have learned about intercultural health facilitators, which term(s) best describe their work: healthcare workers, representatives of the public health system, companions, translators, community leaders, social workers, or something else? Explain and justify your answer.
2. Considering the care work of intercultural health facilitators, propose a different situation or context where this model could work. Why would this model be a good option?
3. The authors say that intercultural facilitators have to "translate the invisible" as part of their work. What is invisible in this case, and what makes it invisible?
4. The authors describe some of the historical factors that have led to health inequities for Indigenous Chileans and recent laws that have changed the relationship between Indigenous peoples and the Chilean state. What do you imagine are some challenges that still need to be addressed to improve Indigenous wellbeing and access to healthcare?

References

Arnold, Lynnette. 2024. *Living Together across Borders: Communicative Care in Transnational Salvadoran Families*. Oxford: Oxford University Press.

Atallah, Devin G., Carlos Contreras Painemal, Lorena Albornoz, Flavio Salgado, Elizabeth Pilquil Lizama. 2018. Engaging Critical Community Resilience Praxis: A Qualitative Study with Mapuche Communities in Chile Facing Structural Racism and Disasters. *Journal of Community Psychology* 46: pp. 575–597. https://doi.org/10.1002/jcop.21960.

Bacigalupo, Ana Mariella. 2016. *Thunder Shaman: Making History with Mapuche Spirits in Chile and Patagonia*. Austin: University of Texas Press.

Bonelli, Cristóbal. 2012. Ontological Disorders: Nightmares, Psychotropic Drugs and Evil Spirits in Southern Chile. *Anthropological Theory* 12(4): pp. 407–426. https://doi.org/10.1177/1463499612469587.

Boric, Gabriel. 2023. Reglamento Sobre el Derecho de las Personas Pertenecientes a los Pueblos Indígenas a Recibir una Atención de Salud con Pertinencia Cultural. https://bcn.cl/3hnyi.

Cayuqueo, Pedro. 2018. *Porfiada y Rebelde es la Memoria: Crónicas Mapuche*. Santiago de Chile: Editorial Catalonia.

Gavilan, Vivian, Patricia Vigueras, Carlos Madariaga, and Michel Parra. 2017. Interculturality, Cultural Traditions and Ethnicities: Three Key Notions to Understand Sanitary Policies in Chile. *Chungara-Revista de Antropología Chilena* 49(4): pp. 477–482.

Guzmán, Jennifer. 2024. Pursuit of Health / Communicative Justice through an Intercultural Health Model in Gulumapu (Chile). In *Language and Social Justice: Global Perspectives*, ed. Kathleen Riley, B. Perley, and I. García-Sánchez, pp. 392–411. New York: Bloomsbury Academic.

Jelves, Ivonne, and José Ñanco. 2004. Experiencia Oficinas Amuldungun y Rol del Facilitador Intercultural. *Actas 5o Congreso Chileno de Antropología*. V Congreso Chileno de Antropología. Colegio de Antropólogos de Chile A. G., San Felipe, Simposio Salud, Cultura y Pueblos Originarios.

Kirmayer, Laurence J. 2012. Cultural Competence and Evidence-Based Practice in Mental Health: Epistemic Communities and the Politics of Pluralism. *Social Science & Medicine* 75(2): pp. 249–256. Available at: https://doi.org/10.1016/j.socscimed.2012.03.018.

Kirmayer, Laurence, Jaswant Guzder, and Cécile Rousseau, eds. 2014. *Cultural Consultation: Encountering the Other in Mental Health Care*. New York: Springer.

Morales, W. and @ISLA.DE.CHILOE. 2024. Interview during AIDS 2024, the 25th International AIDS Conference. Instagram. https://www.instagram.com/reel/C9zXAeQIyDH/?igsh=bjZpcXRlenY5ZmRy.

Paluzzi, J. E. 2004. A Social Disease/a Social Response: Lessons in Tuberculosis from Early 20th Century Chile. *Social Science & Medicine* 59(4): pp. 763–773. https://doi.org/10.1016/j.socscimed.2003.11.039.

Regnum. 2019. *El Hilo Rojo (The Red Thread)*. Accessed on September 22, 2024. https://cinechile.cl/pelicula/hilo-rojo/.

Richards, Patricia. 2013. *Race and the Chilean Miracle: Neoliberalism, Democracy, and Indigenous Rights*. Pittsburgh, PA: University of Pittsburgh Press.

Perley, Bernard. 2024. Inscribing Social Justice through Indigenous Place-Names. In *Language and Social Justice: Global Perspectives*, ed. Kathleen Riley, B. Perley, and I. García-Sánchez, pp. 412–435. New York: Bloomsbury Academic.

Rivera-Cusicanqui, Silvia. 2018. Un Mundo Ch'ixi es Posible: Ensayos desde un Presente en Crisis. Ciudad Autónoma de Buenos Aires: Tinta Limón.

Saravia, Paula Francisca. 2015. Ujuk Usu. Medicine, Tuberculosis and Race among the Aymara of the Border between Bolivia and Chile. PhD dissertation. University of California, San Diego.

Wilson, Shawn. 2008. *Research Is Ceremony: Indigenous Research Methods*. Nova Scotia: Fernwood Publishing.

SECTION 3

COMMUNITY AND COMMUNICABILITY

Editors' Introduction

Some of the most important communication about health happens outside of clinical spaces. Governments debate healthcare policies, officials make announcements about public health, news media pundits and popular influencers vie for attention through dramatic stories about outbreaks of contagious disease or hot takes on the latest health fads. People use social media to find others with similar diagnoses and swap stories, friends and relatives give one another medical advice, adult siblings discuss how to care for their aging parents.

All of these are examples of **communicability**, a term with double meaning. On the one hand, communicable diseases are those which spread from person to person. Communicability also refers to the production, circulation, and reception of knowledge through communication. Scholars use the term **biocommunicability** to refer to the ways that knowledge about health is articulated, how these ideas travel and are taken up, and what the consequences are for health (Briggs and Hallin 2007; Friend 2020).

Certain knowledge or beliefs about health may be particularly "sticky" or easily transmitted to others, while other ideas do not circulate as readily. Biocommunicability draws attention to the role of power in shaping this uneven circulation. Some individuals and social institutions have access to material and communicative resources that allow them to readily disseminate their ideas about health, while others do not have the same platform. For instance, during the COVID-19 pandemic, public officials used their prominent roles to articulate often competing messages about the virus, which circulated through governmental health communication campaigns and the news. Meanwhile, frontline workers who had the highest risk of contracting the disease were less able to disseminate their perspectives about the virus and its impacts. As this example illustrates, biocommunicability can exacerbate existing inequities, marginalizing the perspectives of those who have the least access to economic, political, and social power.

Individuals who feel isolated by health challenges or want to amplify their efforts at health communication often form communities of support. Communities may form around healing methods such as reiki or mindfulness meditation, allowing people to share specialized knowledge and skills. Many such communities coalesce online. Some make valuable contributions to medical knowledge, as when social media groups for COVID long-haulers have provided novel information about common symptomatology. For better or worse, however, the algorithms and affordances of social media platforms shape biocommunicability, causing some ideas to go viral while other, sometimes more valuable information, gets lost in the noise.

The chapters in this section work to advance understanding of biocommunicable processes around the world. Daniel W. Krugman and Mohamed Yunus Rafiq describe the origins and contemporary usage of two different words for cancer in Tanzania, tracing tensions between English-dominant global health and efforts to emphasize Swahili as a decolonial national language. Xochitl Marsilli-Vargas investigates the widespread circulation of psychoanalytic discourse in popular media in Argentina, which has shaped how Argentinians listen to one another. Steven P. Black explores how human immunodeficiency virus (HIV) positive individuals in South Africa confront acquired immunodeficiency syndrome (AIDS) stigma and build a community of support through their use of scientific medical discourse.

References

Briggs, Charles L., and Daniel C. Hallin. 2007. Biocommunicability: The Neoliberal Subject and Its Contradictions in News Coverage of Health Issues. *Social Text* 25: pp. 43–66. https://doi.org/10.1215/01642472-2007-011.

Friend, Julianna. 2020. Sutura 2.0: Queer Biocommunicability and Digital Self-Making in Senegalese eHealth Activism. *Journal of Language and Sexuality* 9(1): pp. 14–47.

7

Kansa, Saratani, and Biocommunicability in Coastal Tanzania

Daniel W. Krugman and Mohamed Yunus Rafiq

A Medical-Linguistic Dilemma in Tanzania

"*Kansa*," Baba Ibrahim started, "go to the hospital, it is only there." We had just sat down at the newsstand on one of the main commercial roads in Bagamoyo, Tanzania, on an already scorching morning. Baba Ibrahim, Baba Ahmed, and Baba Omari were there sipping coffee out of small cups before we arrived. Welcomed into the circle by these three elders, we were served coffee as we introduced ourselves as researchers studying how cancer is understood and talked about in Bagamoyo—a small town 50 miles north of Dar Es Salaam on the Swahili Coast.

After we clarified that we were not doctors, Baba Ibrahim continued: "I do not know much about this. *Kansa* is a nasty bad disease. It cannot be cured. This place, Ocean Road in Dar es Salaam, it is advanced, but it is cursed. Many die there." As we had come to understand, not only was *kansa* not understood by most people we met as "cancer" in a pure biomedical sense, they also utilized a wide range of strategies to make sense of this disease that was increasingly impacting their community and nation. These *wazee*, the term for aged, well-respected men who are addressed in conversation as *baba* "father," made sense of *kansa* through a common strategy—linking the disease to Ocean Road, the widely known national cancer institute in Dar es Salaam.

Baba Ahmed then sharply interjected, cutting Ibrahim off. "*Kaka* 'brother,'" he began, "this place Ocean Road does not treat the *kansa*. They treat *saratani* there, that is what the posters in the hospital say." *Saratani* is another name for cancer in Swahili, the one that is officially recognized by the Tanzanian government. However, throughout our time in Bagamoyo, we found its relationship with *kansa* is contentious and complex.

"No, baba," Ibrahim quickly responded, "*kansa* is the danger. *Saratani* leads to *kansa*, but it is not *kansa*. That hospital over on that side treats *kansa* with equipment from Europe."

"You are embarrassing yourself in front of our guests," Baba Ahmed said, now agitated. "The signs say *saratani*. The news says *saratani*. The government says *saratani*.

Daniel W. Krugman and Mohamed Yunus Rafiq, *Kansa, Saratani, and Biocommunicability in Coastal Tanzania*. In: *Language and Health in Action*. Edited by: Lynnette Arnold et al., Oxford University Press. © Daniel W. Krugman and Mohamed Yunus Rafiq (2026). DOI: 10.1093/9780198933953.003.0007

This *kansa* is a foreign disease. It is here, I have heard of it, but it is not *saratani*. It is very dangerous, but not as much as *saratani*."

"I have heard they are the same," Baba Omari said casually, inserting himself into the conversation for the first time. "I do not know this word *saratani*, but this is what has been said at the hospital. *Saratani* is the swelling, and there are different kinds. *Kansa* is what happens over there [abroad], and could happen here, but *saratani* is here in Tanzania."

The debate deepened. Baba Ibrahim called Omari's claim false and argued that *kansa* and *saratani* were different because *saratani* could be cured and *kansa* could not. Baba Omari stated that *kansa* was any *uvimbe* "swelling" that killed people, but *saratani* had specific types, according to a poster at the regional hospital. They ultimately agreed to disagree after Baba Ahmed tried to launch into a story about a relative who had *saratani* that was not *kansa*, and our conversation moved to other subjects.

Grounded in ethnographic data collected by a team of Tanzanian and US American researchers (2022–2023), this chapter contends with the predicament revealed by this conversation. The biological phenomenon of mutating cells that create tumors on different bodily organs, known as "cancer" in English, has two names—*kansa* and *saratani*—in Kiswahili, the national language of Tanzania and most widely spoken language in Africa. While *saratani* is the official translation of the word "cancer" used by the state and medical system, *kansa*, an adaption of the English word, is much more widely used in everyday conversation. Official documentation and dictionaries define these two words as equivalent terms. Yet, how different people across the Swahili Coast make sense of them is messy, contested, and dynamic. Across Bagamoyo, *kansa* and *saratani* are conceptualized as two completely different diseases with similar symptoms, as two distinct diseases that are connected through a causal relationship, as the same disease originating from different parts of the world, or as different parts of the same larger disease. In short, there is a profound disjuncture between how these two supposedly equivalent terms function in the linguistic ecosystem of Bagamoyo, opening a range of questions about naming disease, translation, and the power to decide the meaning of medical terminology.

Biocommunicability, the ways in which illness, diseases, and public health measures are made known and intelligible in modern society is a key medical-linguistic anthropological idea that helps make sense of this disjuncture between *kansa* and *saratani* and to unravel the complexities of medical nosology. This chapter illuminates the intricacies of biocommunicability and argues that contemporary communication, translation, and conceptualization of medicine, healing, and diseases must be understood as shaped by global politics and historical inequities. In particular, we examine the legacies of nationalism, colonialism, and neoliberal reform. By outlining how larger political projects shaped *kansa* and *saratani*, we show how local medical language is shaped by unequal political economies while foregrounding the real consequences these predicaments create.

Making *Saratani* and the Politics of Biocommunicability

Sitting in front of a bookshelf containing volumes of thick medical texts, Juma, a senior oncologist in Dar es Salaam, told us the origin of the term *saratani* as he remembered it. "Now," he began, "I remember around 1986, the Tanzania Tumor Center, which is what the hospital was called at the time, wanted a Swahili name for cancer. We approached BAKITA with the request." Juma was referring to the former name of the Ocean Road Cancer Institute—the only oncological specialized facility in Tanzania (and Juma's employer) and to Baraza la Kiswahili la Taifa (BAKITA)—a government unit housed at the University of Dar es Salaam that is tasked with producing words in Kiswahili when none are available. He continued, "After pondering, they suggested the word *saratani* to us. It comes from the Arabic word *swaratani*, which means crab." As Juma later established, *saratani* is considered the *official* Swahili word for cancer because it is the name that was created by the people of Tanzania for the people of Tanzania in their own language.

The process of coining a new disease term as Juma outlines is structured by multiple historical trends that characterize the modern world. First, western-derived biomedicine has become the globally dominant way of dealing with health and is largely organized around globalized disease classifications, diagnosis, and treatment. Second, the ideology that a nation-state should have a dominant national language has been naturalized and universalized. Third, nation-states have become dominantly responsible for reinforcing the classification and standardization of diseases through their regulatory control over medical practice and public health. But as scholars Charles L. Briggs and Daniel Hallin point toward through their coining of *biocommunicability* it is the "flows" of medical words and language through society that must be focused on (Briggs and Hallin 2007). As Briggs summarizes later with Mark Nichter, "the production, circulation, and reception of knowledge [is] communicability, and, when it forms part of (bio)medicalized domains, [it is] biocommunicability" (2009:194). Briggs and Hallin establish how discourses of medicine and health are socially constructed by medical and scientific experts who aim to influence the health-related actions and beliefs of the public, and their different "models." These models are ideologically backed logics of how health knowledge should be communicated to the public. Thus, biocommunicability is tied up with broader political projects that, in the end, as Briggs and Hallin suggest, locate the management of populations by the state. Biocommunicable models are thereby used by governments and other state institutions—as well as private media and corporate entities—to influence how biomedical terminology and discourse are understood by people, and thus shape their responses to health information such as pandemic notices or new biomedical advances. This, in the end, is an effort of cultivating **subjects**, or socially acknowledged individuals who think and move through the world in certain ways.

While Briggs and Hallin develop biocommunicability through examining the different biocommunicable models journalists in the United States use to communicate health information to publics, here we are concerned with the political projects *inside* these models and communicative efforts. Dr Juma's description of the Tanzanian government's project to create a *fasaha* "pure" word for cancer in the 1980s is a prime example of how a political program and medical communication can become entangled. Coining the word *saratani* was part of a larger effort of the recently decolonized state to link biomedical communication to the political project of producing decolonial citizens. This project began in 1961 when the Colony of Tanganyika gained independence from Great Britain. Following the idea that nation-states must be unified by a single language, Kiswahili, the most spoken language in the new nation, became a centerpiece of President Julius Nyerere's nationalization effort centered around decolonization, unity, and socialism. From 1962 to 1975, Swahili was "purified" of English words (Whiteley 1969), designated the sole national language, and set up as "a true symbol of the Tanzanian people" that was intended to "mobilize the masses towards Ujamaa and the philosophy of self-reliance (*Kujitegemea*)" (Kishe 2016:4). Alongside *ubuntu*, or, brotherhood, Nyerere's decolonial socialism was built upon this trade language, and the entire nation was reeducated to acquire it (Blommaert 2014; Mugane 2015). Established in 1967, BAKITA became the bureaucratic mechanism to manage this transformation and purification. As James Mdee describes, BAKITA was, and still is, responsible for "standardization of new vocabulary and terms, spelling, and correct usage of the language," for setting "guidelines for coining words for new concepts introduced into Kiswahili and also for standardizing them," and for "advising the government and other public organizations on the correct usage of Kiswahili and to ensure that Kiswahili is used in all governmental business" (1983:109).

In this sociopolitical context and with the spirit of *kujitegemea* (self-reliance), Ocean Road oncologists including Juma requested a "pure" Swahili word for cancer to participate in this national language project, avoiding scrutiny for using the English term "cancer" that was dominant in their space. BAKITA subsequently produced a word based on a particular ideology of what "pure" Swahili is—one based on the idea Arabic is the correct language to draw loan words from. *Swaratani*, the Arabic word for crab that is the basis for *saratan* (cancer), thus became *saratani* in Swahili. A word, created through ostensibly decolonial logic for decolonial nationalism, *saratani* is the product of Tanzanian statecraft. The word represents an effort of biocommunicability that sought to link biomedicine to nationalist sentiments and, through this, produce Tanzanian citizens who thought of themselves as subjects who understand through their seemingly independent African language that they are people no longer ruled by Europe and live in a society that does not borrow from its former rulers.

Assembling the *Kansa/Saratani* Disjuncture

However, as Briggs and Hallin make clear, making health and biomedicine objects, technologies, and knowledges legible through language in the public sphere is incompletely controlled by the biomedical apparatus, state governments, or the media. Not all of the institutions and experts who are in privileged positions to define and disseminate this information seek to circulate the same discourses and understandings (Briggs and Hallin 2007). Further, the people who officialized discourses of biomedical information targets have agency to forge and communicate their own ideas about diseases, therapeutics, and health. Tanzanians have been doing this in regard to the biomedical idea of "cancer" since biomedical knowledge about the disease first arrived in the nation during the colonial period. For decades, the word and idea of biomedical cancer circulated in Tanzania but in a restricted fashion, among Europeans, who were screened and treated for cancer in exclusively white Dar es Salaam hospitals. Later, the English term became familiar among upper-class Tanzanians who worked for the colonial government. It was not until after independence that formerly colonized Tanzanians began to gain access to oncological care, and thus the word circulated among broader populations in higher degrees. By the time Nyerere's socialist government began tracking cancer cases in 1966 and established the nation's first publicly accessible oncological infrastructure at Muhimbili Medical Centre in Dar es Salaam (later transferred to Ocean Road), popular knowledge of cancer in biomedical terms was sparse. As a 1985 article by American physician George Alexander, who worked at Muhimbili, illuminates, "the significance of a diagnosis of cancer in Tanzania can be understood only by knowing the individual who has the disease. Its nature is unknown to the vast majority of people" (Alexander 1985:65). While physicians observed malignant tumors across the nation (Hiza 1976; Manni and Huygen 1990), Tanzanian citizens were left to formulate ideas of cancer largely on their own terms. As a result, they often interpreted encounters with the word "cancer" with non-biomedical sources of knowledge, understanding it as a "foreign" or "white" disease as it was spatially indexed as a disease that happened exclusively in white-only hospitals (Alexander 1985).

Thus, *saratani*—an effort of an explicit kind of biocommunicability linked to decolonialism—entered a medical linguistic context where a word for the disease globalized biomedicine class "cancer" already was circulating, but not widely, and one in which people were formulating ideas of the disease without prominent state or biomedical intervention. The question is, how did *kansa*—the "spontaneously" introduced name (Yambi 2000)—come to dominate the popular lexicon, and why were the two names never effectively linked? The answer is tied to the infliction of neoliberal political-economic and social models in Tanzania. Beginning in the 1980s, in the wake of Nyerere's abdication of the presidency and an economic crisis driven by war with Uganda, the Tanzanian government was forced to take on international loans. These loans required neoliberal changes in government and economic policies: the dismantling of public programs and embrace of open-market capitalism (Aminzade 2013). As part of this neoliberal shift, the Tanzanian government began to break apart and privatize the centralized healthcare system (Kamat 2008). Now reliant upon foreign non-governmental organizations (NGOs) for public health and medical services (Igoe 2003), oncological healthcare for wealthier patients increased as private options for care expanded. However, like other aspects of the healthcare system documented by Kamat (2008), oncological care in the public hospitals utilized by poorer patients lost funding and, thereby, became more unreliable, resource constrained, and overwhelmed as backups increased.

The opening of Tanzania to foreign influence and the ensuing adjustment to a capitalist economy created three entangled issues in Tanzania's contemporary healthcare system, which created the conditions that have given rise to the complex relationship between *kansa* and *saratani*. First, with the increase in foreign influence, particularly from American and British corporations and government agencies, Tanzania and its national Swahili language began to "Anglicize," as English words and grammatical structures became increasingly incorporated into the language (Kishe 1994, 2016). Second, as cancer rates proliferated across the Global South and northern experts began to recognize the underdevelopment of oncological care in the formerly colonized world, the disease became increasingly shaped by a morally charged industry of advocacy, research, and fundraising organized in America (Jain 2013). No longer a "first world disease," the global health industry turned its attention to cancer in the south (Livingston 2012). Finally, governmental efforts toward decolonial nationalism waned, and the related policies and programs that sought to foster *kujitegemea* (self-reliance) declined. No longer seeking to minimize foreign influence and with fewer resources to promote nationalist words, the Tanzanian state shifted from (attempted) tight regulation of Swahili to an approach with limited government intervention. This transition reflects what Briggs and colleagues call the *neoliberal* model of biocommunicability (Briggs and Hallin 2007). Instead of governments and the scientific apparatus having tight control over the health knowledge and dictating its flow, neoliberal governance seeks to promote individual self-help and the resolution of problems through market-oriented thinking and private sector action. In contrast to the logic of *kujitegemea*, which sought to produce citizens who collectively contributed to the Tanzanian nation-state's self-reliance and rejection of colonial influences partially through the medical language they used, the neoliberal model of biocommunicability promotes people deciding what health information to take up—and thereby what words to use—on their own terms.

Thus, while Tanzanians have always formed conceptualizations about cancer from the generally limited information that was available to them, the conditions that shaped what names were seen and interacted with shifted. The two names for cancer now circulated in a moment when dramatic changes to the political and economic landscape of Tanzania caused the linguistic ecosystem to "Anglicize" while the oncological system became more dependent on English-speaking NGOs and private corporations. The visibility of the English word "cancer" thereby increased. Although *saratani* had been integrated into government-sponsored public health notices, hospital registers, and physician vocabulary throughout the 1990s, by the early twenty-first century, usage of "cancer" proliferated with the influx of US American media, international news outlets, increasingly prominent social media platforms, and public health campaigns launched by global health NGOs. Cancer/*kansa*, in short, had not only been circulating more in the national consciousness, but had also gained greater opportunities to become taken up as the term associated with biomedical cancer. Now beholden to private and international influences in healthcare, and competing against global English media, the Tanzanian government was unable to effectively promote the use of *saratani* and the broader decolonial nationalist project it was a part of.

Everyday *Kansa*-Talk in Bagamoyo

Returning now to the newspaper stand conversation with the *wazee*, we can see the historical conditions that structure the conversation and create the confusion between terms for cancer. In debating these meanings among themselves and with us, the elders were drawing from prior instances where they interacted with *kansa* or *saratani*; for instance, hearing "cancer" in an English movie, seeing a public health poster warning about *saratani*, or, most immediately, hearing about a *kansa* diagnosis around town. These three men deployed a plethora of strategies to make sense of these terms that, to them and many others, do not equate to each other and do not directly match scientific-biological understandings of cancer.

These three men, though, only had second or third hand interaction with the disease, thus creating a particular distance of interpretation and, thereby, an ambivalent relation to the disease. For those with cancer diagnoses and their caretakers in Bagamoyo, the stakes of this disjuncture and its effects are much more intense. The story of Bibi Faraja, a beloved grandmother and cancer patient, helped us understand this dynamic. Welcomed into Bibi Faraja's home by her daughter, we sat on the carpet in her living room and broke into the food and milk tea we brought. Bibi Faraja's daughter began by telling us about the lengthy process the family had gone through to get a diagnosis for Faraja's advanced-stage cervical cancer. She recounted the family's struggles to pay for treatment because they did not have state mandated insurance and could not afford the additional costs associated with travel to the specialized cancer hospital in Dar es Salaam due to the lack of employment of the men in the family. Throughout this experience, she explained how differing understandings of *kansa* and *saratani* became an additional hindrance to this long process of oncological screening and care. Having only heard about the dangers of *kansa*, but not the complexities of *kansa* and *saratani* before her diagnosis, Faraja said that she came to understand what *kansa* was and that it was the same as *saratani* only through multiple clinical interactions. Claiming that she and her family never saw and could not find any information that suggested *kansa* and *saratani* were the same. The only way for them to learn about the equivalence of the two names was in their visits to the hospital. According to Bibi Faraja and her daughter, conversations on the streets where *kansa* and *saratani* were theorized in all kinds of different ways only caused them confusion. This terminological confusion made it harder to sort out what disease Faraja actually had. This communicative confusion compounded with common hindrances in oncological care across Tanzania—the family's lack of insurance and insufficient funds to reach Dar es Salaam for treatments, as well as the long queues to see overworked doctors in Bagamoyo. This ultimately delayed Faraja's chemotherapy treatments and, in her daughter's words, it was a miracle Bibi Faraja was still alive.

Doctors in Bagamoyo we spoke to further elucidated what was a common occurrence: the disjuncture of understanding that *kansa* and *saratani* both referred to the same disease among potentially afflicted community members. The clinical encounter, as they explained to us, becomes a space where physicians seek to also "treat" the diseases of misconception and misunderstanding so that patients can receive proper oncological care. Widely envisioning themselves as intellectual superiors entrusted with medical knowledge that they must pass on to uneducated, superstitious patients, doctors in Bagamoyo take on the position of health knower, educator, and disseminator to explain the *kansa-saratani*-cancer relationship to patients who come to the hospitals understanding the terms in ways similar to the *wazee* at the newspaper stand. However, this is a constant uphill battle. As Bibi Faraja explained, not only does this unified conceptualization take time to build, it is constantly muddled by the wider linguistic ecosystem that creates disparate understandings of these names. Most importantly, this understanding puts patients on a long, painful path of chemotherapy that they usually cannot afford and often begins when the disease is already far advanced. While joining *kansa-saratani*-cancer in the minds of patients, doctors simultaneously place patients on an uncertain and expensive journey through the Tanzanian oncological healthcare system that most often ends in death. Thereby, for one Bagamoyo physician clarifying this connection between the three terms seemed like illuminating "a pathway to death" for patients. Rather than seeing his efforts to unite the three terms as significantly improving the lives of his patients, he saw this practice as merely helping them understand a disease that would end in their demise and a long, painful path through a medical system that would most likely not save them.

The Politics of Biocommunicability in a Postcolonial Global System

As Briggs and Hallin chart, modern biocommunicability creates subjects. Close attention to language can help to trace what kind of subjects are being produced in and through public health and medicine, and what ideologies inform their creation. People and institutions inevitably advance different political and ideological projects through biocommunicability: whether it be continued use of *saratani* by doctors despite popular usage of *kansa*, word spreading around town about a new *kansa* diagnosis, or American and British NGOs "sensitizing" people in Bagamoyo to the disease "cancer." The experiences of interacting with the signs *kansa* and *saratani* described in this chapter demonstrate how political projects are intertwined with biocommunicability, and how these projects exist alongside each other in the forms of which words are circulated, seen, and used and which are not. Using medical language—and the implicit choice between unequally influential terms—is never neutral nor does it happen on equal terrain. As demonstrated by the division of *saratani* and *kansa* and the latter's disproportionate ability to circulate over the former, certain medical terms are socially endowed to be seen, taken up, and used more than others. This lopsided selection of one term over others feeds back into larger projects of governance whether the user is conscious of this or not. When *saratani* is not seen or used, the once viable project of Tanzanian decolonial nationalism in the form of biocommunicability is erased. When *kansa* or "cancer" is taken up and used, the Anglicization of Tanzania—which is a key concern in the nation (Kishe 2016)—is advanced. While most of our interlocutors across Bagamoyo also agree that Anglicization is negative, they ardently support Tanzanian cultural independence, and believe in preserving the purity of Swahili, the structuring of how the two terms circulate has led them to dominantly register the Anglicized word over what was supposed to be their *fasaha* term.

What the situation in Coastal Tanzania shows is how biocommunciability unfolds through the everyday ways that people talk about, medicine, health, and disease, and how the inequality of which words, ideas, and discourses are used in this talk is shaped by long historical trajectories. While the coining of the term *saratani* deliberately attempted to link medical language and the provisioning of medical care to the project of decolonial nationalism by the state of Tanzania—and, as we saw, help newly independent Tanzanian citizens to think of themselves as decolonial actors—the global political economy where European languages are the default in scientific, medical, and all other forms of transnational communication was reified and strengthened through neoliberal reform. Paradoxically, *saratani* continues to adorn posters, serve as the standard term for medical record keeping, and be widely used every day by doctors in a society where decolonial culture, linguistic purity, and Tanzanian nationalism through Swahili are still widely supported. Yet, backed by a powerful western global health industry and social system dedicated to fighting the disease, as well as English-language media, *kansa* has become the dominant name for the disease among the people.

Briggs and Hallin make clear how models of biocommunicability are "multiple, competing, and contradictory," which means that people "confront multiple sources of information and competing forms of reception" (2007:61). What we add to this is the idea that no matter how multiple or diverse these competing forms of information are, the struggle to understand and live with cancer in Bagamoyo nonetheless occurs on an unequal playing field. In the realm of medical terminology, as well as many other facets of 21st-century globalized society and life, power still resides with the languages of formerly colonizing states and the biocommunicable models they create and promote. The case of *saratani*/*kansa* demonstrates how certain words or discourses that are backed by powerful institutions and systems on other continents can come to dominate nationalist and local programs.

These linguistic dynamics, it must be remembered, unfold in conjunction with a material colonial political economy that renders oncological healthcare in Tanzania as underdeveloped. As the story of Bibi Faraja and the physician's morbid perspective on this linguistic issue tell, these competing ideological, subject-making projects merely shape the experiences of healthcare within a severely limited health system. This is not to suggest that either the issues of oncological healthcare or its communication in Tanzania would be solved if a single term for cancer was used. It is to establish the fact that a formerly colonized nation attempted to create an independent biocommunicable program on their own terms that was subsequently thwarted by neoliberalization that benefits formerly colonizing nations and now creates a linguistic environment that renders oncological care more confusing and inaccessible.

Conclusion

What medical words get used? Which biocommunicable models hold power? What political projects are advanced, and who benefits and loses through the political economy of medical terminology? By tracing how *saratani* and *kansa* circulate in Tanzania, this chapter turns attention toward the unequal political economy of biocommunicability. Defining the terms of disease, illness, and treatment is a political act, and in this modern era, disproportionate power over communicating health and medicine is latently held by the former colonizing world. While public health communication advocates commonly point to Indigenous or non-western words as solutions to this problem—assuming that these languages are more relevant to people—the case of cancer in Bagamoyo shows how this notion can be counterproductive. It is the colonially derived word, *kansa*, that dominantly indexes the biological disease of cancer, not the *fasaha* (pure) Swahili word *saratani*. Thus, insistence on a less familiar name for cancer may compound confusion about the disease. Ultimately, what the disjuncture between *saratani* and *kansa* demands is a broader attention to the political economy of medical language and who gets to create it. In other words, a more just health communication in Tanzania and beyond, one built upon agency and sovereignty, cannot be achieved without dismantling the latent ability of biocommunicable regimes from elsewhere to have power over other subject-creating projects.

Questions for Reflection and Discussion

Reflection Questions

1. Can you think of any other examples where terminology contributes to confusion about medical issues?

2. Are there any national or local language policies at work in your own society? If you know of such policies, what political goals do they reflect? If you are not aware of such policies, why do you think that might be?

Looking In: Small Group Discussion Questions

1. What are the histories of these two words for cancer: *saratani* and *kansa*? How did each word enter into use in Tanzanian society?
2. What is biocommunicability? Provide a definition in your own words and identify some examples from the chapter or other contexts.
3. What is a "subject," as this term is used here? How does biocommunicability create subjects? Explain using the examples from the chapter.
4. What is the neoliberal model of biocommunicability? In the Tanzanian case, how is this model tied to political and economic shifts and changes to health care provision?

Looking Out: Large Group Discussion Questions

1. What are the consequences of the use of two terms (*saratani* and *kansa*) and their complex relationship for oncological care in Tanzania? How are histories of colonization and current postcolonial realities reflected in and perhaps reproduced by these two terms?
2. How is biocommunicability tied to political economic inequality? How is it tied to the nation-state?
3. Given the situation of *kansa* and *saratani* presented, what would it mean to decolonize medical language? If it is not simply enough to prioritize "local" language in biomedical spaces, then what is a solution?
4. As Krugman and Rafiq ask, can there be biocommunicability without harmful forms of subject making? Is it possible to disseminate medical and health information across large populations without it favoring the biases, interests, and control of the powerful?

References

Alexander, G. A. 1985. A Survey of Traditional Medical Practices Used for the Treatment of Malignant Tumors in an East African Population. *Social Science & Medicine* 20: pp. 53–59. https://doi.org/10.1016/0277-9536(85)90311-9.

Aminzade, Ronald. 2013. Neoliberalism and the Transition from State Socialism to Capitalism. In *Race, Nation, and Citizenship in Postcolonial Africa: The Case of Tanzania*, pp. 245–275. Cambridge Studies in Contentious Politics. Cambridge: Cambridge University Press. https://doi.org/10.1017/CBO9781107360259.012.

Blommaert, Jan. 2014. *State Ideology and Language in Tanzania.* Second and revised edition. Edinburgh: Edinburgh University Press. https://doi.org/10.1515/9780748675814.

Briggs, Charles L., and Daniel C. Hallin. 2007. Biocommunicability: The Neoliberal Subject and Its Contradictions in News Coverage of Health Issues. *Social Text* 25: pp. 43–66. https://doi.org/10.1215/01642472-2007-011.

Briggs, Charles L., and Mark Nichter. 2009. Biocommunicability and the Biopolitics of Pandemic Threats. *Medical Anthropology* 28: pp. 189–198. https://doi.org/10.1080/01459740903070410.

Hiza, P. R. 1976. Malignant Disease in Tanzania. *East African Medical Journal* 53: pp. 82–95.

Igoe, Jim. 2003. Scaling up Civil Society: Donor Money, NGOs and the Pastoralist Land Rights Movement in Tanzania. *Development and Change* 34: pp. 863–885. https://doi.org/10.1111/j.1467-7660.2003.00332.x.

Jain, S. Lochlann. 2013. *Malignant: How Cancer Becomes Us.* Berkeley, CA: University of California Press.

Kamat, Vinay. 2008. This Is Not Our Culture! Discourse of Nostalgia and Narratives of Health Concerns in Post-Socialist Tanzania. *Africa* 78(3): pp. 359–383. https://doi.org/10.3366/E0001972008000223.

Kishe, Anne J. 1994. The Englishization of Tanzanian Kiswahili. *World Englishes* 13(2): pp. 185–201. https://doi.org/10.1111/j.1467-971X.1994.tb00306.x.

Kishe, Anna J. M. 2016. English Influence on Kiswahili: The View of Language Purists. *Journal of Linguistics and Language in Education* 5(1): pp. 1–21.

Livingston, Julie. 2012. *Improvising Medicine: An African Oncology Ward in an Emerging Cancer Epidemic.* Durham, NC: Duke University Press.

Manni, J. J. and P. L. Huygen. 1990. Head and Neck Cancer in Tanzania in Comparison with the Netherlands. *East African Medical Journal* 67: pp. 162–171.

Mdee, James S. 1983. The Policy of Adapting Loan Words in Kiswahili as Conceived by BAKITA: A Critique. *Multilingua* 2(2): pp. 109–112.

Mugane, John M. 2015. *The Story of Swahili.* Athens, OH: Ohio University Press.

Whiteley, Wilfred H. 1969. *Swahili: The Rise of a National Language.* London: Routledge.

Yambi, Josephine. 2000. Planned and Spontaneous Vocabulary Expansion in Tanzanian Kiswahili. *Studies in Linguistic Sciences* 30(2): pp. 209–222.

8

The Circulation of Psychoanalytic Discourses Beyond the Clinic in Buenos Aires

Xochitl Marsilli-Vargas

Introduction

In Buenos Aires, practicing psychoanalysts and psychologists are often invited to discuss different aspects of Argentine society on TV talk shows and in newspaper editorials. Their expertise is considered relevant to understanding Twitter exchanges between politicians, the behavior of celebrities, the Argentine national character, and many other matters. In this way, discourses of mental health and wellbeing pervade everyday life (see Brotherton 2020; Dagfal 2009; Plotkin 2001; Visacovsky 2009). Indeed, it sometimes seems as if, for the inhabitants of Buenos Aires, any social or political problem is amenable to an analysis in terms of unconscious motives and Freudian notions of the id, the ego, and the superego. The language of psychology and psychoanalysis has even spread into commercial advertising and is used in television commercials to market a wide range of goods and services (van Roekel 2018).

Psychoanalysis is a methodology for treating mental disorders that emerged in the late nineteenth century in the clinical practice and writings of Austrian psychiatrist Sigmund Freud. It is a form of therapy that emphasizes unconscious mental processes, especially the repression of painful memories and everyday experiences. This repression is seen as the cause of different mental health ailments that manifest in neurosis, disassociation, panic attacks, and so on. Psychoanalysis is undergirded by a belief about language: that people's words convey meanings other than the overtly obvious ones. It is the task of the analyst to bring to light the real, yet hidden, meanings that lurk below the surface of the patient's talk. To do this, Freud introduced a technique of listening that he referred to as "floating attention" in which, instead of focusing on the semantic significance of the words, the analyst attempts to *resonate* with the talk of the patient. Through this, the analyst can hear what the unconscious is saying, identifying repressed memories and drives behind the patient's talk and action. This idea, that words invoke in the expert listener different meanings

Xochitl Marsilli-Vargas, *The Circulation of Psychoanalytic Discourses Beyond the Clinic in Buenos Aires*. In: *Language and Health in Action*. Edited by. Lynnette Arnold et al., Oxford University Press. © Xochitl Marsilli-Vargas (2026).
DOI: 10.1093/9780198933953.003.0008

and affective states, is the basis of psychoanalysis, and as my research shows, it has permeated many social contexts outside of clinical settings in Buenos Aires.

As an example illustrating the extent to which psychoanalysis appears in everyday discourse, consider the primary elections in Argentina, held in 2023. The independent ultra-right-wing candidate Javier Milei got the highest number of votes (30%), worrying many who wanted to preserve progressive social programs that Milei aimed to eliminate. A few days after the election, psychoanalytic interpretations began to proliferate in media outlets as experts attempted to explain how such a sinister character had managed to become so popular. Indeed, a few months before in *Página 12*, a left-leaning newspaper, the psychologist Claudia Messing had analyzed this situation through what she calls the *unconscious symmetrization of family bonds*, that is, the infantile stage in which the child challenges the parents when given instructions (e.g., "Get down from there, because you are going to fall!" "Let me be! I can do it!") in order to contest the asymmetry of power between child and parent (Messing 2023). Messing suggested that Milei, being openly libertarian, awakens among some Argentineans a desire for absolute freedom (libertinism), in which there are no limits on action and no expectation that one should think about the consequences of action for others. In particular, Messing suggests that Milei's message resonates for those young men who have never challenged parental authority and so have not achieved the symmetrization of family bonds. Focusing on the resonance that Milei's last name can produce if interpreted as "mi-ley" (my law), Messing suggests that the words Milei uses in his daily rants sound different to his followers, and that these words resonate with their experiences in a particularly effective way.

Whether Messing's analysis is correct or not, the example shows just how pervasive and persuasive the discourse of psychoanalysis has become for many people in Buenos Aires. This type of interpretation is very common in Argentina and many examples of such analysis can be seen, not only in newspapers and news programs, but also in various media. This results in what many scholars call *la cultura psi* (psy culture), a culture in which talk about internal, subjective states figures prominently in contexts not usually considered part of the medical field, including politics in this case.

The big question that many scholars and others have long asked is: why? Why are psychoanalytic discourses so prevalent in Argentina? The World Health Organization estimated that in 2016, Argentina had the highest percentage of psychologists in the world: 222.6 per 100,000 inhabitants. These numbers are very high, especially when compared to other countries. For instance, the country that follows Argentina is Costa Rica with 142 (per 100,000 inhabitants). The United States comes in fourteenth place with 31.1 psychologists per 100,000 inhabitants (see Figure 8.1). In Buenos Aires, statisticians, making a conservative estimate, came out with a much higher number: 786 psychologists per 100,000 inhabitants (Alonso and Klinar 2016), suggesting that Buenos Aires is the city with the most psychologists per capita in the world.

It is difficult, perhaps impossible, to know why there are so many psychologists and psychoanalysts in Argentina. In this chapter, however, rather than answering

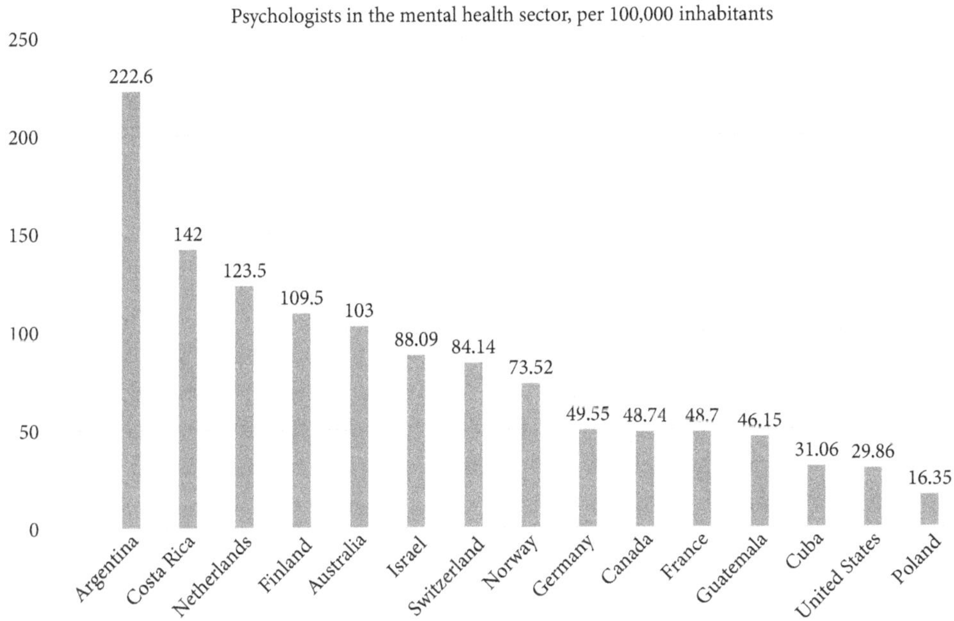

Fig. 8.1 Psychologists in the mental health sector, per 100,000 inhabitants.
Graphic display created by author of data from WHO 2015–2017.

the *why*, I am interested in exploring the *how*. Specifically, I seek to understand how psychoanalytic discourses circulate outside of the clinical setting. As the Milei example illustrates, psychoanalytic modes of interpretation are widely diffused far beyond the clinic. The question, then, is how this happens. How do the interpretive techniques, expert forms of knowledge, and descriptive vocabularies of psychoanalysis travel beyond the clinic? How do such ways of making sense become normalized such that their appearance in everyday life is widely accepted by people who are not themselves psychoanalysts? By focusing on the reproduction of discourses of mental health and wellbeing that are inserted into contexts far removed from their origin, we can better understand how these discourses are able to infiltrate everyday practices.

Consuming Psychoanalytic Discourse

I am a linguistic anthropologist and was trained in ethnographic methods in Mexico and the United States. As an undergraduate student, I studied with Roger Bartra at the National School of Anthropology (ENAH) in Mexico City and, under his influence, became interested in the anthropology of mental health, especially what Bartra referred to as melancholia (Bartra 1992). Later, as a PhD student at the University of California, Berkeley, I knew I wanted to conduct my own research in this area and found, in Argentine psychoanalysis, a unique form of therapeutic discourse. My book, *Genres of Listening: An Ethnography of Psychoanalysis in Buenos Aires* is based on the six years of ethnographic research I conducted as a graduate student. This research involved interviewing psychoanalysts and their patients, attending meetings of the Multi-family Psychoanalytic Therapeutic Community at the Association of Psychoanalysts of Argentina (APA), and participating in everyday life and conversations during mealtimes, gatherings of friends, and special occasions such as birthdays, weddings, celebratory parties, and so on.

One of the most important ways that psychoanalytic discourse circulates is through commercial advertisements on television and in other media. In these ads, central ideas from the psychoanalytic tradition are deployed in comic ways in an effort to induce consumer desire for a product and so to increase sales. Such commercial uses of psychoanalytic discourse act in two significant ways. On the one hand, they assume that the intended audience has some familiarity with the terms and key ideas of psychoanalysis. At the same time, such ads also extend the social domain of psychoanalysis as more and more people are exposed to it.

In the case of psychoanalysis in Buenos Aires, both consumers and producers of psychoanalytic discourses are responsible for its circulation and dissemination. The boundaries between "authoritative" discourse of experts (psychologists) and the "lay" representation of these discourses in ads are not as fixed as in other fields (Briggs 2005, Briggs and Hallin 2007). To see how this plays out, let's look at this Andes (2009) beer commercial produced in Argentina (see Figures 8.2 and 8.3).

Psychoanalyst/psychologist

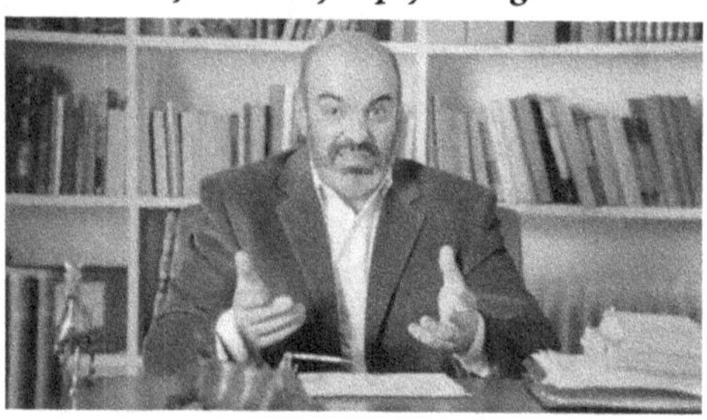

Fig. 8.2 Screenshots of psychoanalyst/psychologist from Andes commercial.

Friend

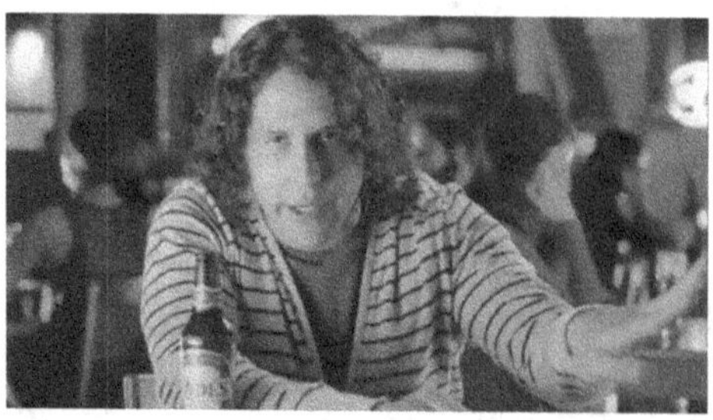

Fig. 8.3 Screenshot of friend from Andes commercial inside a bar.

Andes is known for creating many advertisements in which the psychoanalytic encounter is invoked in a humorous and often sexist way. This ad begins with the voice of a man posing the following question: "My girlfriend doesn't turn me on anymore ... What should I do?" Immediately afterward we see a psychoanalyst, represented as a bearded man sitting at a desk in front of a full bookshelf, responding to the man's question. The commercial then cuts to a different setting: a bar where a young man with long hair, an open white and black hoodie, and blue t-shirt, with an Andes beer in his hand, responds to the same question. The ad cuts back and forth between both settings three times as shown in Example 8.1.

Example 8.1 Dialogue from Andes commercial

Exchange 1: Psychologist	*Exchange 2: Friend*
El estrés en el trabajo, la rutina, atentan contra las relaciones de pareja. Lo importante es, alimentar la relación	Déjala.
(Stress at work and the daily routine threaten a couple's relationship. The important thing is to nurture the relationship,)	(Leave her.)
tener momentos íntimos, buscar cosas nuevas, jugar más,	Fuera bagarto.
(to have intimate moments, to look for new things, to play more,)	(Bye, reptile.)
reencontrarse el uno con el otro.	Corta: no calienta, se cambia.
(to find each other again.)	(It's simple: if she doesn't turn you on, replace her.)

The ad closes with the following slogan: "A friend is a psychologist without a diploma. It's just how we are."

Here we see that the practice of psychoanalysis—the highly ritualized and private contract between a psychoanalyst and an analysand—is represented in a creative way in the Argentine media. Psychoanalysis as a clinical practice entails a relationship between an analyst and an analysand. Here I do not use the term patient because it suggests passivity, nor the term client, which suggests a merely commercial transaction. **Analysand** is the preferred term in psychoanalysis because it indicates that the person undergoing psychoanalysis is participating actively in the analytic practice. As Gabriel Rolón, one of the most famous psychoanalysts in Argentina stated in a recent interview with journalist María Laura Santillán (2022):

> Un médico puede jubilarse y no deja de ser médico. Pero un analista si deja de atender deja de ser analista porque uno es *analista de*. Si no hay un alguien, no sos analista. El analista se constituye y se actualiza a cada instante en el acto de analizar.

> A doctor can retire and still be a doctor. But if an analyst stops seeing people, he stops being an analyst, because one is an *analyst of.* If there is no analysand, there is no analyst. The analyst is constituted in the act of analyzing.

So, according to Rolón, psychoanalysis is a practice that needs to be performed in order for the analyst to exist.

The characters in the Andes commercial are obvious stereotypes. In one scene, we have a well-dressed man speaking in a formal register using one long sentence with complex syntax. In the other, we find a young man speaking in extremely short sentences, using slang (e.g., *fuera bagarto* (bye reptile)) and responding to the intimate question posed at the beginning of the commercial in an overtly sexist way. The common understanding that those who have received formal training—psychologists—are more informed and qualified to help with personal issues, as opposed to a friend who can only provide a personal opinion, is reversed in the Andes ad. This is seen in the claim that a friend *is* a psychologist, albeit one without a title. The ad then challenges familiar assumptions about who is authorized to speak. To say that the friend is a psychologist without a diploma is to cast doubt on the very foundations of expertise that psychoanalysis is built upon.

In this example, the psychoanalytic relation between analyst and analysand is both stereotyped (in the figure of the doctor) and ironicized (in the figure of the friend who is also a "psychologist"). Through these two figures, a form of clinical talk is transformed from a use value (the cure) to a commodity (a service) which has an exchange value. Anthropologist Asif Agha calls the process by which discourse is commodified in this way **mediatization**. As he puts it: "to speak of *mediatization* is to speak of institutional practices that reflexively link processes of communication to processes of commoditization" (Agha 2011:163). In the context of the Andes commercial, we can see how discourses about wellbeing and establishing healthy relationships get mediatized, serving as the means by which a commodity like beer is branded and advertised. In other words, in this example, the use value of therapy (wellbeing) is transformed into an aspect of the exchange value that the beer company mobilizes to sell their commodity. Mediatization need not always involve the media, although this is one of the most common ways that communication gets linked to commoditization today. In this example, however, both are relevant as the beer company is using the medium of a TV commercial.

Let us consider another commercial for CAR ONE (2015) mechanical services, in which an economic transaction is thematized and satirized. Here, the analyst is likened to a dishonest mechanic and psychoanalytic techniques are compared to the replacement of automotive parts. Interestingly, in this case, it is the specialized, esoteric quality of the psychoanalytic vocabulary that is foregrounded, which suggests that this jargon is akin to the unfamiliar terms used by mechanics to explain the exorbitant cost of repairs. Once again, the commercial both assumes and extends familiarity with this way of speaking.

The commercial begins with a woman sitting in a chair in a waiting room. A door opens and the analyst, depicted as a formally dressed bearded man in his 50s, comes through the door, followed by a casually dressed young man in his early 20s. The woman stands up and asks, “So, how was the test? What have we got? An engineer like his father?” The psychoanalyst answers, patting the young man’s back: “Good, good. Ramiro will tell you all about it.” Ramiro tells the woman “Mom, I’ll wait for you outside,” and leaves the room. The woman and the psychologist then have the following exchange:

Example 8.2 Car One commercial

(01)	Woman:	Bueno, ¿qué te debo?	So how much do I owe you?
(02)	Psychologist:	Bueno, del test en si son 600, pero ya que estaba le hice otras cosas. ¿Si? Había un tema ahí con el super yo, un ruidito, vos no notaste nada?	Let’s see, the test itself is 600 [pesos], but while I was doing it, I did some other things. Right? There was a problem with the superego. A little noise, you didn’t notice anything?
(03)	Woman:	No.	No.
(04)	Psychologist:	Le arreglé eso, son 400 más. Y después encontré unos miedos que no eran originales. Se los saqué, les pusc los originales, el fracaso, la muerte. Así barato son 200 más.	I fixed that, there’s 400 more. And then I found some fears that were not original. I took them out and put in the original ones: failure, death. A reasonable rate is 200 more.
(05)	Woman:	Pero yo te lo traje solo por el test.	But I only brought him in to have the test.
(06)	Psychologist:	Si, pero ¿sabes qué? Si yo te lo doy así, en un mes me lo traes de nuevo. No, con esto hasta los treinta, te olvidás. Además vos calculá, ¿no? Si se te rompe el super yo, se te termina rompiendo el ello, el yo, le tenés que cambiar los objetivos, la personalidad, te termina haciendo catarsis por ahí. Vos haceme caso a mí, llévatelo así y mírale de vez en cuando la figura paterna que anda medio suelta.	Yes, I know, but if I gave him back to you like this, you’d bring him back in a month. Now with what I have done, you can forget about it until he is thirty. Think about it this way, when the superego breaks down, the id breaks down too, so you have to change the self, the goals, the personality, and it ends up being a catharsis over there. Listen to me, take him like this and take a look at his father figure, which is a little loose, from time to time.
(07)	Woman:	Puede ser.	It could be.

(08) Psychologist:	Son 1200.	It's 1200.
(09) Woman:		(opens her checkbook)
(10) Psychologist:	¿Factura vas a necesitar?	Do you need a receipt?
(11) Woman:	Eh, no.	Uh, no.
(12) Psychologist:	Dame 1100.	Give me 1100.

The commercial closes with a black screen with the text: "Fortunately, psychologists are not like mechanics. Fortunately, our mechanics are not like other mechanics. *CAR ONE* Mechanic Services."

In the CAR ONE example, we see the use of many psychoanalytic terms: superego, id, self, catharsis, personality, father figure. When specific knowledge is inserted into mass media, the duration, scale, and proximity of the event changes (Agha 2011). This helps us identify the connections (semiotic chains) that certain words evoke in the listener, indicating how concepts travel and how information generated long ago—Freud's first book on aphasia was published in 1891—is recontextualized in a new context: a television commercial for mechanical services. The discourse of psychoanalysis circulates in part because the consumers created through these forms of commercial exchange continue to disseminate and recycle it. In other words, when people watch such ads, they find them funny or at least attention getting, and may share them with friends or otherwise take them up. As a result, when advertisers deploy psychoanalytic discourses, they use a language that is tied to ideas and concepts that go back to Freud, but which are nevertheless recognized by a large part of the population in Buenos Aires.

In the CAR ONE ad, the psychoanalyst acts like a sleazy mechanic, providing a variety of unnecessary and unwanted services. Moreover, when discussing the young man with his mother, the analyst refers to him as if he were discussing a car whose parts are worn out. Concepts such as *ego* and *id* are objectified, characterized as things in the world that can be observed, adjusted, put in and taken out, and so on. This is a form of **recontextualization**, in which words are taken from their original context and used in another setting. Recontextualization allows expert psychoanalytic terminology to infiltrate social spheres beyond the clinical setting. What the analysis of these commercials shows, then, is that psychoanalytic discourse is incorporated into processes of commodification and market exchange, and is thereby both transformed into a popularized image of itself and made to circulate both through various media channels (such as television, and YouTube) and along with the commodities with which it becomes associated such as beer and car mechanic services.

Genres of Listening

In my research, I have come to understand the circulation and mediatization of psychoanalytic discourses in Buenos Aires as the result of a social way of listening based on psychoanalysis, what I call a **genre of listening**. I define a genre of listening as a relatively stable and partially conventionalized frame of reference by which listeners contextualize interaction and in relation to which they organize their behavior. The psychoanalytic tradition has developed distinct techniques of listening specially adapted to this context. In the clinical setting, an attentive listener (the analyst) will suspend attention to the referential meaning of the patient's words and instead try to resonate with the patient's talk in order to connect with unconscious discourses. This genred form of listening has a structure in which the meanings of words are **polysemic**, acquiring different meanings depending on the context in which those words are uttered. The therapeutic foundation of psychoanalysis therefore involves a particular way of listening that involves hearing the submerged meanings in what people say, the unconscious messages that a speaker conveys without intending to do so. Whether speakers do in fact convey such unconscious messages is irrelevant to my argument (or, put another way, nothing hangs on the question of whether psychoanalysis is science or pure fiction). The psychoanalytic genre of listening assumes the existence of such messages and meanings, and thus establishes them as objective social facts.

Genres of listening are learned, and in Buenos Aires, people have learned to use the psychoanalytical genre of listening in spaces far beyond the clinic. *Porteños*, as the inhabitants of the city are called, have developed a kind of "psychoanalytic ear" which hears not the fixed meaning of words, but rather the resonances they generate and the interpretations they evoke. To understand how this process works, think about music. Have you ever heard a commercial song on the radio that you don't necessarily like, but its constant repetition somehow penetrates your sensory sphere and you find yourself unexpectedly humming it to yourself? Something similar happens with discourses that circulate widely in different contexts. The resonances that accumulate from listening to a particular song or discourse over and over again imprint themselves on our minds and we begin to understand the world through that particular lens. The same thing happens with political discourse, where the listener of political propaganda begins to repeat an idea or policy that they have heard many times. Repetition creates contagion, through the resonance of words and sounds, which in some cases have a clear reference; but sometimes they do not. So it is "the music in the words" (Marsilli-Vargas 2022), the resonances, that cause the humming: one finds oneself repeating sounds, melodies, and discourses without being fully conscious of it. The more one hears a particular genre of music, the easier it is for a song to get stuck in one's head.

In Buenos Aires, people are always asking about the "real motives" that certain words convey to the listener. That is, in Buenos Aires there is a culture of listeners who have learned to listen to the resonance and polysemic meaning of words outside of the clinical setting.

During my ethnographic fieldwork, I witnessed many interactions in which Porteños used this psychoanalytic genre of listening in casual encounters: among gatherings of friends, at bars, while waiting for the bus, etc. Some I recorded; some I wrote down afterward from memory. This next example was one that occurred during a dinner at a friend's house in Buenos Aires. Here Emilia, a woman in her early 30s, is complaining to Manuel and Carmen, both in their 40s, about Ana, a friend who got back together with her ex-boyfriend. Emilia vehemently opposed this decision.

Example 8.3 Conversation among friends

(01) Emilia:	¡Ya estoy cansada de hablar sobre Ana! Además no le hace caso a nadie. ¿Podemos cambiar de tema?	I am tired of talking about Ana! Besides, she doesn't follow any advice. Can we change the subject?
(02) Manuel:	Es una amiga ¿no? Uno tiene que bancarlos aún cuando sean unos pelotudos.	She is a friend, right? One should support [friends] even if they are morons.
(03) Carmen:	Me sorprende escuchar que digas eso Emilia. Me gustaría entender ¿qué es lo que estás tratando de decir? A lo mejor tocó alguna fibra en la que te reconoces. ¿Porqué te molesta tanto?	I'm surprised to hear you say that Emilia. I would like to understand what it is that you are trying to say? What do you mean by that assertion? Perhaps it touched a fiber in which you recognize yourself. Why does it bother you so much?
(04) Emilia:	Y qué se yo, todos hemos pasado por lo mismo. Pero tenés razón, no se qué me pasa.	What do I know? We all have done stupid things. But you are right, I don't know what's happening.
(05) Manuel:	Pon atención a lo que dices.	Pay attention to what you say.

In this example, Carmen implies that Emilia's words "uncover" meanings other than the one she explicitly articulated of disagreement with Ana's choice. These words suggest that Emilia is unaware of the real motives of her actions and feelings, so Carmen's intervention is justified. As this example shows, Porteños often use this genre of listening to enact certain kinds of social relations with their interlocutors. Here we see that it is not only speaking but also listening that can performatively act in the world. This genre of listening has a source in psychoanalysis that the listener may or may not be aware of. The commodification of psychoanalytic discourses in the media supports the acquisition of this genre of listening, as Porteños are exposed to these discourses across a wide range of contexts, from TV ads to Twitter feeds, from political commentary to newspaper cartoons. Although there is no way to concretely measure the specific impact of this mediatization of psychoanalytic discourse on the broader presence and circulation of the genre of psychoanalytic listening throughout Buenos Aires and Argentina, its prevalence in social spheres far outside the clinic suggests that this mediatization and the development of the genre of listening in different social contexts are intertwined.

The prevalence of psychoanalytic listening as a genre of listening in Argentina has important implications for how key areas of social organization are enacted and maintained. This includes the way people formulate knowledge and assign authority, how they portray themselves as political actors, and how they engage in conversations across class, gender, and racial differences. Psychoanalytic listening draws extensively on modern ideas of the self as the expression of an abstract, autonomous, and unique individuality, characterized by the presence of psychological depth that is knowable only through various kinds of expert knowledge (including, of course, psychology). Recognizing the way these ideologies of the self are deployed through this genre of listening reveals that listening can be vital to the reproduction and dissemination of such social ideas.

Listening is key to the reproduction and circulation of any discourse. How people listen is determined by their social position (e.g., brother, worker, philosopher), the context (e.g., inside a church, listening to music at home, comforting a despondent friend), and the ideas they attach to sounds, which in turn depend on their histories. This dynamic creates different genres of listening that guide behavior in particular ways (e.g., auscultation, a mechanic listening to a broken car, a lawyer, a music tuner, etc.). Similarly, nurses are trained to listen to their patients in an especially caring way, and a doctor's "bedside manner" involves a special kind of attentive listening. Because listening is a ubiquitous social activity, such genres shape the way members of a group relate to one another. By focusing on how people listen to each other, we can gain a deeper understanding of social interaction that goes beyond the analysis of talk alone.

Conclusion

In Argentina, television advertisements and other forms of mass media provide a powerful vehicle for the dissemination and circulation of some key elements of psychoanalytic discourse, carrying these ideas and practices beyond the clinical setting and into the domain of everyday life. Studying the process of mediatization allows us to see how health discourses get taken up and adapted, how they travel beyond the contexts in which they originate and are transformed as a result. In Argentina, psychoanalytic discourses are routinely invoked in political discussions and are understood to provide genuine and profound insight into otherwise mysterious events and processes. The popularity, indeed normalization, of psychoanalytic discourse in Buenos Aires is no doubt linked to the very high numbers of practicing psychologists among the Argentine population. But the intensive circulation of these discourses cannot be explained simply and solely by reference to the development of psychoanalysis as a profession. As we saw in the example of the beer and car insurance ads, the roles of "psychologist" or "psychoanalyst" on the one hand,

and of "lay person" on the other, are not entirely discrete ("a friend is a psychologist without a title"). Rather, expert producers of psychoanalytic discourses (psychologists) regularly become consumers of these discourses, as when reading a newspaper article about Milei. Both producers and consumers also disseminate psychoanalytic discourse, circulating ideas (about the role of the unconscious, for instance) and practices (ways of asking questions, of listening, etc.). Analyzing this movement in terms of mediatization reveals how these ideas and practices become commodities that can be bought and sold and from which profit is derived. I have suggested that these processes of circulation and commodification are made possible by a specific genre of listening. In everyday conversation in Buenos Aires, such as in Example 8.3, this genre of psychoanalytic listening is ubiquitous and, for Porteños, mostly unremarkable. It is these mundane social interactions that shore up the mediatization of psychoanalysis beyond the clinic.

Question for Reflection and Discussion

Reflection Questions

1. What media have you seen about therapy, psychoanalysis, or mental healthcare in general? How might these media examples have influenced your understanding of mental healthcare?
2. Think about the last time you discussed a problem with a friend. Did you stick to a surface level interpretation or did you look for hidden meanings?

Looking In: Small Group Discussion Questions

1. What is mediatization? Provide a definition in your own words and identify some examples from the chapter or other contexts.
2. What are genres of listening? Provide a definition in your own words and identify some examples from the chapter or other contexts.
3. Choose one of the media examples discussed in the chapter. How does this example demonstrate the role of mediatization in producing Argentinian psy-culture?
4. Why is it important to consider listening as part of studies of language and communication? How is listening a form of communication?

Looking Out: Large Group Discussion Questions

1. What factors have contributed to the circulation of psychoanalytic discourse beyond the clinic in Argentina?

2. How do discourses related to health and wellbeing become commodities? What are the effects of this commodification?
3. What kinds of tools are needed to do an ethnography of listening/reception? How must you consider your own identity and background to do this kind of work?

References

Agha, Asif. 2011. Meet Mediatization. *Language and Communication* 31: pp. 163–170.

Alonso, Modesto M., and Doménica Klinar. 2016. Los psicólogos en Argentina. Relevamiento cuantitativo 2015. VIII Congreso Internacional de Investigación y Práctica Profesional en Psicología XXIII Jornadas de Investigación XII Encuentro de Investigadores en Psicología del MERCOSUR. Facultad de Psicología, Universidad de Buenos Aires, Buenos Aires. https://www.aacademica.org/000-044/371.

Andes. 2009. Mi novia ya no me excita … ¿Qué hago? [My Girlfriend Doesn't Turn Me on Anymore … What Should I Do?]. Accessed July 28, 2024. https://www.youtube.com/watch?v=OQ95Zu4cERE.

Bartra, Roger. 1992. *The Cage of Melancholy: Identity and Metamorphosis in the Mexican Character*. New Brunswick, NJ: Rutgers University Press. (Originally published as *La jaula de la melancolía. Identidad y metamorfosis del Mexicano*. Grijalbo, 1987).

Briggs, Charles L. 2005. Communicability, Racial Discourse, and Disease. *Annual Review of Anthropology* 34(1): pp. 269–291.

Briggs, Charles L., and Daniel C. Hallin. 2007. Biocommunicability: The Neoliberal Subject and its Contradictions in News Coverage of Health Issues. *Social Text* 25(4): pp. 43–66.

Brotherton, Sean. 2020. Armed against Unhappiness: Psychoanalytic Grammars in Buenos Aires. *Medical Anthropology Quarterly* 34(1): pp. 99–118.

CAR ONE. 2015. Por suerte, los psicólogos no son como los mecánicos. Por suerte nuestros mecánicos no son como otros mecánicos [Fortunately, Psychologists Are Not Like Mechanics. Fortunately, Our Mechanics Are Not Like Other Mechanics]. https://www.youtube.com/watch?v=6DR8FCl-zq4&t=17s.

Dagfal, Alejandro. 2009. *Entre París y Buenos Aires. La invención del psicólogo (1942–1966)*. Buenos Aires: Editorial Paidós.

Marsilli-Vargas, Xochitl. 2022. *Genres of Listening: An Ethnography of Psychoanalysis in Buenos Aires*. Durham, NC: Duke University Press.

Messing, Claudia. 2023. Dónde cala el discurso "libertario" en la subjetividad actual. Aportes para la comprensión del fenómeno Milei [Where Does the "Libertarian" Discourse Fit into Current Subjectivity? Contributions to the Understanding of the Milei Phenomenon], *Pagina12* (Online), June 19. https://www.pagina12.com.ar/563084-aportes-para-la-comprension-del-fenomeno-mileii.

Plotkin, Mariano Ben. 2001. *Freud in the Pampas: The Emergence and Development of a Psychoanalytic Culture in Argentina*. Stanford, CA: Stanford University Press.

Santillán, María Laura. 2022. Gabriel Rolón con María Laura Santillán. "Estoy cansado de ver sufrir gente a la que le dijeron. Si vos querés, podés." *Infobae*, November 26. Accessed July 28. https://www.infobae.com/reportajes/2022/11/20/gabriel-rolon-con-maria-laura-santillan-estoy-cansado-de-ver-sufrir-gente-a-la-que-le-dijeron-si-vos-queres-podes/.

Visacovsky, Sergio E. 2009. La constitución de un sentido práctico del malestar cotidiano y el lugar del psicoanálisis en la Argentina. *Cuicuilco* 16(45): pp. 51–79.

van Roekel, Eva. 2018. Traumatic Home: Argentinian Victimhood and the Everyday Moral Comfort of Trauma. *Ethos* 46: pp. 537–556.

9

Facing HIV Stigma with Scientific Medicine in a Bio-Speech Community in South Africa

Steven P. Black

Introduction

This chapter is about the Thembeka choir, a Zulu gospel choir comprised of individuals living with human immunodeficiency virus (HIV). This choir sang together for ten years, from 1999 to 2009 in Durban, South Africa. The group was a vibrant beacon of hope at a time when funerals were being held every week, patient-activists were in the streets protesting for government-subsidized acquired immunodeficiency syndrome (AIDS) treatment, and rampant HIV stigma threatened the wellbeing of those diagnosed with the virus. I conducted ethnographic fieldwork with the Thembeka choir for nine months in 2008. I video recorded rehearsals and performances, interviewed group members and others living with HIV, spent time with group members as they went about their lives, and wrote fieldnotes nearly every day about these experiences. I documented the ways that the choir sang, joked, and told stories about HIV together.

In this chapter I focus on singing and joking about HIV. I examine how the Thembeka choir was able to be a cohesive group despite marginalization within the world of global health, difficulties stemming from illness experiences, and the push and pull of stigma. And I discuss how group members engaged with English medical concepts and terminology as they worked together as a support group, an activist organization, and a performance troupe. For reasons that are largely beyond the scope of this chapter, I use the term "scientific medicine" to refer to what other anthropologists may call "biomedicine" or "western medicine." In doing so I am *not* making any claim that only this tradition of medicine and no other is scientific in the broad sense of being evidence based, nor that this tradition of medicine is always fully rational or evidence based. Instead, I use "scientific medicine" to refer to the cultural tradition of medicine whose historical antecedents were established in the Mediterranean (the Hellenic world) through dialogue with the Middle East, India, and beyond, later developing during colonization through the exploitation and abuse of colonial subjects and, sometimes, the appropriation of their medical traditions (Greene et al. 2013; see also Said [1978]1994, Wolf 1982).

Steven P. Black, *Facing HIV Stigma with Scientific Medicine in a Bio-Speech Community in South Africa*. In: *Language and Health in Action*. Edited by: Lynnette Arnold et al., Oxford University Press.
DOI: 10.1093/9780198933953.003.0009

Scientific medicine was a powerful force for choir members partly because it was associated with prestige and money that flowed from aid and global health organizations in the US and Europe. But it was also powerful because it named and identified the HIV pathogen while also providing successful treatments that improved the lives of HIV positive individuals like the choir members. This chapter discusses the distinctive power of scientific medicine for group formation and maintenance, not just for this choir in South Africa but for many places, people, and cultural contexts in which scientific medicine shapes people's experiences with and responses to illness.

The HIV Epidemic and the Thembeka Choir in Historical Context

By the year 2000, about 20% of South African adults were living with HIV (the virus that causes AIDS). This was the highest proportion of infected persons to population size in the world (in comparison, in 2008 the US infection rate was about 0.019% [Centers for Disease Control and Prevention 2010]). While there were many reasons for the rapid rise in infections, one point stands out among the rest: the AIDS epidemic gained full force just as the country was in the final years of the struggle against Apartheid. Apartheid was a form of minority rule inspired by segregation and the Jim Crow South in the United States. It was fully instituted in 1948 after a colonial period (1800s to early 1900s). The Dutch had colonized the Cape Town area and migrated inland, referring to themselves first as *boers* (farmers), then *voortrekkers* (pathfinders) and Afrikaners (Africans). The English had focused their efforts on the east coast (including the founding of the port city of Durban). They also brought a substantial population of South Asian indentured migrants to that area (primarily for work on sugar cane plantations).

During Apartheid, a minority of white South Africans maintained power through economic inequities, political oppression, and state-sanctioned violence. Apartheid rigidly classified Black South Africans by their ethnic affiliation, which included the use of African languages such as isiZulu and isiXhosa, and racialized others as Indian (of South Asian ancestry), "Coloured" (of mixed ancestry), and white (of European ancestry). Many Indian South Africans and some white South Africans spoke English as a first language, especially in the city of Durban. Most Apartheid government officials spoke Afrikaans (a language derived from Dutch), and many Coloured South Africans also spoke Afrikaans. Language was an important part of the Apartheid project. For instance, in the 1970s the Apartheid government forced all South Africans to use Afrikaans as the language of instruction in schools. This sparked a student protest that became violent when police started shooting Black South African children—the Soweto uprising.

In 2008 in Durban (when I conducted fieldwork), many Black South Africans viewed Afrikaans to be a language of oppression. While also a colonial/European language, English tended to be viewed more neutrally by those with whom I worked, perhaps because Apartheid had been so closely associated with Afrikaans in particular (in comparison, see Chapter 7, this volume). isiZulu was spoken by the majority of Black South Africans living in the city and surrounding areas (the area had been part of the Zulu kingdom prior to colonization). Note that I was instructed by research participants to say "isiZulu" to refer to their language; "Zulu" is actually a word that can take many different prefixes (e.g., *phezulu* means "above" while AmaZulu means the Zulu people, literally "the people of heaven").

South Africans felt the impacts of Apartheid long after it ended in 1994. Though a middle-income nation, the country soon had the highest level of income inequality in the world. Apartheid also cast a long shadow over South African healthcare. While the country had a public health system, this system was seriously underfunded. There was a better resourced private healthcare system, which was often utilized by those with the means to do so. Within this context, post-Apartheid inequality fueled the AIDS epidemic. Economic possibility drew many migrants both from rural areas of South Africa and other African nations—migrants who were often young men who were either unmarried or far from their partners for extended periods of time (Farmer 1999; Hunter 2005). As HIV/AIDS spread, the new South African government was focused primarily on rebuilding the nation economically, socially, and politically.

In this context, the Thembeka HIV support group was established at the HIV clinic of a privately run Christian hospital (note that the name of the choir and research participants mentioned are pseudonyms, in accordance with University of California, Los Angeles [UCLA] Institutional Review Board [IRB] approved research protocol and agreements with research participants). In 1998, Black isiZulu-speaking women began meeting at the hospital to make traditional Zulu beadwork with the goal of selling these crafts to help pay for medical treatment. Singing while working was embedded into the fabric of Zulu culture. So, the women in the support group sang as they did their beadwork. This led a social worker to suggest that they form a choir. Over the next ten years, the Thembeka choir would become known among members of the global health /international aid community, touring abroad six times (to the US and Great Britain) to raise money for the clinic.

One thing that choir members needed to pay for was anti-retroviral medications (ARVs). ARVs had been proven to be an effective treatment for AIDS. However, the World Health Organization (WHO) had made the unethical utilitarian declaration that ARVs were too expensive for treating poor people (Hanna and Kleinman 2013:25). Even after the WHO reversed course on this issue in the early 2000s, the government of South Africa—led by President Thabo Mbeki—refused to authorize the distribution of ARVs in the country's public health system. Instead, Mbeki suggested that people could support their immune system by eating certain foods and getting exercise (famously this included eating beetroot, earning Health Minister Tshabalala-Msimang the nickname "Dr Beetroot"). For a full discussion of the complex reasons for President Mbeki's refusal, see Fassin (2007). In response, South Africans living with HIV created the Treatment Action Campaign (TAC) in 1998. Throughout the 2000s, the TAC organized protests and filed court cases that forced the South African government to start providing ARVs in 2004. Many Thembeka choir members were part of the TAC, something that shaped their perspective on HIV activism (see also Robins 2006, 2008).

Durban: A Global Health City

The Thembeka choir was based in the city of Durban, a vibrant port on the Indian Ocean (the largest port in southern Africa). Durban was also an epicenter of the HIV epidemic in South Africa. In the metropolitan area, infection rates were estimated at close to 30% (Shisana et al. 2009). Durban had a population of about three million people, many of whom identified as ethnically Zulu and who spoke isiZulu. Many residents, including choir members, also spoke English, regularly using the language in encounters with monolingual English speakers and code mixing, deftly switching between English and isiZulu even in single phrases and sentences, with bilingual speakers.

Durban was a major hub for global health and international aid interventions, with the International AIDS Conference convening there in 2000 (and again in 2016). Despite the near-constant stream of challenges and tragedies punctuated by regular funerals for residents who died from AIDS, life went on in the city; and some found a great deal of support and community in groups comprised of people living with HIV. Support was especially important in the context of pervasive HIV stigma in the country in the early 2000s (Niehaus 2007; Roberts 2006). People who revealed their HIV status were sometimes ostracized, kicked out of familial homes, beaten, and in some cases even killed. In this context, the community and services offered by the hospital support group and the choir could be quite literally life saving.

Key Term: Bio-Speech Community

A **bio-speech community** is a group that is formed both through language use and through group members' sense of identity as people whose embodied (physical) selves are different from others'. Thembeka choir members thought of themselves as living with the HIV pathogen inside them, and understood themselves to be changed through the use of ARVs and other clinical treatments. In theory, this kind of community may form through engagement with other traditions of medicine (e.g., Zulu herbalism), but my work with the choir leads me to think that the distinctive power of contemporary clinical medicine to act on human bodies makes bio-speech community formation much more likely.

With the term "bio-speech community" I am linking theory from linguistic anthropology and medical anthropology. **Speech community** is a classic linguistic anthropology concept that describes how a community may form when three criteria are fulfilled: group members must share a verbal repertoire (in other words, speaking the same language varieties); speakers must have frequent contact with one another; and they must have shared ways of using language and understanding these uses (Gumperz 1972). Research shows that this definition works especially well for small, tight-knit groups who live in the same town, village, or neighborhood. Still, communities may form even when one or more of these criteria are not met, as long as the groups share something else in common—for instance, watching/listening to the same media, sharing ethnic identification, and using the same conventions for how to tell stories (even when doing so in different languages) (Falconi 2011; Morgan 2001; Spitulnik 1996).

Medical anthropologists have also developed a model of community formation. This model, **biosociality**, draws from the work of Michel Foucault ([1961]1965), a French sociologist and philosopher who produced a highly influential analysis of the history of medicine. As scientific medicine has developed, it has wielded incredible power; and this power has led people to sometimes view themselves and their bodies through an increasingly medicalized lens, shaping people's fundamental experiences of self and society. Historically, as scientific medicine began to diagnose human difference (especially pathological genetic difference) and to intervene to alter that difference, people increasingly identified with their diagnoses and sometimes even formed communities based on a particular diagnosis. This sense of social connection rooted in diagnosis/intervention is termed biosociality (Rabinow 1992). Over the past fifty years the scientific approach to medicine has led to unprecedented and unparalleled advances in the ability of medicine to exert power over people, healing by identifying and altering the very cells and even genetic material of the human body. It is now common for people to understand an illness not as a moral or religious failing but as a mechanistic biological failure or invasion of the body. And people sometimes form social groups based on a shared medical diagnosis (e.g., support groups for people living with diabetes; online groups for people who have long COVID) (Guell 2011; Hunt and Koteyko 2015).

Though not often mentioned, language and communication play a defining role in the creation of these biosocial groups. The idea of a bio-speech community combines the concepts of biosociality and speech community to show how medical terms and concepts often provide the glue that holds these groups together. The examples that follow illustrate how this works.

Language(s) and Explanations of Illness in the Thembeka Choir

One of the Thembeka choir's key way of using language related to HIV/AIDS was singing about the virus. Below are lyrics from a song composed by members of the Thembeka choir. I recorded the song at a choir rehearsal in 2008 held in a group member's garage (I video recorded choir rehearsals and performances as well as a birthday party and a wedding). I transcribed and translated this and other recordings with two transcription assistants—a choir member and an isiZulu-speaking student at the University of KwaZulu-Natal.

This song's lyrics identify some of the ways that South Africans avoided saying "HIV." These are terms that many South Africans regularly used, but group members felt that the phrases were stigmatizing. The song was composed and performed to create a sense of support and solidarity in the face of pervasive stigma and to educate others about why these commonly used words and phrases were stigmatizing.

Example 9.1 Song lyrics

(01) Abanye bahlekisa ngayo	Some are joking about it
(02) Bayibiza ngeqhoks	They are calling it "high heels"
(03) Bayibiza ngamagama amathathu	They are calling it "a three letter word"
(04) Abanye bayibiza nge TB	Some are calling it TB
(05) Abanye bayibiza ngedliso	Some are calling it poisoning [by witchcraft]

In line 02 of these lyrics, *iqhoks* ("bayibiza nge**qhoks**") is the isiZulu word for "high heels." The *q* is an alveolar click consonant, one of three click consonants in isiZulu. The word mimics the sound of high heels on a hard surface and points toward gender stereotypes. High heels were associated with ideals of femininity—and in particular, with a "western," American, and/or non-African femininity; and some South Africans erroneously blamed the high prevalence of HIV in the country on inaccurate perceptions of women's sexual promiscuity, which they linked to this stereotype of femininity.

In line 03, "a three letter word" refers to the three letters of the HIV acronym. In line 04, TB is an acronym for tuberculosis. Pulmonary TB (tuberculosis of the lungs) was a disease of epidemic proportions in South Africa that predated the end of Apartheid. During that time, it was especially common among Black South African miners who worked for gold and diamond mines in hazardous conditions with poor air quality and working in close quarters (Packard 1989). In the 2000s, it was one of the most common of several opportunistic infections—illnesses that impacted people living with HIV because the virus reduced their immune system's ability to fight off infections. In line 05, *idliso* (*bayibiza nge***dliso**) describes poisoning by "witchcraft." Sometimes, isiZulu speakers might visit a *sangoma*—a Zulu spiritualist (sometimes referred to in derogatory fashion as a "witchdoctor"). Some people believed that HIV infection could result from actions taken by a *sangoma*. However, choir members felt that attributing HIV infection to a supernatural cause led to fear, ignorance, and blame.

Both men and women choir members rejected the idea that HIV infections were caused by the promiscuity of women—in fact, it was men who were sometimes expected to have more than one girlfriend as part of a stereotypical Zulu masculinity, and thus logically could be considered to be more promiscuous (Hunter 2005, 2007). Group members recognized the link between TB and HIV but understood this link in terms of the scientific medical model of opportunistic infections. In addition, group members forcefully rejected the idea that HIV could be caused by a *sangoma* or Zulu herbalists.

The Hidden Meanings of English and isiZulu for Naming Illnesses

Instead of the euphemistic terms showcased in the song, choir members insisted on using scientific medical terms and visiting clinics for any health issues related to HIV. They used English medical terminology whether they were speaking in English or in isiZulu. In most cases, isiZulu terms were available and were even sometimes used in scientific medical contexts, but these terms had hidden connotations.

One example of these hidden connotations was the isiZulu word for TB. In 2008, I worked with choir members on a community outreach board for a major scientific study that was examining the effects of taking TB medication at the same time as ARVs. At one of the board's meetings, I collected a copy of a flier that provided information in English and isiZulu about TB and its connections to HIV/AIDS. The English version of the flier says:

> What is TB?
> TB is an infectious disease spread by coughing, sneezing and singing.

While the isiZulu version of the same flier says:

> Siyini isifo sofuba?
> Isifo sofuba yisifo esithelelanayo esibhebhethekiswa ukukhwehlela, ukuthimula nokuphefumula umoya onegciwane ongena emaphashini.

The headline of the isiZulu flier asks, "Siyini isifo sofuba?" (what is TB?) or (what is sickness of the lungs?). *Siyini* can be translated as "what." Here and elsewhere, *isifo sofuba* is offered as a translation of TB ("is TB"). However, the term can also mean something broader in isiZulu. Literally, it means sickness of the lungs, and it may refer to a range of afflictions related to breathing. In Zulu herbal medicine, *isifo sofuba* was connected to an explanation of illness in which a person could become ill from breathing in air or dust that was disturbed or carried on what might be considered a bad wind (Ngubane 1977). It is possible that the creators of the flier decided to attempt to redefine the isiZulu term and to instead link it with scientific medicine. However, there is a danger associated with this strategy: people may instead read the flier and understand the use of *isifo sofuba* in terms of the explanations provided by Zulu herbal medicine. Choir members avoided this danger by using the English term "TB" whether speaking in English or in isiZulu. This use of English medical terms, even when speaking isiZulu, was part of how the choir created and maintained itself as a bio-speech community.

Joking about HIV

One example of this use of the English "TB" comes from a moment of joking between two choir members before a choir rehearsal began. Many stigmatizing ways of discussing HIV in South Africa relied on humor (or what some people perceived as humorous). Choir members' awareness of this stigmatizing humor was articulated in line 01 of the song discussed earlier, "abanye bahlekisa ngayo" (some are joking about it). When choir members joked about HIV, they accomplished two things. First, they turned stigmatizing humor on its head by joking about stigma. Second, they were able to display their level of comfort with their own and others' HIV positive statuses without discussing it outright.

One day, while preparing for choir rehearsal two group members—Bongiwe (a vocalist) and Ndumiso (a drummer)—were moving things around the garage where rehearsal would be held. Bongiwe was sweeping dust out of the garage, when she got to a bench and was uncertain whether or not to move the bench elsewhere Bongiwe asked,

Example 9.2 Transcript of choir rehearsal (English terms noted in bold)

(01)	Bongiwe:	Sima lapha vele?	Is [the bench] supposed to be here?
(02)	Ndumiso:	Yah sima lapha. Noma uzosidonsa uhamba naso.	Yeah, it's supposed to be here. Or you'll drag it and go [home] with it.
(03)	Bongiwe:	Hayibo. Ngiyaphuquza mina.	Hey no. Me, I'm making dust.
(04)	Ndumiso:	Sizoba ne**TB.**	We will get **TB.**
(05)	Bongiwe:	Kade ngingashaneli bengini phathisa ngethi—ehh. nge**TB.**	I wasn't sweeping, I was just infecting you with—ehh, with **TB.**
(06)	Ndumiso:	Mmm.	Mmm.

Bongiwe and Ndumiso's playful exchange depended on shared understanding of three things. First, they were playing with their knowledge of the Zulu herbalist explanation of *isifo sofuba*—the idea that one could get sick with TB by breathing bad air. The idea here was that Bongiwe's sweeping would lead to Ndumiso breathing something that might cause *isifo sofuba*. Second, the two were relying on knowledge of the scientific medical explanation of opportunistic infections (in which people living with HIV could be infected by TB). They implied that Ndumiso was especially susceptible to TB because he was HIV positive. Finally, they were sharing a moment of recognition that they were both living with HIV (calling attention to themselves as people living with HIV without saying so outright).

This joking was successful because the two choir members used the English scientific medical term "TB" (in bold, lines 04 and 05), alluding to scientific medical explanations of HIV, TB, and opportunistic infections, while simultaneously critiquing the Zulu herbal medical understanding of the relationship between *isifo sofuba* and sweeping dust. In doing these three things, Bongiwe and Ndumiso reinforced their shared sense of being part of a distinct group of people who were living with HIV, who communicated about HIV in specific, shared ways utilizing scientific medicine (e.g., singing together; joking together), and who understood HIV/AIDS and their own HIV infection within scientific medical frameworks for explaining illness. Together, they were reinforcing/maintaining a bio-speech community.

Why Bio-Speech Communities Matter

The Thembeka choir community mattered—for group members, for the communities in which choir members lived, for others living with HIV in Durban, for global health organizations operating in Durban, and for scientific medicine as a whole. For group members, the choir was a source of support in a context where individuals had to navigate the challenges of being diagnosed and living with a chronic or terminal illness in a context of widespread stigma. Joking and singing about HIV relieved stress and affirmed support for one another, and the use of scientific medical terminology emphasized that they were dealing with an explainable, treatable disease rather than some moral or spiritual failing. After choir rehearsal, group members then returned to home communities, in some cases acting as pillars of support for friends and neighbors who were living with HIV.

Many group members were also participants in scientific medical studies on HIV/AIDS being conducted in Durban. The community outreach board I mentioned earlier was just one example. Choir members were not passive patients in these studies—they were patient-activists who used their detailed knowledge of scientific medical models of HIV to participate in conversations with researchers about how to best carry out the studies in question and, in some cases, to help recruit volunteers for these studies. In these and other efforts, the Thembeka choir contributed to the field of global health. At the same time, they were marginalized within that field. They did not have degrees in medicine or public health that would have led global health specialists to recognize them as central contributors to the design and implementation of health interventions. Still, they used musical performance to find ways to engage with global health leaders as they sang about HIV (e.g., as a performing group at medical conferences, on tour to the US and the United Kingdom).

Some scholars have described the twenty-first century as "the age of biomedicalization" (Moyer and Nguyen 2016). What this means is that in the twenty-first century, scientific medicine has dramatically expanded its reach into many different realms of human life. Often, researchers write about this in terms of how scientific medicine constrains people's possibilities for thought and action. But the example of the Thembeka choir demonstrates how scientific medicine can also open up new spaces for sociality and creativity. Choir members' use of scientific medicine as an explanation of their illness—and as the basis for a new understanding of themselves as individuals and as a group—was linked to new possibilities and resources associated with the power and authority of scientific medicine. The Thembeka choir, and the idea of bio-speech communities more generally, demonstrates how people sometimes harness the creative potential of scientific medicine's global and often-expanding power.

Questions for Reflection and Discussion

Reflection Questions

1. What communities are you part of? What brings these communities together? What kinds of interests or practices do they share, including language?
2. Think about your experience, or that of loved ones, with social stigma (related to an illness or condition, an identity, an action, etc.). What role did language and communication play in constructing (or reducing) that stigma? Was humor or avoidance involved? If so, how?

Looking In: Small Group Discussion Questions

1. What is "scientific medicine"? Why does the author use this term instead of other terms? Why is this particularly relevant to the context of HIV/AIDS in South Africa?
2. What is a bio-speech community? Provide a definition in your own words and identify some examples from the chapter or other contexts.
3. What is the connection between scientific medicine and bio-speech communities?
4. When are English medical terms used by the Thembeka choir, and when are isiZulu words or phrases used? Why? What does this code switching accomplish?
5. How does the concept of a bio-speech community help us understand how the Thembeka choir was produced as a community through language?

Looking Out: Large Group Discussion Questions

1. Singing, joking, and storytelling were key parts of the Thembeka choir's shared linguistic practices. What do these types of communication share in common that might have made them good ways for group members to communicate about HIV in the context of stigma? Do you think that these types of communication are as effective in communicating to their friends and family?
2. What would need to change in the practice of global health for the contributions of communities like the Thembeka choir to be more fully recognized?
3. How might the idea of bio-speech communities be applied to another group of people who have organized around a shared illness or condition? What is the role of scientific medicine in this community?
4. What ethical considerations do anthropologists make about research when it concerns a stigmatized subject? What publication practices do researchers follow when publishing research about stigmatized communities?

References

Centers for Disease Control and Prevention. 2010. HIV Surveillance Report, 2008, Vol. 20. Atlanta, GA.

Falconi, Elizabeth. 2011. Migrant Stories: Zapotec Transborder Migration and the Production of a Narrated Community. Unpublished dissertation. University of Michigan, Ann Arbor MI.

Farmer, Paul. 1999. *Infections and Inequalities: The Modern Plagues*. Berkeley, CA: University of California Press.

Fassin, Didier. 2007. *When Bodies Remember: Experiences and Politics of AIDS in South Africa*. Berkeley, CA: University of California Press.

Foucault, Michel. [1961]1965. *The Birth of the Clinic: An Archaeology of Medical Perception*. New York: Vintage.

Greene, Jeremy, Marguerite Thorp Basilico, Heidi Kim, and Paul Farmer. 2013. Colonial Medicine and Its Legacies. In *Reimagining Global Health: An Introduction*, ed. Paul Farmer, Jim Yong Kim, Arthur Kleinman, and Matthew Basilico, pp. 33–73. Berkeley, CA: University of California Press.

Guell, Cornelia. 2011. Candi(ed) Action: Biosocialities of Turkish Berliners Living with Diabetes. *Medical Anthropology Quarterly* 25(3): pp. 377–394.

Gumperz, John. 1972. The Speech Community. In *Language and Social Context*, ed. P. P. Giglioli, pp. 219–231. Harmondsworth: Penguin.

Hanna, Bridget, and Arthur Kleinman. 2013. Unpacking Global Health: Theory and Critique. In *Reimagining Global Health: An Introduction*, ed. Paul Farmer, Jim Yong Kim,

Arthur Kleinman, and Matthew Basilico, pp. 15–32. Berkeley, CA: University of California Press.

Hunt, Daniel, and Nelya Koteyko. 2015. "What Was Your Blood Sugar Reading This Morning?" Representing Diabetes Self Management on Facebook. *Discourse and Society* 26(4): pp. 445–463.

Hunter, Mark. 2005. Cultural Politics and Masculinities: Multiple-Partners in Historical Perspective in KwaZulu-Natal. *Culture, Health and Sexuality* 7(4): pp. 389–403.

Hunter, Mark. 2007. The Changing Political Economy of Sex in South Africa: The Significance of Unemployment and Inequalities to the Scale of the AIDS Pandemic. *Social Science and Medicine* 64: pp. 689–700.

Morgan, Marcyleina. 2001. The African American Speech Community: Reality and Sociolinguistics. In *Linguistic Anthropology: A Reader*, ed. Alessandro Duranti, pp. 74–94. Malden, MA: Blackwell.

Moyer, Eileen, and Vinh-Kim Nguyen. 2016. Is the 21st Century the Age of Biomedicalization? *Medicine Anthropology Theory* 3(1): pp. i–vii.

Ngubane, Harriet. 1977. *Body and Mind in Zulu Medicine: An Ethnography of Health and Disease in Nyuswa-Zulu Thought and Practice*. New York: Academic Press.

Niehaus, Isak. 2007. Death Before Dying: Understanding AIDS Stigma in the South African Lowveld. *Journal of Southern African Studies* 33(4): pp. 845–860.

Packard, Randall. 1989. *White Plague, Black Labor: Tuberculosis and the Political Economy of Health and Disease in South Africa*. Berkeley, CA: University of California Press.

Rabinow, Paul. 1992. Artificiality and Enlightenment: From Sociobiology to Biosociality. In *Incorporations*, ed. J. Crary and S. Kwinter, pp. 234–252. New York: Zone Books.

Roberts, Sandra Jane. 2006. Countering Stigma: Collectively Counselling an AIDS Identity. In *Globalisation and New Identities: A View from the Middle*, ed. P. Alexander, M. C. Dawson, and M. Ichharam, pp. 171–190. Johannesburg: Jacana Media.

Robins, Steven. 2006. From "Rights" to "Ritual": AIDS Activism in South Africa. *American Anthropologist* 108(2): pp. 312–323.

Robins, Steven. 2008. *From Revolution to Rights in South Africa: Social Movements, NGOs and Popular Politics After Apartheid*. Pietermaritzburg: University of KwaZulu-Natal Press.

Said, Edward. [1978]1994. *Orientalism*. New York: Vintage Books.

Shisana, Olive, Thomas Rehle, Leickness Chisamu Simbayi, Khangelani Zuma, Sibusiso Jooste, Victoria Pillay-van-Wyk, Nokuthula Mbelle, Johan van Zyl, Warren Parker, Nompumelelo Zungu, Sibusiso Pezi, and the SABSSM III Implementation Team. 2009. *South African National HIV Prevalence, Incidence, Behavior and Communication Survey, 2008: A Turning Tide among Teenagers?* Pretoria: Human Sciences Research Council.

Spitulnik, Debra. 1996. The Social Circulation of Media Discourse and the Mediation of Communities. *Journal of Linguistic Anthropology* 6(2): pp. 161–187.

Wolf, Eric. 1982. *Europe and the People Without History*. Berkeley, CA: University of California Press.

SECTION 4

LANGUAGE AND ENVIRONMENT

Editors' Introduction

Discussions about health and the environment often treat human bodies as bounded entities that move through an environment, as if humans were separate from the ecosystems where they live. These framings neglect the many ways that humans constitute a dynamic part of nested environments across large and small scales. Humans impact and are impacted by the environment, for example through practices of extraction, cultivation, pollution, and conservation, all of which affect food and water supplies, the spread of pathogens, and climate change. In addition human bodies are, themselves, environments, with interactions among internal systems and complex interrelationships that extend beyond the body. For instance, scientists who study microbiome health point out that human beings are "symbiotic assemblages of human cells and microorganisms," shaped by myriad environmental factors (Benezra 2021:511). The boundaries between body and environment are therefore porous and this has profound significance for health.

Environmental impacts on health are not limited to the natural world or even the built physical environment. Human wellbeing is also profoundly influenced by social, cultural, political, and economic environments where poverty and discrimination operate and produce health inequities. In their efforts to address such intractable problems, global health institutions have sometimes framed health as a human right and argued for a more equitable distribution of medical resources. While these ideas have had some meaningful impacts, other deeply rooted ideas in the global geopolitical environment have posed obstacles to their realization. Dominant assumptions about who counts as human, for example, are underpinned by racialized models that center whiteness (Smalls 2020). And narrow definitions of citizenship generate categories of people who are viewed as undeserving of medical care, at the same time as they reinforce conceptualizations of health as a privilege and medicine as a commodity (Willen 2012).

Across domains, language practices shape how people understand and interact with the multiple overlapping natural and social environmental systems that shape their health. Additionally, language can be an important tool in the work of environmental health justice. If both ecosystems and communication involve multilevel interactions that occur among organisms and other actors in the environment, then thinking about them together can lead to a productive reimagination of health, disease, and healing as operating across different scales of magnitude, time, and place.

The chapters in this section explore how language is central to the ways that social, political, and material environments shape human health. Shohet and Schmidt show how structural inequalities and systems of oppression can cause and exacerbate kidney disease, as well as how patients on dialysis narrativize these experiences. Harvey brings environmental science and ethnographic methods together in order to study how infrastructure, resident knowledge, and public health messages shape perceptions about water safety and risk in rural Guatemala. Faudree traces the social and scientific history of one medicinal plant, *xka pastora*, showing how global pharmaceutical exploitation involves narrative reframing and the silencing of Mazatec indigenous environmental stewardship.

References

Benezra, Amber. 2021. Microbial Kin: Relations of Environment and Time. *Medical Anthropology Quarterly* 35(4): pp. 511–528.

Smalls, Krystal A. 2020. Race, SIGNS, and the Body. In *The Oxford Handbook of Language and Race*, ed. H. Samy Alim, Angela Reyes, and Paul V. Kroskrity, pp. 233–259. Oxford: Oxford University Press.

Willen, Sarah S. 2012. How Is Health-Related "Deservingness" Reckoned? Perspectives from Unauthorized Im/Migrants in Tel Aviv. *Social Science and Medicine* 74(6): pp. 812–821.

10

"I'm still here!"

Listening to African American Silences and Narratives of Life on Dialysis in Boston

Merav Shohet and Insa M. Schmidt

Many Americans remember the COVID-19 pandemic as a time of crisis, when lives were disrupted, put on hold, and for many, ended altogether. It was a time of loss and uncertainty, when life as we knew it seemed to have stopped. But is that how everyone experienced the pandemic? At Boston Medical Center (BMC), an urban hospital in the Northeastern United States serving some of the area's most marginalized, poor, and racialized patients, this was not the case. How is this possible?

First, consider the fact that many of the BMC patients we worked with were people of color who endured not only a painful chronic disease known as **end-stage kidney disease (ESKD)** but also faced ongoing **structural racism**, or the institutional ways that racial discrimination is built into society (American Medical Association 2021). Robust scholarship and media sources document how the racism embedded in interlocking social systems has had historic and continuing negative impacts on the health of individuals and communities of color in the United States (e.g., Alexander 2010; Anderson et al. 2014; Davis 2019; Duvernay and Moran 2016; Hannah-Jones 2020; Kendi 2016; Schmidt et al. 2023; Wakeel and Njoku 2021). Is it any surprise, then, that for these patients, structural racism profoundly shaped their experiences of ESKD?

Second, consider ESKD and its treatment. Also called "renal failure" or "kidney failure," ESKD progresses when people's kidneys cannot filter out the excess fluid, salt, and waste that their body accumulates as they eat and drink. This is fatal unless the ill person travels to a clinic every few days to be hooked up to dialysis machines that will "wash out" their "dirty" blood and then infuse them with cleaned-up blood. The process of dialysis accomplishes in just twelve hours spread over three days what human kidneys normally do daily around the clock. Often, it causes painful muscle cramps, itchiness, blood pressure fluctuations, headaches and dizziness, nausea and vomiting, and it weakens patients' immune systems while increasing their risk for other diseases. These effects were what Rodney Jones and Christopher Gordon (both pseudonyms), along with the other patients we interviewed, endured weekly, many for years.

Merav Shohet and Insa M. Schmidt, *"I'm still here!"*. In: *Language and Health in Action*. Edited by: Lynnette Arnold et al., Oxford University Press. © Merav Shohet and Insa M. Schmidt (2026). DOI: 10.1093/9780198933953.003.0010

By the time we asked Rodney to compare pandemic-related difficulties with the other challenges he’d mentioned suffering over his lifetime—including discrimination, incarceration, limited education and job mobility, divorce and family estrangement, homelessness, food insecurity, and feeling like a “guinea pig” under medical trainees’ care—we were no longer surprised by his answer: “It was not the same, but problems are problems, you know, and one problem ain’t no bigger than the other one.” With this succinct dismissal, Rodney articulates what we heard from most patients: the pandemic was essentially just one more thing in their long litany of problems. Their narratives minimized the importance of the COVID-19 pandemic not because it was not challenging, but because its impact was dwarfed in comparison to the combined, chronic assault of the structural racism and terminal illness they confronted over their lifetime.

This chapter introduces a micro-analytic approach to analyze the narratives that BMC dialysis patients recounted in their interviews. We focus here on the narratives of one of our early interviewees, Mr. Gordon, to show how paying attention not just to the surface content of stories, but also to their narrative structure and the silences embedded in them, provides key insights into people’s experience in their broader social context. We argue that such listening to what is at stake for patients, and understanding this in relation to the sociocultural, economic, and political forces that shape their lives, can be particularly helpful not only for scholars, but for practitioners and policy makers. We begin with a brief introduction to our study and to Mr. Gordon, followed by further discussion of kidney disease and its treatments, and our initial assumptions, which he led us to reevaluate.

Our Pandemic Syndemics Kidney Failure Study

Our study, conducted from December 2020 through August 2021, was designed to understand the harmful effects of the pandemic on BMC dialysis patients and to trace their sources of support (Shohet et al. 2023). This collaborative research included Merav Shohet, a medical and linguistic anthropologist of mixed Ashkenazi and Mizrahi Jewish origins, and Insa M. Schmidt, a white nephrology (kidney disease) researcher, licensed as a clinician in Germany. As a team of researchers with biomedical and linguistic anthropological expertise, we drew on our respective skills in the audio-recorded remote interviews we conducted with twenty BMC patients. Eighteen self-identified as Black / African American, one Latinx, and one Vietnamese American. Eleven of the patients were men and only three worked full time. Most patients were unable to work due to illness-related disability.

In December 2020, we interviewed Christopher Gordon, a disabled Black / African American man who at the time was 55 years old and had been on dialysis for about twenty-one years. His demographic characteristics and the themes in his narrative correspond to those of most of the patients we interviewed, although of course there is variation. One striking, and yet in retrospect unsurprising, finding that emerged was that while the pandemic exacerbated patients' hardships and poor health, they did not view it as a crisis. Echoing Rodney's statement, the pandemic was simply "one more thing" to add to the burden of living with a debilitating chronic terminal illness while enduring structural racism that compounded the adversities that patients faced. We also found that patients' supportive social networks and religious orientation played important roles in staving off despair. In short, in contrast with popular culture depictions that portray the miraculous nature of medical technologies and professional medical expertise in saving lives, patients instead pointed to the *social* roots of their suffering and highlighted how relatives, friends, and God shaped the quality of their lives and the timing of their death.

In Mr. Gordon's narratives below, he prioritizes "listening to my body" and trusting in God over any particular doctor or technology. In this way, he also deflects the pervasive anxiety that accompanied the pandemic, minimizing the role of COVID or impending death in his life; instead, he presents himself as uniquely positioned to accept and convey God's blessings. Yet Mr. Gordon's story is less an unrealistically optimistic account of triumphant survival than one where he at once connects structural violence to ill-health, while paradoxically also aligning with biomedical accounts and tropes of Black masculinity that privilege unattainable individual agency and control over one's life.

Kidney Failure and Its Treatments

Mr. Gordon described dialysis as follows: "Dialysis is a cruel thing, and the machine is a cruel machine. It doesn't keep you alive, it just keeps you from dying quicker." He was right. Dialysis does not heal damaged kidneys, but it does keep patients alive, at a cost. Dialyzed patients report feeling drained, often for the rest of the day and even the next day, by which point it is practically time to go back to the dialysis center and start the process again. Perhaps worse, dialysis also requires adherence to strict dietary restrictions and typically results not only in feeling awful for much of the week, but also, consequently, it leaves patients unable to work and earn a wage, and less than fully able to take care of themselves and their loved ones at home, which can lead to further financial insecurity and stigmatization.

Sadly, the only alternative to dialysis, aside from hospice and end-of-life care, is to receive a kidney transplant. These come from a living donor, such as a relative or friend who must undergo a rigorous process to determine if they are a good match, or from a deceased (usually anonymous) donor, or a matching seller on the black market. Sources for a "spare" kidney are scarce, and like dialysis, may extend one's life, but do not provide a cure.

A donor kidney, while portrayed by many as a miracle or a new lease on life (Ikels 2013; Kaufman 2015; Sharp 2014), often takes years to procure, and even once transplanted, can lead to a range of social and physical vulnerabilities. Moreover, transplant patients must remain under regular healthcare surveillance and take daily immunosuppressant medications to ensure that their body does not reject the donated kidney. These required lifelong immunosuppressive medications are expensive and, by definition, leave patients more vulnerable to infection and disease since they weaken (by "suppressing") their immune system, meaning patients' health and wellbeing remain compromised. Finally, because patients are only eligible for a transplant if they are deemed stable and healthy enough, transplantation is out of reach for most ESKD patients, even if they desire it. The vast majority therefore begin on dialysis, rightfully bitter. Like Rodney bluntly put it, medicine, inflected by racism, is stacked against them: "Black people end up never getting their kidney. And that's why we end up dying."

Kidney Disease, Structural Violence, and Pandemic Syndemics

Given this background, many researchers and medical professionals expected the COVID-19 pandemic to bring magnified hardship to ESKD patients. To sustain their lives, most patients had no choice but to break social isolation rules and travel to their local dialysis clinic three times a week, leaving them more vulnerable to becoming infected by the virus. This alone might lead scientists to expect a magnified crisis in the lives of patients. Further, as economically disadvantaged and racialized people of color, BMC's patients faced many additional challenges due to structural and systemic oppression. In launching our study, then, we immediately turned to the lens of syndemics to help us understand what impacts the pandemic could have.

Syndemics is a concept originally developed by critical medical anthropologist Merrill Singer (Singer et al. 2021). It is used as a shorthand way to describe how multiple social and biological conditions interact to exponentially magnify each one's harmful effects. The idea of syndemics goes beyond that of comorbidities, which focuses exclusively on how physical conditions cluster together. It is not just that diabetes, hypertension, and CKD (the precursor to ESKD) often cluster together, or that diabetes and hypertension often lead to CKD and ESKD. Rather, the concept of syndemics is explicitly political, revealing how, when combined with poverty, both the patients' suffering and their economic conditions worsen. Structural racism further exacerbates suffering: not only because racialized populations are often excluded from economic advancement and various forms of care, but also because the continual stress from racism depletes their physical (bodily) resources and ability to combat illness and negatively impacts their health. So, for instance, food and housing insecurity can be both the effects and causes of illness, and these conditions are magnified by racial discrimination compounded by ill-health. Adopting the lens of syndemics thus reveals how health is profoundly impacted by aspects of the social, political, and economic environment that are often not treated as relevant to healthcare.

Narrative Insights

Working at BMC, we expected the COVID-19 pandemic to interact in precisely these harmful ways with already marginalized and stigmatized patients, to cause even more suffering and harm. To understand how BMC patients were experiencing this syndemic intersection, we attended to both their illness concerns and to how they *narrated* their concerns—what we call their **narrative features**. We drew on previous work on patients' narratives of illness and recovery (Capps and Ochs 1995; Garro 2003; Mattingly 2010; Mattingly and Garro 2000; Samuels 2018, 2019; Shohet 2007, 2018) to help identify important narrative features to analyze and track how patients positioned themselves and others in their stories. For example, do narrators portray themselves as agents (the main actor in control) or the grammatical patient in the narration (the person to whom things happen and on whom others act)? What sort of moral stances do they take: who is portrayed as "good" or "bad," and who is to "blame" or held "responsible," for example?

We also attended to the structure of patients' narratives. For example, are stories structured as linear progressions with a clear beginning, middle, and end; or are they "sideshadowing narratives" (Shohet 2021), whether moving back and forth in time, or circular, with no clear beginnings or endings, since they meld together and repeat as cycles? Finally, what might we learn from various forms of silences within narratives? These could include pauses, cut-offs, and subject changes, which may point to topics left unsaid or avoided.

In this chapter, we show that this linguistic anthropological lens provides insights into a person's life and what is at stake for them as they navigate illness in a context of syndemics. This analytic framework enriches and nuances more content-based research that focuses exclusively on what people say and ignores the details of *how* they say it. Paying attention to language can direct us in productive ways to address medical racism and broader societal ills, as we demonstrate here with excerpts from Mr. Gordon's interview. We conclude that this lens reveals how human suffering is caused by both disease and adverse social environments while also demonstrating the complex consequences of the coping mechanisms that patients adopt.

Suffering and Resilience in Mr. Gordon's Narrative and Silences

Medical anthropology has shown that, whereas biomedical clinicians focus on diagnosing and treating diseases (pathologies in the body), patients' illness experiences (how sickness stems from and impacts broader aspects of their lives) are no less important (Kleinman 1988). Mr. Gordon oscillated at first between these. He provided the biomedical explanation of renal failure as caused by (seemingly apolitical) "high blood pressure" but also told us about how illness both pervaded and stemmed from his marginalized positionality.

For instance, at the beginning of the interview, when we asked about his occupation, he recounted that he had lost his job in construction years ago, as soon as he was diagnosed with ESKD, pointing to the disease's deleterious effects on life and livelihood. We followed up by asking him the open-ended question, "How did that come about?" Mr. Gordon responded first with the most immediate circumstances of his diagnosis, alluding to the fact that financial pressures were already part of his life before illness.

He recounted one holiday weekend when he had intended to earn extra cash by working overtime but had stopped in at BMC to renew a prescription. A master storyteller, Mr. Gordon uses repetition and parallel structure with the logical connector "so" ("So I went ... So when they ...") and builds suspense with interjections like, "you know what? You know what was the next thing?" to ensure listeners are paying attention. Whether reliving the moment or to draw his audience closer to his experience, he narrates his dialogue, thoughts, and feelings in detail, using direct reported speech (quoting himself and the clinical staff):

> So I went around to urgent care to take my blood pressure,
> and they were taking a long time. [...]
> So when they came back, [...]
> They said, "Mr. Gordon?"
> I said,—you know what? You know what was the next thing? [...]
> My kidneys failed on Memorial Day. [...]
> So I was anxious to leave it all,
> Cause I was like, "C'mon, I gotta go to work
> and make me some holiday money, I gotta go."
> She [the clinician] was like, "Mr. Gordon, I'll tell it to you just like it is:
> if you leave this office right now, you'll be dead by tomorrow."

Mr. Gordon then went on to tell us, with wonder in his voice, as though the event of over twenty years ago continues to perplex him, how he found himself in the hospital, having gone down from a healthy 235 pounds to 160 pounds in just a month. But rather than continuing to narrate the biomedical aspects of his disease, at this point, he paused and pointed out his exceptionality, emphasizing that unlike most dialysis patients who typically suffer edema (swelling due to water retention in one's body tissues), he did not:

> I never blew up, like people blow up when they're on dialysis, they get that fluid. [...]
> I just—
> I pushed through it,
> I pushed through it, [...]
> And next thing you know I was in the hospital with kidney pain.

By displaying Mr. Gordon's narrative clauses line by line on the page, we can see the poetic structure of his account, which is filled with repetition and voice play common in the rhetorical repertoire of Black communities (Smitherman 1977). Through this, Mr. Gordon frames himself as the hero overcoming pain ("I just—I pushed through it"), only to be felled by illness, as though taken by surprise ("next thing you know I was in the hospital"). This exemplifies what Sherman James (1994) calls **John Henryism**: an active approach for responding to prolonged adversity through superhuman efforts. James developed this framework as a way of understanding how Black men tended to respond to intersecting health challenges and structural racism, naming it after one of his patients and also an American folk hero who represents Black masculine strength but also labor exploitation. Subsequent scholarship has shown that the pressure and burden of "pushing through" can be so overwhelming that it deteriorates the person's physical health (Robinson and Thomas Tobin 2021). Through the use of this trope, Mr. Gordon's narrative thus conveys, without saying it, how his adherence to oppressive ideals of Black masculinity led to poor health.

So far, this is a story of the tragedy of illness that upturned Mr. Gordon's life: "That changed my whole life ... My whole life." With kidney failure, he was no longer "an outgoing guy" and instead became "too weak to even do anything." As he goes on to catalogue the surgeries and other difficulties he has endured, we were struck by what he remained silent about: any challenges of living with renal failure during the closures and prevaccination period of the pandemic. Indeed, the interview went on for nearly five hours and was not confined to Mr. Gordon's dramatic descent to illness or most recent surgery. A linguistic anthropological attunement to the unfolding flow and narrative strategies within participants' interviews reveals which segments they mark linguistically as significant, regardless of whether they explicitly name them as such.

Contrast the above segments about his diagnosis to how Mr. Gordon talked about the onset of the pandemic and its consequences for him. He begins his response by minimizing COVID as an event, saying laconically, "A lot of things are off track." Asked to elaborate, he again rhetorically minimizes the pandemic using the mitigators "well actually" and "it's just" as he frames COVID as merely contributing to already established routines continuous with his underlying illness: "Well actually, it's just, the mask, wearing a mask, you know." In contrast with the tale of a life-changing diagnosis (the kidney failure), after this minimal response, Mr. Gordon shifts the focus to how COVID affected not him, but others, again using a mitigator: "It's just, it's just messed with a whole lot of people's lives."

Later in the interview, when we ask Mr. Gordon how the pandemic affected his care, he insisted that his routine has been left relatively intact and that he remained self-sufficient and in control. He grammatically marks himself as full of agency (the capacity to act) by using the first person pronoun followed by present tense, active verbs:

Yeah, the docs haven't changed.
I mean, we get new nurses,

we get new techs come in,
but like I said, [...]
I stick myself,
so they don't do anything for me.
I stick it in
and I control the machine bars,
my blood pressure,

Through this framework, Mr. Gordon established himself as someone in control of his illness experience. Here, the self-reliance of John Henryism is an empowering trope, mobilized to depict his sense of ownership over his treatment. Again and again, it became notable how quickly Mr. Gordon abandoned the topic of COVID in favor of portraying himself as master of his chronic disease, even as he acknowledges help from his kin ("I got my sister, and I got my daughter, and my fiancée, my son even helps"). Not all patients articulated this degree of self-sufficiency, but the message that COVID had altered but did not dramatically change dialysis routines echoed throughout our interviews with patients.

The above analysis illuminates how Mr. Gordon's narrative strategies convey his experience of kidney failure itself as the major crisis of his life, whereas the pandemic appears more minor: a nuisance rather than a turning point for him. He spends far more time discussing his diagnosis and uses rhetorical devices that invite listeners to pay attention to its significance. At the same time, he linguistically minimizes any changes that may have resulted from the pandemic that upturned others' lives. His relative silence and topic shifts when we ask about COVID are indicative of this stance.

True, silences could alternatively be read as signs of repression—a reluctance to talk about topics that are too painful or forbidden in other ways (see Dragojlovic and Samuels 2021; Shohet 2023; Trouillot 1995; Weller 2017). But Mr. Gordon's narrative moves suggest otherwise: that the COVID pandemic is not traumatic but, rather, simply not all that interesting. For example, he mentioned a recent trip he took to visit relatives in a southern state, which surprised us given the demands of dialysis. In response to our expression of surprise, he reminded us of his motto to listen to his body and told us that he only went for a few days and even went to an amusement park. Such narrative moves led us to realize that the additional challenges presented by the pandemic were less relevant for patients, even though this was what research funders wanted to hear about. Instead, the close analysis of narrative features revealed that the experience of chronic illness exacerbated by structural inequalities and racism were what mattered most to Mr. Gordon and most of the BMC patients we interviewed.

The Social Roots of Disease in Mr. Gordon's Narrative

In his narrative, Mr. Gordon described the violence and racism that he has faced. He explicitly depicted these experiences as root causes of his chronic stress, anger, and consequent ill-health. Early in the interview, he told us that high blood pressure led to his illness. During our second session, he more explicitly attributed this hypertension to his experiences of racism.

In contrast with COVID-19, about which he did not elaborate, Mr. Gordon told us in vivid detail about Boston's anti-Black violence during his childhood. For example, recalling his first day being bused to a white neighborhood school in the 1970s, he recounted how "White Caucasian people" harassed him and his peers with "rakes and golf clubs." They threw "bricks and bottles" while shouting at him and his Black classmates to "go back home," using the n-word. He continues, using direct reported speech:

> So, we got to the school,
> the police were rushing us and getting us into the school
> and I was like, "What the hell? What's going on?"
> You know, and I was like, shocked

Remarking on the dissonance between being happy to be in school, and the life-changing "shock" he felt, he explains:

> as the day went on, I just stopped focusing on school.
> But even though I was probably happy to be in school [...]
> the thought in the back of my mind was,
> "What's gonna happen when I leave the building?"
> It changed my life.

This account implicitly counters tropes of police as protective or racist stereotypes of Black children as uninterested in school. In addition, Mr. Gordon here uses the same phrase ("it changed my life") that he used to describe the impact of his diagnosis with kidney failure. This linguistic parallel suggests a connection between his experience of racism and his experience of illness. He elaborates this syndemic intersection in a subsequent monologue replete with repetition and parallel structure that outlines his growing insights about the relationship between the stress of racism and its ill effects on health:

> when we were babies,
> we didn't really notice shit going on
> until we got old enough to see what was going on,
> what was really going on. [...]
> It put a scar on me [...]
> Because as I started going through high school and stuff,
> and I was angry.
> I guess all this tied into kidney failure.
> So, I grew up a little aggressive, you know,

He waffles at this point (using "I think" rather than "know"), as though uncomfortable admitting his anger and aggression, but then articulates a direct connection:

And I think what anger is,
anger, it raises your blood pressure.
Yes, I look back on my life now on what the reasons,
or some of the reasons why my blood pressure stays so high,
and how I used to live.

We were struck by Mr. Gordon's insight and the linear way in which he structured his story, tying cause and effect directly, from anti-Black white racism to anger and stress, to ill-health. Through this account he articulated not just a medical cause for his illness, but also a **political etiology**, or the social and political causes of disease (Hamdy 2008). For Mr. Gordon, the social environment of anti-Black racism, financial stress, and injustice led to debilitating illness.

Managing Syndemics through Faith

How do individuals facing such pernicious syndemics respond? In Mr. Gordon's narratives, his faith in God was central to his response (see also Mack, Chapter 13 in this volume). He highlighted the blessings and even sense of mission and belonging that his faith provided, which is consistent with the centrality of the Christian church in Black communities and their attendant linguistic practices (Smitherman 1977).

Faith and church communities have been central to many Black-led struggles for racial justice. Space constraints preclude a fuller discussion, but consider just the following excerpt, in which Mr. Gordon narrates himself as God's messenger ("I'm a testimony"; "There's something that God wants me to do") and concludes that his fate is ultimately decreed by God ("Only God knows when it's time") when discussing the relation between his faith, illness, and the dramatic violence he's survived:

I'm a testimony.
My life is a testimony. [...]
every time I just bounce back
and I know that's the power of God.
There's something that God wants me to do that I haven't done yet.
And that's why I'm still here, surviving with this, twenty years.
I've been shot twice.
See I lived,
I got stabbed in the chest.
I've had more—
I'm still here!
See, when it's your time to go, ain't nobody can tell you that.
Only God knows when it's time.

Throughout his story, Mr. Gordon positions himself less as a victim than as a faithful believer actively involved in advocating for himself and overcoming severe difficulties, with God as his beacon and backer. This reflects once again the positive, self-reliant John Henryism approach, through which Mr. Gordon asserts a sense of agency in his life in the face of the syndemics of structural racism and ESKD.

Conclusion: Syndemics Exceed the Pandemic

Narrative analysis illuminates how the type of "crisis" that patients like Mr. Gordon face is not terminal and bounded, but chronic and enduring. Racism, poverty, and kidney failure all work hand in hand to exacerbate each one's harmful effect. This syndemic was not initiated nor substantively changed by the pandemic. Attention to narrative features and to silences provides additional insights into which social dimensions matter most for each patient, and how (see Shohet and Samuels 2024). Such insights can be used to help practitioners and policy makers better listen to what is at stake for those under their care or whom they want to aid. Part of such listening involves reading in between the lines to assemble the resources, attitudes, and demeanors needed to alleviate the societal and medical evils and ills that patients chronically face. This work includes understanding how the seemingly protective attitude of John Henryism, when confronting structural racism, often leads to poorer health.

We suggest, based on close listening to dialysis patients' narratives and silences, that addressing suffering requires structural changes in society and coordinated, preventative, and maintenance care. Such an integrated approach could be more effective than simply tackling the individual symptoms of specific illnesses that add to racialized and marginalized ESKD patients' ongoing life struggles. Forging effective alliances with patients will involve learning how to listen, to detect and then mobilize frameworks that are meaningful to them. Thus, closer attention to social environments and the narratives and silences that illuminate them is a crucial part of a long-term, ongoing struggle to dismantle racist structures and battle the social and bodily ills they produce.

Questions for Reflection and Discussion

Reflection Question

1. How have you or someone close to you dealt with long-term illness or chronic conditions? How was language used in discussing care with medical professionals, friends, or family? What was silenced?

Looking In: Small Group Discussion Questions

1. What is structural racism? Provide a definition in your own words and identify some examples from the chapter or other contexts.
2. What are syndemics? Provide a definition in your own words and identify some examples from the chapter or other contexts.
3. What are narrative features? Provide a definition in your own words and identify some examples from the chapter. How does a micro-analytic narrative approach contribute to attempts to understand the lived experiences of patients with kidney failure?
4. What is John Henryism? Based on the examples from Mr. Gordon's narrative, how might it be both helpful and harmful to individuals?

Looking Out: Large Group Discussion Questions

1. How does the chapter utilize the concept of syndemics to discuss the effects of COVID-19, racial and economic disparities, and chronic illness on patients? In what ways does this perspective shift understandings of the pandemic's impact?
2. Imagine you are a case manager working at BMC and you have been assigned a 62-year-old Asian American woman who has been diagnosed with ESKD. Your job is to help the patient manage her chronic illness. Using the chapter as a model, (1) design a set of interview questions that would allow you to understand the complexities of her illness experience; and (2) discuss the analytical approaches you can employ to analyze your interview data.

Acknowledgments

We thank the participants of the study, as well as the editors of this volume and our UROP student researchers Nicole Nguyen, Merilyn Amponsah-Asamoah, Margaret Farr, Guhan Venkatesan, and Xin (Landy) Guo for help with transcription and coding. The study was funded by the Social Science Research Council / Wenner-Gren Foundation (grant SSRC-4393), the Boston University Center for Innovation in Social Science (CISS) faculty research pilot grant, and the Boston University INSPIRE (Innovation Stimulus Pilot in Renal) award.

References

Alexander, Michelle. 2010. *The New Jim Crow Mass Incarceration in the Age of Colorblindness*. New York: New Press.

American Medical Association. 2021. What Is Structural Racism? https://www.ama-assn.org/delivering-care/health-equity/what-structural-racism.

Anderson, Kim, James Collins, Richard David, Michael Lu, Camara Jones, Fleda Jackson, Mona Phillips, and Carol Hogue, dirs. 2014. *Unnatural Causes: Episode 2, When the Bough Breaks*. San Francisco, CA: Kanopy Streaming.

Basso, Keith H. 1970. "To Give up on Words": Silence in Western Apache Culture. *Southwestern Journal of Anthropology* 26(3): pp. 213–230.

Capps, Lisa, and Elinor Ochs. 1995. *Constructing Panic: The Discourse of Agoraphobia*. Cambridge, MA: Harvard University Press.

Davis, Dána-Ain. 2019. *Reproductive Injustice: Racism, Pregnancy, and Premature Birth*. Anthropologies of American Medicine. New York: University Press.

Dragojlovic, Ana, and Annemarie Samuels. 2021. Tracing Silences: Towards an Anthropology of the Unspoken and Unspeakable. *History and Anthropology* 32(4): pp. 417–425. https://doi.org/10.1080/02757206.2021.1954634.

Duvernay, Ava, and Jason Moran, dirs. 2016. *13TH*. Netflix.

Garro, Linda C. 2003. Narrating Troubling Experiences. *Transcultural Psychiatry* 40(1): pp. 5–43. https://doi.org/10.1177/1363461503040001001.

Hamdy, Sherine F. 2008. When the State and Your Kidneys Fail: Political Etiologies in an Egyptian Dialysis Ward. *American Ethnologist* 35(4): pp. 553–569. https://doi.org/10.1111/j.1548-1425.2008.00098.x.

Hannah-Jones, Nikole, dir. 2020. *Untold. 1619: The Legacy of Slavery in America*. Londonderry: Makematic.

Ikels, Charlotte. 2013. The Anthropology of Organ Transplantation. *Annual Review of Anthropology* 42(1): pp. 89–102. https://doi.org/10.1146/annurev-anthro-092611-145938.

James, Sherman A. 1994. John Henryism and the Health of African-Americans. *Culture, Medicine & Psychiatry* 18(2): pp. 163. https://doi.org/10.1007/BF01379448.

Kaufman, Sharon R. 2015. *Ordinary Medicine: Extraordinary Treatments, Longer Lives, and Where to Draw the Line*. Durham, NC: Duke University Press.

Kendi, Ibram X. 2016. *Stamped from the Beginning: The Definitive History of Racist Ideas in America*. New York: Nation Books.

Kleinman, Arthur. 1988. *The Illness Narratives: Suffering, Healing, and the Human Condition*. New York: Basic Books.

Mattingly, Cheryl. 2010. *The Paradox of Hope: Journeys through a Clinical Borderland*. Berkeley, CA: University of California Press.

Mattingly, Cheryl, and Linda C. Garro. 2000. *Narrative and the Cultural Construction of Illness and Healing*. Berkeley, CA: University of California Press.

Robinson, Millicent N., and Courtney S. Thomas Tobin. 2021. Is John Henryism a Health Risk or Resource?: Exploring the Role of Culturally Relevant Coping for Physical and Mental Health among Black Americans. *Journal of Health and Social Behavior* 62(2): pp. 136–151. https://doi.org/10.1177/00221465211009142.

Samuels, Annemarie. 2018. "This Path Is Full of Thorns": Narrative, Subjunctivity, and HIV in Indonesia. *Ethos* 46(1): pp. 95–114. https://doi.org/10.1111/etho.12194.

Samuels, Annemarie. 2019. *After the Tsunami: Disaster Narratives and the Remaking of Everyday Life in Aceh.* Honolulu: University of Hawaii Press.

Schmidt, Insa M., and Sushrut S. Waikar. 2021. Separate and Unequal: Race-Based Algorithms and Implications for Nephrology. *Journal of the American Society of Nephrology* 32(3): pp. 529–533. https://doi.org/10.1681/ASN.2020081175.

Schmidt, Insa M., Merav Shohet, Mariana Serrano, Pranav Yadati, Hanni Menn-Josephy, Titilayo Ilori, Nwamaka D. Eneanya, Emily C. Cleveland Manchanda, and Sushrut S. Waikar. 2023. "Patients' Perspectives on Race and the Use of Race-Based Algorithms in Clinical Decision-Making: A Qualitative Study." *Journal of General Internal Medicine* 38(9): pp. 2045–2051. https://doi.org/10.1007/s11606-023-08035-4.

Sharp, Lesley Alexandra. 2014. *The Transplant Imaginary: Mechanical Hearts, Animal Parts, and Moral Thinking in Highly Experimental Science.* Berkeley, CA: University of California Press.

Shohet, Merav. 2007. Narrating Anorexia: "Full" and "Struggling" Genres of Recovery. *Ethos* 35(3): pp. 344–382. https://anthrosource.onlinelibrary.wiley.com/doi/10.1525/eth.2007.35.3.344.

Shohet, Merav. 2018. Beyond the Clinic? Eluding a Medical Diagnosis of Anorexia through Narrative. *Transcultural Psychiatry* 55(4): pp. 495–515. https://doi.org/10.1177/1363461517722467.

Shohet, Merav. 2021. *Silence and Sacrifice: Family Stories of Care and the Limits of Love in Vietnam.* Berkeley, CA: University of California Press.

Shohet, Merav. 2023. Silenced Resentments and Regrets: Aging in a Changing Kibbutz. *American Anthropologist* 125(4): pp. 896–899. https://doi.org/10.1111/aman.13921.

Shohet, Merav, Nicole H. Nguyen, Lauren D. Stern, Sushrut S. Waikar, and Insa M. Schmidt. 2023. Structural and Psychosocial Challenges among Underserved Patients Receiving Hemodialysis During and Beyond the COVID-19 Pandemic: A Qualitative Study. *Kidney Medicine* 5(11): 100717. https://doi.org/10.1016/j.xkme.2023.100717.

Shohet, Merav, and Annemarie Samuels. 2024. Revisiting and Revisioning Silence and Narrative in Psychological Anthropology. In *Innovations in Psychological Anthropology*, ed. Rebecca J. Lester. New York: Routledge. https://doi.org/10.4324/9781003311713-7.

Singer, Merill, Nicola Bulled, Bayla Ostrach, and Shir Lerman Ginzburg. 2021. Syndemics: A Cross-Disciplinary Approach to Complex Epidemic Events Like COVID-19. *Annual Review of Anthropology* 50: pp. 41–58. https://doi.org/10.1146/annurev-anthro-100919-121009.

Smitherman, Geneva. 1977. *Talkin and Testifyin: The Language of Black America.* Boston, MA: Houghton Mifflin.

Trouillot, Michel-Rolph. 1995. *Silencing the Past: Power and the Production of History.* Boston, MA: Beacon Press.

Wakeel, Fathima, and Anuli Njoku. 2021. Application of the Weathering Framework: Intersection of Racism, Stigma, and COVID-19 as a Stressful Life Event among African Americans. *Healthcare* 9(2): p. 145. https://doi.org/10.3390/healthcare9020145.

Weller, Robert P. 2017. Salvaging Silence: Exile, Death and the Anthropology of the Unknowable. Anthropology of This Century 19. http://aotcpress.com/articles/salvaging-silence/.

11

Water Everywhere, but Is It Safe to Drink?

Risk, Perception, and Public Health in Guatemala

T. S. Harvey

In memory of Dr Paul S. Auerbach, physician, friend, and inspiration

A world of clear water, brilliant-edged, still one would want more, one would need more ...

("The Poems of our Climate," Wallace Stevens 1942; Bloom 1980)

Introduction

To the naked eye, the blue waters of Lake Atitlán, a splendid volcanic crater lake in the heart of Guatemala's western highlands, are a clear and brilliant aquatic world (Figure 11.1). Yet today these same clear waters, reaching depths of over 1,000 feet and covering more than 49 square miles, are contaminated and not fit for human consumption. An estimated 100,000 residents in the surrounding lake towns, mostly Tz'utujil and Kachikel Maya (Indigenous) peoples, depend on the lake as their primary source of water for drinking, bathing, and washing, and another 250,000 rely on it for transportation, and commerce. It is easy to understand how they would want more.

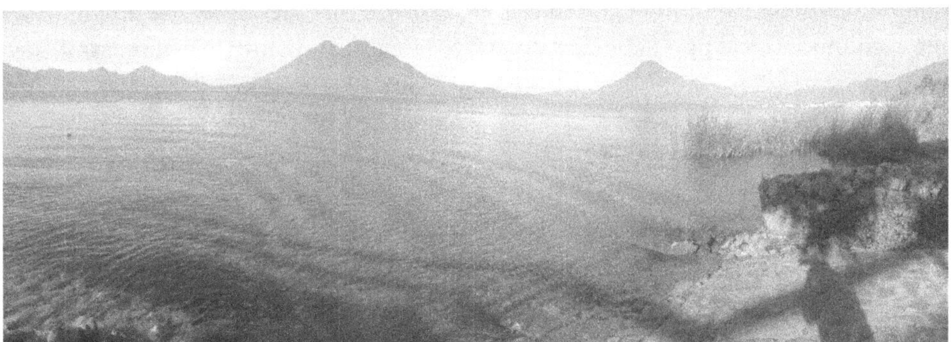

Fig. 11.1 Lake Atitlán from the shores of Panajachel, Department of Sololá, Guatemala. Photograph by the author.

T. S. Harvey, *Water Everywhere, but Is It Safe to Drink?*. In: *Language and Health in Action*. Edited by: Lynnette Arnold et al., Oxford University Press. © T. S. Harvey (2026). DOI: 10.1093/9780198933953.003.0011

What is more difficult to "see," however, is the lake's contamination, episodic toxicity, and risk to human health and aquatic life (Rejmánková et al. 2011). This is what the lake's clear appearance conceals for much of the year. The precarious water conditions result from environmental degradation that has both anthropogenic (human) as well as natural causes, spanning decades (Harvey 2012). From the commonplace to the catastrophic, demographic pressures, agriculture, deforestation, erosion, and the destruction of a wastewater treatment plant in Panajachel in 2005 by Hurricane Stan all contribute to a range of unsafe water conditions. Compounding these problems is the production of an estimated 45,500 cubic meters of wastewater in the Lake Atitlán basin daily, of which only about 20% gets treated (Ferráns et al. 2018).

Inhabitants of towns along the shores of Lake Atitlán who rely on its water want, and in fact need, more than clear water. They need clean water, a term that is defined by the United States Geological Survey (USGS) as "water that will not harm you if you come in contact with it." The transdisciplinary research on which this chapter is based shows that at Lake Atitlán, clean water is, at once, *apparently* everywhere and perplexingly nowhere. Herein lies an underinvestigated paradox and problem not only for the populations surrounding Lake Atitlán, Guatemala, but millions of others in similar environmental, systemic, and infrastructural situations around the globe, as well as those working to reduce the risk of waterborne disease.

What are the public health implications for understanding and managing the potenital risk of waterborne disease in a context where presumably "clear" sources of water are neither clean nor safe to drink? Further, for individual daily health decision making, what happens when the water that people drink doesn't come from the sources they think or have the safeguards in place that they might reasonably assume it does? This chapter explores the answers to these public health questions through close attention to language. I argue that, in any given context, identifying health risks involves context-specific attention both to what appears to be safe to drink or eat, and the way that natural and built environments shape public perceptions about these conditions. Interdisciplinary work that includes close attention to the accounts of local populations is crucial to efforts to ameliorate health risks.

Water as a Health Issue

Before presenting data from my collaborative research in the Atitlán Basin, some background information concerning the epidemiological and global health implications of water is in order. To start with a basic premise of global health, clean water is neither too much to want nor too much to ask. It is an irrefutable human need. The United Nations (UN) General Assembly officially recognizes "the human right to water and sanitation" (UNHRC 2010), and in its concomitant Sustainable Development Goals (UNDP n.d.; 2014), the organization declares that "everyone has the right to sufficient, continuous, safe, acceptable, physically accessible and affordable water for personal and domestic use." However, there is still no universally accepted or maintained standard for drinking water globally.

There is widespread awareness that clean water is not available in many parts of the world. For example, the Centers for Disease Control (CDC) official guidance to US travelers is to "avoid contaminated water during travel." US college students, to take one example, are often told ahead of international travel, some variation of "Don't drink the water. The natives can, but it'll make you sick." Underlying this admonition, partially echoed in the CDC's official guidance to US travelers is an implicit acknowledgement of two things. On the one hand, the existence of unequal access to clean water globally and on the other, albeit indirectly, a normalization of understandings about who does and does not "need" clean water for health. A more generous interpretation, equally revealing, is that it is simply a reminder to US students, who are accustomed to drinking "treated" tap water, that they cannot necessarily do that in other parts of the world. But this also functions to remind them, not so indirectly, that they live in a more "advanced" nation.

Such views inadvertently naturalize the structural violence of unequal access to clean water globally. By **structural violence** I refer to the sorts of "social arrangements that put individuals and populations in harm's way"; they "are structural because they are embedded in the political and economic organization of our social world; they are violent because they cause injury to people" (Farmer et al. 2016). In the context of Lake Atitlán, Guatemala, structural violence involves inadequate water and sanitation systems, built environments, policies, and habitation patterns that expose the lake to non-point source pollutions (run-off), and ecosystems that intersect with infrastructures to expose populations (people, animals, and plants) to the risks of torrential rain, hurricanes, droughts, landslides, and earthquakes. By contrast, **health equality** would be expressed and evidenced by the provision of the same standard of care, or in this case, water safety standards, everywhere and to everyone, regardless of and responsive to differences in geographical location, cultural context, and histories of inequality. The road to the goal of health equality, however, often must pass through **health equity**. In the case of water safety, this means identifying and addressing existing inequalities and securing different resources for different populations according to their context-specific needs and challenges. Taking the UN's position that access to clean drinking water is not only a human need but also a human right, lack of access to safe drinking water reveals social arrangements in which some people are presumed to be somehow less vulnerable to waterborne disease, or worse still, as Farmer might have put it, are not considered "human enough to have that right."

Globally, as of 2022, an estimated 1.7 billion people were using contaminated drinking water sources. In global public health, the greatest drinking-water risk to human health is by far the consumption of water contaminated with fecal coliform (WHO 2023). The term fecal coliform refers to pathogens or disease-causing organisms that are present in the feces of humans and other warm-blooded animals. Regular testing for coliform bacteria is essential for public health and is relatively inexpensive, but testing alone does not ensure or provide clean water.

Public works infrastructures are almost always necessary to ensure clean water, since clean sources of water for drinking that are naturally free of harmful contaminants are rare. Instead, water treatment plants are usually needed to regularly test for microbial contamination and provide water purification.

One of the characteristic health consequences of drinking contaminated water is diarrhea. Although short stints of diarrhea are not typically dangerous to otherwise healthy adults, repeated or ongoing exposure to contaminants can lead to chronic diarrhea, which can be extremely dangerous. Globally, diarrhea is still the leading cause of preventable death among children in the developing world, making its reduction and prevention a global priority. This study argues that this goal is complicated in some contexts by the presence of clear water that is perplexingly not clean.

Study Overview

A World Bank report on global health inequality found that 55% of the population of Guatemala was living in poverty and more than half in extreme poverty, making the population among the most underserved globally with respect to clean water and sanitation. These figures persist despite the country having the largest economy in Central America in terms of population (over seventeen million people) and economic activity (a gross domestic product (GDP) of US$92.7 billion in 2022). Causes of contemporary poverty include, but are not limited to, legacies of European colonialism, western interventionism, a thirty-six-year civil war, genocide, discrimination, political instability, economic inequality, and infrastructural vulnerability to climate change. According to the World Health Organization (WHO), in Guatemala, "diarrheal diseases accounted for 7% of deaths and 8% of disability-adjusted life years among children under 5 years of age," resulting "in approximately 30% of Guatemalan children suffering from diarrhea, about 35% in rural areas and 25% in urban centers" (Vásquez and Aksan 2015).

Against this public health backdrop, I assembled a multidisciplinary, international research team to develop a collaborative project that would support multisectoral (government, non-government, community, and scientific) efforts aimed at reducing the risk of waterborne disease at Lake Atitlán. The impetus for this research comes from my long-term involvement as a researcher, community organizer, and public health collaborator in Guatemala. Trained as a linguistic and medical anthropologist, I have worked for more than two decades with Maya communities on a range of health- and environmental-related issues, including Maya intracultural therapeutic care, cross-cultural biomedical clinical interactions, environmental health and social justice, waterborne disease, and risk communication in disaster management and crisis response.

The study's design used what is called a **One Health** approach. The CDC broadly describes the One Health framework as "a collaborative, multisectoral, and transdisciplinary approach—working at the local, regional, national, and global levels—with the goal of achieving optimal health outcomes recognizing the interconnection between people, animals, plants, and their shared environment" (CDC 2025). Our study adopted and elaborated on this approach to investigate waterborne disease with a focus on prevalence and transmission at the intersections of water, animals, food, society, and health communication. In alignment with One Health, the research team for the study, by design, included underrepresented Indigenous and non-Indigenous Guatemalan scientists, physicians, governmental and non-governmental environmental organization partners, community leaders, and Maya stakeholders from the Lake Atitlán area. As a Spanish and Maya speaker, I worked with this team of partners and collaborators on every aspect of the project from community outreach and data collection to analysis and information sharing.

One primary method used for the transdisciplinary study was water collection and testing. Local Guatemalan field researchers, trained in environmental science and anthropological methods, collected over one hundred water samples from households across a range of socioeconomic and demographic groups. Samples were collected across all geographic sectors of Santiago Atitlán, a city located on the shores of Lake Atitlán. The samples were collected in sterile (disposable) lab bottles, incubated in a clean and temperature-controlled environment at 44.5 degrees Celsius, and tested for bacteria (e.g., E coli or Escherichia coli) using Watersafe test kits (see Figure 11.2). These tests are calibrated to US Environmental Protection Agency (EPA) reliability standards. Pairing the results from the water sample testing with Geographic Information System (GIS) mapping, we were able to precisely map the geographic distribution of municipal water determined to be contaminated with fecal coliform throughout the town. Results from the water testing were analyzed and shared with collaborating Guatemalan environmental scientists at El Centro de Estudios del Mar y Acuicultura (CEMA), at the Universidad de San Carlos in Guatemala City, as well as with the team's wilderness medicine expert at Stanford University.

In addition to documenting the presence of contaminated water in the community, members of the research team conducted over 250 in-depth ethnographic interviews with town residents in order to identify and understand people's perceptions of the risk of waterborne disease. These interviews and our follow-up consultations with local stakeholders were conducted in each participant's language(s) of choice: Tz'utujil or Kachikel (Maya languages) or Spanish. To transcribe the audio recordings of these interviews, I worked together with Maya research assistants who were native speakers of the respective languages of each interview.

To analyze study data I drew on James Gibson's landmark theory of "affordances" (Gibson 1986) from the field of psychology to interpret our findings regarding the distribution of water contamination and local risk perception surrounding water sources, safety, and water use (drinkability). The aim was not only to better understand risk and vulnerability in the wider context of global public health and waterborne disease, but also to create a transdisciplinary framework that could help reduce them.

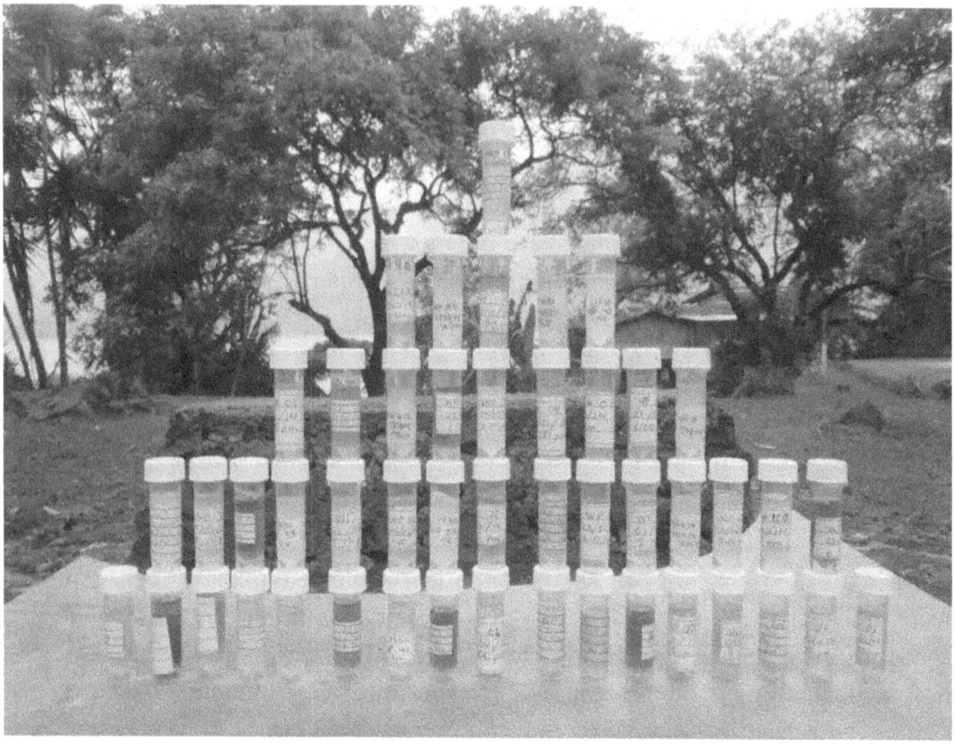

Fig. 11.2 One set of community water samples tested using "Watersafe testkits."
Photograph by the author.

Before presenting the findings from our research, in the next section, I describe a recent historical case of a dangerous algal bloom in the lake. My focus in this section is on the language that was used in a health communication campaign that authorities launched in response to the environmental crisis. The recommendations and language from this campaign may have shaped local perceptions and expectations about water in unintended yet consequential ways.

Health Communication during a Water Contamination Crisis

Two years prior to our study, a massive cyanobacteria bloom carpeted 76% of Lake Atitlán and miles of shorelines in a dense, lentil soup-like mat of bacteria (see Figure 11.3). Cyanobacteria are a group of bacteria distinct from but often linked to cyanoHABS, i.e. cyanobacterial harmful algal blooms that "threaten people, animals, or the environment" (CDC 2009:2). This bloom exposed thousands of people who depend on the lake as a primary water source to a poorly understood and mismanaged environmental health crisis.

Public health officials working at Lake Atitlán during the cyanobacteria bloom of 2009 posted hundreds of flyers instructing the public on how to obtain safe drinking

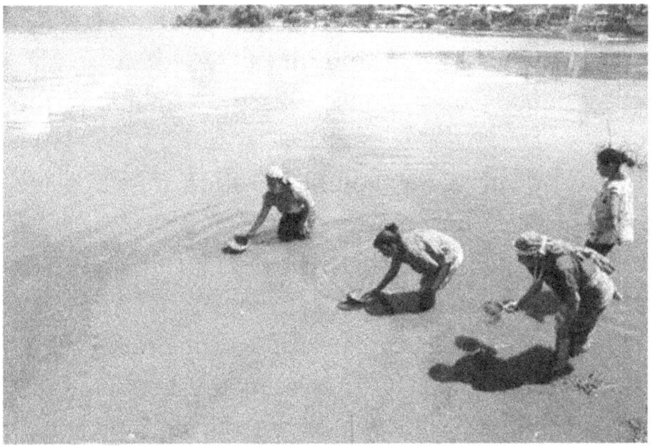

Fig. 11.3 Tz'utujil Maya women wading into a cyanobacteria bloom in Lake Atitlán, Guatemala. Photograph Prensa Libre.

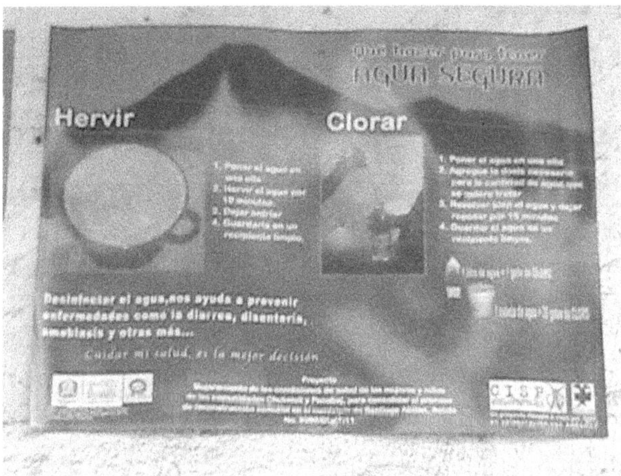

Fig. 11.4 Public health poster, Lake Atitlán, "What to Do in Order to Have Safe Water."

water during the height of the crisis. The now infamous poster entitled "Qué Hacer Para Tener Agua Segura" (What to Do to Have Safe Water) contained dangerously inaccurate recommendations (see Figure 11.4).

Wrongly assuming that the cyanobacteria could be treated as other common pathogens like fecal coliform in water, the officials who designed the posters urged residents to use conventional methods of home water purification, to boil water and chlorinate it by adding bleach. Under most circumstances, the purification methods described in the poster would have been good public health advice. However, given the microbiology of cyanobacteria, if followed, the methods listed would amplify rather than eliminate the potential health risk to residents. According to research in toxicology, boiling or chlorinating water containing cyanobacteria kills the bacteria, but because cyanotoxins can either attach themselves to the outside of cyanobacteria or exist within them, boiling and chlorinating water can also release cyanotoxins, actually increasing the amount of free toxins in the water (Hitzfeld, Hoger, and Dietrich 2000) and, consequently, amplifying the health risk of drinking it.

In addition to this and other risk communication missteps around waterborne disease during cyanobacteria outbreaks on Lake Atitlán (Harvey 2012), one public health message to local populations that was successful to a fault was the idea that visibly dirty water, untreated, was not drinkable. People were given to understand that visibly dirty, murky, or cloudy water was unsafe. Unfortunately, one unintended and inaccurate conclusion that people may have deduced from this health communication was that visibly clear water was a reliable sign of clean, drinkable water. The linguistic/semantic relationships of analogy and antonymy are helpful for illustrating a potential cognitive pathway for this rationality. If "unclear" or otherwise "murky" equals "undrinkable," then people may be inclined to expect an analogous relationship to exist between the antonyms, that is, the idea that "clear" equals "drinkable."

Water Sources, Water Contamination, and Water Perceptions in Santiago de Atitlán

Lake Atitlán is the primary water source for most residents of Santiago de Atitlán. Water from the lake reaches homes via a municipal infrastructure, pump stations, holding treatment tanks, and a network of pipes. Residents refer to this piped water as "running water" and routinely utilize it for drinking, cooking, and in many households, bathing. Notably, this system differs from those in some neighboring towns, where water is piped into homes from municipal wells.

Results of the water sample analysis from our study revealed that 75% of the household water supplies in Santiago de Atitlán tested positive for fecal coliform (see Figure 11.5). This high rate of contamination reveals that the majority of town residents at the time of the study were being exposed to disease-causing contaminants whenever they used water from the faucets in their homes or from private and public *pilas*, wash basins with running water.

My analysis of interviews with city residents revealed local ways of speaking (Hymes 1962) and perceptions about the risks associated with water sources and water use. Initially, some of the interviewees' statements seemed contradictory, but on closer examination these apparent contradictions revealed important patterns. My interpretation of interviewees' responses was aided by thinking in terms of perception, adapting aspects of James Gibson's theory of affordances in order to think about how visual appearances and language shape the action possibilities (i.e., choices) that are associated with water.

The exchange in Example 11.1 represents a typical response to one of our interview questions about risk.

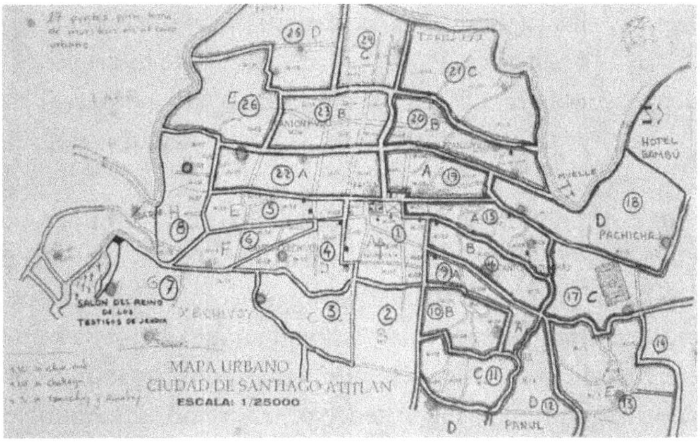

Fig. 11.5 Map documenting contaminated household water sources in Santiago de Atitlán.

Example 11.1

(01)	Researcher:	K'ol k'yiwaal k'aan ja ya' tap nataj?	Does drinking the water pose any risk?
(02)	Respondent:	Majon naq ri' yival rk'an ja ya' taq nataaj chaqaa maj'on nokrtz'ilata.	There is neither risk to drinking the water nor does it have any effect.

This interviewee's response, and many others like it, might at first suggest that people were unaware of water contamination. However, our hundreds of ethnographic interviews on Maya perceptions of the risk of waterborne disease in Santiago Atitlán were also replete with what amounted, for outsiders, to head spinning contradictions that seemed to resist straightforward interpretations. Example 11.2 is emblematic of these complexities and their would-be illogicalities, illustrating the kinds of difficult and reasoned assessments that vulnerable populations have to make daily in evaluating whether the water that is available to them may be safe or unsafe to drink.

Example 11.2

(01)	Researcher	Ab'aar tzara kolwa ja ya'nataj i naq xub'an xwanqerpa?	Where do you get the water that you drink and where does it come from?
(02)	Respondent	Utz nataj majo'on tziil chik qanaq chupaam ja qa ya' kitjoon je ch'uu je chikopa kitjoon lee nataj chick tee nuya je yub'ilaal.	The water is good to drink because there is no trash in the lake. Also, the animals drink the water. We have drunk the water, and there are no illnesses.

(03) Researcher	Jaa ya' rixin tinamit tz'utujil qas utz nataj?	Is the water of Lake Atitlán safe to drink?
(04) Respondent	Majoon utz ta pik kola chik je' tiziil chapaam.	No, because it is contaminated.

This deceivingly straightforward exchange, taken from an ethnographic interview conducted between two Maya-speaking townspeople (without the presence of foreign researchers), points to the local use of a range of evaluative measures to reach an empirically and sensorially informed assessment about whether a source of water is drinkable. Note that the respondent (interviewee) identifies four kinds of evidence used to assess drinkability: (1) the absence of trash and/or turbidity in the water (clarity); (2) observation of animals unharmed by drinking the water; (3) a past history of having drunk water from the source; and (4) the absence of the experience of illness after consumption.

A final interview excerpt (Example 11.3) illuminates one of the key reasons why town residents often considered water to be safe.

Example 11.3

(01) Researcher:	Ab'aar tzara kolwa ja ya'nataj i naq xub'an xwanqerpa?	Where do you get the water that you drink and where does it come from?
(02) Respondent:	Kintaj ya' rxinn pa chorro (agua potable).	I drink water from the faucet, potable water.

This response demonstrates that local Maya residents' perceptions of the risk of waterborne disease was informed by the infrastructure of piped water. Piped water from household *chorros* (faucets), commonly referred to as "running water" was locally understood as a "secure source," and as such, considered drinkable (potable). That is, because it was piped, it was considered not only clean but not lake water at all. This conflation is highlighted though not mirrored, cross-culturally, in the North American distinction between so-called "fresh" water and salt water, where the "fresh" is not indicative of it being potable but rather it having negligible salinity levels, similar to Spanish use of *agua dulce* (sweet) and *agua salada* (salt) water.

Discussion

From a risk-perception point of view, how is it possible to make sense of the many local observations that asserted that the lake water was at once safe to drink and yet contaminated? Given that our findings from water testing indicated that water contamination was pervasive in Santiago de Atitlán, a reductive interpretation of this perceptual complexity might conclude that indigenous Mayas simply misunderstand the risk of waterborne disease. It is important, however, to resist jumping to conclusions and to reject the temptation of defining what is not familiar—the would-be illogicalities of "Native" risk perceptions—as merely the product of "local" ignorance, illiteracy, or worse, a fault or feature of Indigenous culture. Such judgments relegate unfamiliar ways of knowing and being in the world to residual categories of "backward," lacking, and or otherwise underdeveloped.

Instead, a close linguistic and cultural analysis of interviewee responses and of public health and environmental communication in the Lake Atitlán region suggests several intersecting reasons why residents sometimes perceived the water in their homes and in the lake as safe and other times as unsafe.

One reason stems from the unreliable indicator of water clarity and the ways that health communication in the region has historically invoked ideas of dirtiness or murkiness in warnings about unsafe water. Adapting aspects of Gibson's ecological approaches to visual perception to the analysis of waterborne disease risk perception, our study considered the *apparent* and overwhelmingly imposing visual clarity of Lake Atitlán, as both a perceived property of the water and an aspect of the environment. We further considered how this appearance provided observers, who relied on the lake for life and livelihood, with a number of apparent "affordances" and "action possibilities" or choices. Chiefly among those with which we have been concerned here is the perception that "clear water," in particular, as a substance contrasted with, for example, murky or dirty water, *appears* clean. The lay observation of a perceived distinct contrast between "clear" and murky or dirty water was important to understanding local perceptions of risk in the context of Lake Atitlán.

Another factor influencing local perceptions of risk and safety stemmed from the fact that lake water reached most households in Santiago de Atitlán via municipal pipes. The conflation of water clarity and low risk or drinkability was compounded by the infrastructure used to pipe "clear," yet un- and/or undertreated water into homes and public *pilas*. Piped or so-called "improved water sources," then, seem to afford the public presumption of drinkability, in part because pipes and faucets are indices of human intervention (construction and technology), and in a fundamental way appear protected from outside contamination.

Seen through the lens of perceptions of "clear" water flowing through pipes, the once perplexing responses of local Maya peoples to the study's ethnographic questions about whether or not they drink lake water become clearer. Locals reported that they did not drink the water from Lake Atitlán because, in their words, "it is contaminated," but they did drink household (piped) water from their *chorros* faucets because "there is neither risk to drinking the water nor does it have any effect." The public health messages that urged residents to *not* drink lake water during the cyanobacteria outbreak, over legitimate concerns of waterborne disease, sadly missed the mark and the ethnography of risk communication revealed the reasons. Interviews show that most people thought that public health messages concerning lake water did not apply to them because they were not aware that the piped household water that they were drinking came from the lake rather than municipal wells, as is the case in some nearby towns.

Maya communities at Lake Atitlán, Guatemala, are not alone in their complex perceptions and sometimes contradictory behaviors surrounding perceptions of water safety, which as we have alluded, could unintentionally induce vulnerability and public health risk.

To consider the breadth of the problem, we need only consider the inconspicuous role that "piped" water plays in the WHO's evolving definition of "secure water sources" or "improved water sources." While terms like these may describe legitimate infrastructural improvements and the expansion of access, they are not necessarily synonymous with the availability of safe water supplies. Like the striking visible appearance of water clarity at Lake Atitlán for much of the year, and its link to local perceptions of "clear" as "clean" with which we began this chapter, I contend that discourses and assumptions surrounding "piped water," as part of the "built" rather than the "natural" environment, may lead millions of people worldwide to inaccurate conclusions concerning water safety and therefore drinkability.

"Piped water," where infrastructural inequalities exist, does not necessarily correlate to improved water quality. When the water running through pipes is untreated, undertreated, or otherwise contaminated, the fact that it is piped (protected from contamination en route) may mean very little to human health. Barring viable alternative information and sources, untreated piped water (and dilapidated infrastructures in general) can amount to a perception of drinkability that increases rather than reduces a population's risk and vulnerability.

Furthermore, when access to piped water is used uncritically as a poverty diagnostic or as an indicator of health equity, it can mask rather than reveal infrastructural inequalities. When official documents, for example, refer to "piped water" as an "improved water source" it may be wrongly equated with "access to clean drinking water." This can lead to such apparently positive but misleading statements as "91% of the population [had] access to improved drinking water" and "53% of the population [in Guatemala had] access to improved sanitation" (World Bank 2018). In these cases, the descriptor "improved" fails to account for actual water safety (drinkability). Understanding structural violence, not only theoretically but contextually, as in this case, requires identifying the social arrangements that cause harm. In this context, "the cultural history" (Viniegra-Velázquez 2008) of waterborne disease, includes not only environmental degradation and infrastructure inequality (Harvey 2012) but also institutional language, categories, policies, and practices that conceal this structural violence (Harvey 2015).

Conclusion

Our findings about water safety and risk perception in Santiago de Atitlán are important beyond the context of this Guatemalan town. Access to safe water is one of the most pressing global health issues today, and it is not a problem that is confined to countries that are characterized as "developing." In many places, piped water coming out of the faucets in people's homes is not safe to drink. Consider recent examples of Flint, Michigan (2014) and Jackson, Mississippi (2022) in the United States. Both crises involved threats to public health by way of household drinking water. In Flint, the problem was caused by lead in drinking water that leached from old pipes, while in Jackson, water quality and safety of drinking water was impacted by aging infrastructure and untreated water. The fact that water in both of these cities was piped (presumably improved) helped to afford the public a perception of clean water, when in fact it was not, inadvertently increasing the public's vulnerability to the risk of waterborne disease caused by neglected infrastructure (and linked to structural inequalities).

This observation on perception is also powerfully expressed in the existential philosophy of Jean Paul Sartre who, in his book, *Being and Nothingness*, notes that the reality of any given phenomenon, "remains relative because its 'appearing' necessarily implies someone to whom it appears. [...] It does not indicate, behind its shoulder some true being, a being that is itself the absolute" (Sartre 2018:2). Applied to this case, Sartre's observation is a helpful reminder that because "clear" water appears "clean," whether it actually is or not, people are likely to consider it drinkable until it is understood or experienced otherwise.

In the same way that water clarity (in nature) can wrongly imply cleanliness and drinkability, (in practice) untreated and undertreated "tap water" or even "fresh" water piped into homes and made available in public space can suggest to the public that these sources have been improved (made drinkable). In this scenario, it is the built human environment (pipes and faucets) that can unwittingly induce a false sense of water security, reducing the precautions that people might otherwise take to protect their health with water sources not presumed to be safe for drinking.

The research presented in this chapter brings together environmental science, an affordance framework, and innovative interdisciplinary methods for understanding and mapping the complex risk of waterborne disease. This approach has the potential to advance public health understandings of how the complex relationships between risk perception and physical environment can come together in what Gibson (1986) called 'action possibilities' (clues in the environment that point to possibilities for action) that inform decision-making and behaviors. By seeking to develop better frameworks for understanding and predicting complex global public health problems today, we will be better able to disrupt the processes that produce them, reducing risks and vulnerabilities, and improving health tomorrow. Notably, the problems of infrastructure inequality and lack of access to clean drinking water cannot be solved by improvements in how researchers study public perceptions of risk alone, or even through improvements in risk communication, though these are critically important. If clean water is to be a human right that is afforded to everyone, it must become a global responsibility, secured, maintained, and delivered by a universally accepted standard for everyone, everywhere.

Acknowledgments

This research was conducted with funding and support from an Environmental Protection Agency (EPA) Cooperative Agreement Grant and a Fulbright Award from the International Institute of Education (IIE).

Questions for Reflection and Discussion

Reflection Questions

1. What public health messaging or popular media discussions have you seen about contaminated water or food where you live? If you have not seen such messages, why do you think this might be?
2. Have you ever been told to avoid drinking the water in a place you lived or visited? If so, how did you access drinking water while you were there? What precautions did you take, and what resources were required for you to get clean water?

Looking In: Small Group Discussion Questions

1. What is structural violence and what are its impacts on health? How do the issues of contamination and access to drinking water in Guatemala illustrate structural violence and its health consequences?
2. What is health equality? What about health equity? Define and contrast these terms in your own words. Come up with an example of each with regards to water safety protocols.
3. What is the One Health framework? How can this perspective, when combined with social science research, help to identify how the environment and cultural understandings of the environment shape disease risk, prevalence, and transmission?
4. What messages about "clean water" were included in public health communication during the cyanobacteria bloom at Lake Atitlán? How might these messages have impacted people's risk perception related to water?

Looking Out: Large Group Discussion Questions

1. What specific observations and beliefs do people in the Lake Atitlán region rely on to assess whether water is clean and safe to drink? How do these understandings inform their perceptions of the risk of waterborne disease? What do these patterns suggest about how people in different settings might approach the problem of evaluating water and food safety?

2. Rather than dismissing Mayan Guatemalans' understandings of risk as illogical or uneducated, this chapter takes these understandings seriously. What do these local understandings reveal about the language that global health agencies use in official reports, for example describing piped water systems as "improved water sources"?
3. What are the benefits of using transdisciplinary methods to study health hazards, for example designing a study that combines water sample testing, mapping, and ethnographic interviews?

References

Bloom, Harold. 1980. *Wallace Stevens: The Poems of Our Climate*. Ithaca, NY: Cornell University Press.

CDC (Centers for Disease Control). 2009. Harmful Agal Blooms. Facts about Cyanobacteria and Cyanobacterial Harmful Algal Blooms. http://www.cdc.gov/hab/cyanobacteria/pdfs/facts.pdf.

CDC. 2025. About One Health. One Health, July 3. https://www.cdc.gov/one-health/about/index.html.

Farmer, Paul, Bruce Nizeye, Sara Stulac, and Salmaan Keshavjee. 2016. Structural Violence and Clinical Medicine. *Understanding and Applying Medical Anthropology* 3(10): pp. 336–343. https://doi.org/10.1371/journal.pmed.0030449.

Ferráns, Laura, Serena Caucci, Jorge Cifuentes, Tamara Avellán, Christina Dornack, and Hiroshan Hettiarachchi. 2018. *Wastewater Management in the Basin of Lake Atitlán: A Background Study.* United Nations University Institute for Integrated Management of Material Fluxes and of Resources (UNU-FLORES).

Gibson, James J. 1986. *The Ecological Approach to Visual Perception*. Mahwah, NJ: Lawrence Erlbaum Associates.

Harvey, T. S. 2012. Cyanobacteria Blooms: Maya Peoples between the Politics of Risk and the Threat of Disaster. *Medical Anthropology* 31(6): pp. 477–496.

Harvey, T. S. 2015. Muddying the Waters: Protection, Public Participation, and Ambiguity in the Language of Pollution in the Great Lakes. *Culture, Agriculture, Food and Environment* 37(2): pp. 107–115.

Hitzfeld, Bettina C., Stefan J. Höger, and Daniel R. Dietrich. 2000. Cyanobacterial Toxins: Removal during Drinking Water Treatment, and Human Risk Assessment. *Environmental Health Perspectives* 108(suppl 1): pp. 113–122.

Hymes, Dell. 1962. The Ethnography of Speaking. *Anthropology and Human Behavior* 13(53): pp. 11–74.

Rejmánková, Eliška, Jiří Komárek, Margaret Dix, Jaroslava Komárková, and Nancy Girón. 2011. Cyanobacterial Blooms in Lake Atitlan, Guatemala. *Limnologica* 41(4): pp. 296–302.

Sartre, J. P. 2018. *Being and Nothingness: An Essay in Phenomenological Ontology*. London: Routledge.

United Nations Human Rights Council (UNHRC). 2010. *Resolution on the Human Right to Safe Drinking Water and Sanitation.* Geneva: UNHRC; Resolution A/HRC/RES/15/9.

UNDP (United Nations Development Programme). n.d. Sustainable Development Goals. Accessed July 25, 2025. https://www.undp.org/sustainable-development-goals.

UNDP. 2014. *Human Development Report 2014—Sustaining Human Progress: Reducing Vulnerabilities and Building Resilience.* New York: UNDP.

Vásquez, William F., and Anna-Maria Aksan. 2015. Water, Sanitation, and Diarrhea Incidence among Children: Evidence from Guatemala. *Water Policy* 17(5): pp. 932–945.

Viniegra-Velázquez, Leonardo. 2008. La historia cultural de la enfermedad. *Revista de Investigación Clínica* 60(6): pp. 527–544.

WHO (World Health Organization). 2023. Drinking Water. https://www.who.int/news-room/fact-sheets/detail/drinking-water.

World Bank. 2018. Key Findings of the Water Supply, Sanitation, and Hygiene (WASH) Poverty Diagnostic Guatemala. https://thedocs.worldbank.org/en/doc/693261528124154204-0090022018/render/Draftwpdgtinfo.pdf.

12
Introducing *Xka Pastora*, One of the World's Newest "Drugs"

Paja Faudree

Meet a Magical Plant

Let me begin with stories.

Or, rather, let me tell a story then open the door to another.

These stories concern a plant sometimes called "magic mint" (Figure 12.1).

But people also use other names to denote the plant, including *Salvia divinorum*, its scientific name. In everyday language in the US and elsewhere, people sometimes call the plant simply "salvia," even though the genus *Salvia* has nearly 1,000 species that are widely used as ornamental plants and culinary herbs.

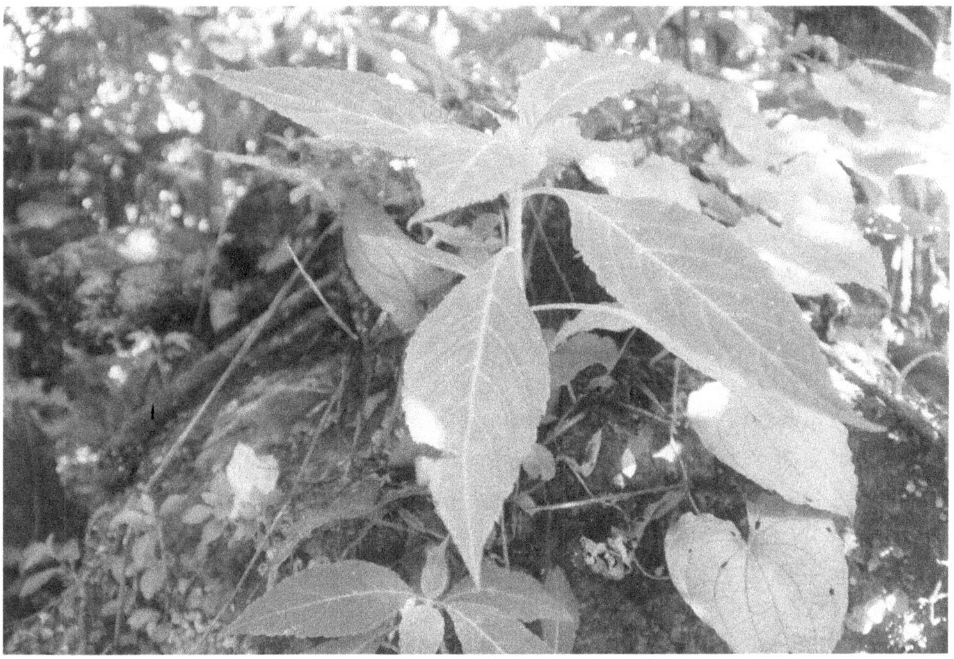

Fig. 12.1 *Xka pastora* growing in the Sierra Mazateca.
Photo: Paja Faudree.

Paja Faudree, *Introducing Xka Pastora, One of the World's Newest "Drugs"*. In: *Language and Health in Action*. Edited by: Lynnette Arnold et al., Oxford University Press. © Paja Faudree (2026). DOI: 10.1093/9780198933953.003.0012

A few things, though, set this salvia apart from others. It is psychedelic, containing psychoactive substances that affect the human nervous system by inducing altered states of consciousness ("trips") and may involve visual and auditory changes ("visions" or "hallucinations"). Other psychedelics include LSD, mescaline, psilocybin, and ayahuasca. The wider category of psychoactive drugs includes not only illegal drugs like cocaine and heroin but also legal ones such as alcohol, nicotine, and caffeine. Some psychoactive substances, including salvia, are recreational "street drugs" in some forms (e.g., heroin) but medical treatments in others (e.g., morphine) (Courtwright 2001). The effects from ingesting salvia are short-lived but extremely intense, and forms of the plant are now used by young people and others in countries across the world. This context gives salvia's history broader relevance—and shows why people who have never heard of the plant, let alone used it, can benefit from learning more about it.

Another unique aspect of the plant is that it is endemic only to one spot on the globe: the Sierra Mazateca, a mountainous region of Oaxaca, Mexico. Although the plant was largely unknown outside the Sierra prior to 2000, it is now sold worldwide as a recreational drug. In fact, the plant is also called "the YouTube drug" thanks to the prevalence and popularity of online "trip videos" that feature users smoking the plant. Additionally, biomedical researchers are actively exploring its pharmaceutical potential. Its psychoactive molecule, salvinorin A, is one of the most powerful naturally occurring psychedelics, twenty times more potent than psilocybin and comparable in strength to LSD. That and other distinctive qualities make analyzing the plant doubly promising for pharmacological researchers who hope to develop novel—and patentable—pharmaceuticals and treatments based on the molecule. Emerging research indicates its derivatives could one day treat such maladies as chronic pain, arthritis, inflammation, mood disorders, anxiety, schizophrenia, Alzheimer's disease, gastrointestinal dysfunction, malignant brain tumors, and substance abuse.

I begin with the story about how scientists first learned of the plant. Though that tale is the most widely known, other stories about the plant offer a radically different perspective. Those include the second of the stories I mentioned, which provides a very different way of narrating the life of this humble plant and the people who have long cared for it, just as the plant has taken care of them. Not widely known outside the Sierra, this story is one I know only because I lived in the region for several years as an ethnographer. While scientists refer to the plant as *Salvia divinorum* and recreational users call it "salvia," Sierra people identify the plant with the name they've used as far back as anyone now living can remember: *xka pastora* (pronounced "shkah pah-STOH-rah") or "leaf of the Shepherdess." Their name is linked to other language usage that differs dramatically from the discourses that outsiders use. For example, to people from the Sierra, the plant isn't an "it" but a "she": a female earth spirit who guides her human interlocutors toward the truth.

When I talk about the plant, I use the Sierra name, *xka pastora.* I also use feminine pronouns to reflect what people in the Sierra shared with me and to honor their perspectives, as the people who have cared for and learned from the plant for so long. This view is also supported by my reading of scientific research. Many botanists believe *xka pastora* is a cultigen—meaning she was created through "artificial selection." Agriculture and other forms of domesticating the natural world depend upon such deliberate human actions, which have produced animals like dogs, cows, and chickens; and crops like wheat, corn, peas, peanuts, and rice. Scientific research also tells us that *xka pastora* rarely produces seeds. Instead, she tends to reproduce vegetatively (through asexual "cloning" rather than sexual reproduction) and survives today primarily because humans purposefully grow her. This research clearly implies that people from the Sierra are fundamentally responsible, at multiple levels, for the plant's existence today.

However, scientists and others writing about *xka pastora* never tell her story that way. They skip right over the fact that Sierra people not only birthed the plant but have also cared for and protected her for centuries, even when faced with brutal repression dating back to colonial era Inquisition trials, during which the Catholic Church used violence to prevent Indigenous people from continuing traditions it considered heretical. Church authorities were particularly savage in attacking people who used psychoactive plants (Chuchiak 2012).

I use the name *xka pastora* and otherwise mirror how people from the Sierra talk about her to help repair the damage caused when outsiders renamed the plant. Though it might appear simple and innocuous, that act of renaming was profound; it produced significant changes not just in how people talk but also in the tangible world. In renaming the plant, outsiders changed *xka pastora* herself: converting her from a plant that—to people from the Sierra—was a living being, worthy of reverence and love, into a mere object. By renaming her, outsiders also erased her ties to the people in her birthplace and homeland.

This is an example of what I call **discursive violence**: ways of talking about things that produce harm. Note "discursive" is the adjectival form of discourse; and while "discourse" can mean many things, I use it to indicate forms of communication, oral or written, that may also include non-verbal elements such as visual images. In aiming to mitigate discursive violence, I try to recover how people in the Sierra engage with *xka pastora*. This process advances what I call **discursive transformation**: forms of communication intended to change the world around us by correcting problematic discourses that advance injustice. I call the plant *xka pastora* to make visible the central place of the Sierra's people in the plant's past and present, to provide a history that critiques existing public stories, and to help reverse the ways Sierra people are regularly erased from stories about their plant.

When juxtaposed against each other, these different ways of engaging with the plant through language illustrate a central point of this essay: that stories create the world. As a poet once wrote, "The universe is made of stories, / not of atoms" (Rukeyser 2006:675). The tales we tell about "drugs" and other commodities—or those we tell in the name of "advancing science"—create the things we are talking about as particular realities, as specific objects. Such stories also create us as subjects: as particular kinds of people with specific identities. But this positive, meaning-generating force of stories is also inalienably linked to its negative side: stories can also be agents of violence, weapons that hurt people and destroy realities.

Many widespread discourses—including claims about scientific discovery that are often accepted uncritically—are full of the violent erasures we see in the most common stories about *xka pastora*. The "discovery" of the plant shows how the production of "scientific knowledge" is intimately linked to extractive, colonial, profit-driven practices, including those central to the pharmaceutical industry and to biomedicine in general. Though we rarely think about them in these terms, the ways we talk about scientific and medical truth depend on systematic erasures and distortions: forms of discursive violence with profound material effects that can harm people in tangible ways.

Discursive Violence in the "Discovery" of *Salvia divinorum*

One of the most widely circulating stories about *xka pastora* concerns how she became known to science. The history of biomedicine is full of such tales of "discovery"—a word I place in quotation marks to invite a critical reading. The term invokes the fifteenth-century "Doctrine of Discovery," a legal and moral cornerstone of colonialism. It contended that lands not inhabited by Christians were available to be "discovered" and possessed such that the inhabitants could be converted to Christianity, thereby saving their souls. That doctrine provided the justification for European colonization of the Americas and beyond, including the United States' own western expansion.

The tale of *xka pastora's* "discovery" is linked to another story—a different but related "discovery" that also took place in the Sierra Mazateca. That earlier story involves psilocybin-containing "magic mushrooms," which grow across the Sierra. The history of their "discovery" is an important frame of reference for Sierra people, who understand outsiders' interest in *xka pastora* through this prior encounter with extractive colonialism.

In the mid-twentieth century, researchers "discovered" that people from the Sierra were using psilocybin mushrooms ritually (e.g., Johnson 1939). This was stunning news. Although Indigenous people throughout what is now Mexico and Central America had practiced mushroom ceremonies for centuries before Europeans arrived, most historians thought the Catholic Church had brutally eliminated those traditions during the colonial era. For many years, this "discovery" of living psychedelic mushroom traditions was known mostly to a small number of scholars. However, amid the counter-culture movement and Psychedelic Revolution, the "discovery" of psychoactive mushroom use was trumpeted in popular publications that sparked global interest (e.g., Wasson 1957). The resulting attention thrust the Sierra and its people into the international spotlight for the first time, and hippies flocked to the region by the busload throughout the 1960s and 1970s in search of its now-famous mushrooms.

Stories about the "discovery" of the mushrooms—and the uncritical dissemination and praise of those stories in the decades since—constitute discursive violence. Broadcasting news of the Sierra's secret and closely guarded traditions had pervasive and powerful material effects for the region's people. While the mushroom trade provided new economic opportunities for some Sierra people, it also induced myriad forms of social trauma, including deep divisions among local people about whether it is right for the mushrooms and rituals to be treated as commodities: things that can be bought and sold through capitalist consumer markets. Popular tales of "discovery" erased the central role that generations of Sierra people had played in learning about and perfecting use of the mushrooms, in defending and renewing that knowledge despite colonial and ongoing threats.

The arrival of mycotourists—my term for mushroom seekers—continues to this day. The more recent commercialization of *xka pastora* builds on this sixty-year history of mycotourism in the Sierra. Commerce in both plants has been stoked, in turn, by the recent "renaissance" in psychedelic medicine. After several decades during which psychedelic research was largely prohibited, it is now resurgent across the world and makes headlines almost daily (Hadar et al. 2023). Amid enthusiasm about psychedelics, tales of "discovery" involving the Sierra's "magic plants" are once again reaching wide audiences who consume them uncritically. This extends the pattern whereby for decades outsiders have talked and written about the region and its people in ways that exoticize them on the one hand and erase their achievements on the other. Earlier tales about the mushrooms established a narrative template through which more recent stories about *xka pastora* perpetuate discursive violence (see Faudree 2015).

The public history of *xka pastora's* "discovery" is not as widely known as that of the mushrooms, but likewise it has been reproduced and disseminated countless times. The author of the most sensationalist writings about the mushrooms subsequently learned about another psychedelic plant that Sierra people use. In 1962, he and other researchers ingested the plant in ceremonies with local people and took away specimens used to classify the plant as a novel species (Epling and Játiva-M. 1962). In the articles they published about the "discovery," they bestowed upon the plant a scientific name, *Salvia divinorum*. In that act of discursive violence, the new name publicly supplanted those that for centuries people in the Sierra had used for her.

But the erasures at the center of *xka pastora's* public history go beyond the change in her name. Almost all published accounts offer at most a brief mention of her past that rarely strays beyond a single sentence. For example, the opening passage from a widely cited, historically important article advancing scientific knowledge about *xka pastora* reads as follows: "*Salvia divinorum* is used by the Mazatec Indians of northeastern Oaxaca, Mexico primarily for its psychoactive effects which aid in ritual divination" (Siebert 1994:53). That boilerplate blip of recognition radically obscures what generations of Sierra people achieved by keeping this remarkable plant alive, and what their labor should entitle them to in the present.

Furthermore, the discursive strategy used in that article is pervasive. It is deployed so uniformly in scientific literature about *xka pastora* that most authors merely rephrase or repeat verbatim the same vague characterizations; sometimes, they get even the basic facts in that one sentence wrong or reproduce the same typographical errors. The few publications offering more context generally jump straight to the plant's "discovery" in the middle of the twentieth century. Through this robust discursive pattern, *xka pastora's* past becomes almost entirely reduced to the history of her appeal to scientific researchers from outside the Sierra.

These habitual ways of talking establish **discursive grooves**: communicative templates that foster specific habits for discussing and interacting with the plant and the people who care for her. Discursive grooves obscure the distance between reality and representation by distorting perception and tacitly shaping how people interact with the world. Put differently, discursive grooves suppress other narratives about reality. The story I discuss in the next section is one such example: a discourse about *xka pastora* that has been forced into the shadows by the boastful and widely repeated assertions made by those who claimed to have "discovered" her.

Before I turn to that story, let me dwell briefly on the material entailments of the most common discursive grooves surrounding *xka pastora*. Established ways of talking about the plant, particularly those advancing scientific knowledge, fundamentally decontextualize her. They dehistoricize and depeople her, stripping her of ties to the people with whom she has lived in shared communities of care since her birth. This decontextualization is essential to the profit-making machinery of the pharmaceutical industry. Through such extractive practices, companies claim ownership in the form of patents over the drugs they develop from *xka pastora*. Companies extract promising medicinal plants from their original contexts; and from those decontextualized plants they extract the molecular substrates for new drugs (see Hayden 2003).

But the extractions aren't just material: at every level, these physical practices are entangled with discursive ones as well. The discourses that researchers and pharmaceutical companies use for plants like *xka pastora*—stories presenting the plants as "products of nature," free from prior claims of ownership or moral obligation, cleansed of any recognition of the labor required to create or protect them—are precisely what makes their physical extraction possible, both legally and ethically. The stories researchers tell about *xka pastora* enable them to pluck her from her context, erase her history, and dismiss as irrelevant the social matrix that surrounds and supports her. That process, in turn, makes it possible to turn the plant into a commodity ripe for consumption and rich in potential to reap profits.

The financial stakes are considerable. One *Forbes* journalist claims that "The psychedelic drug market is projected to soar to $7.2 billion by 2029" (Adams 2023). Even though access to psychedelics remains highly restricted or illegal in countries across the world, several multinational psychedelic companies are already valued above $100 million dollars each. One of the largest, atai Life Sciences, is notable for its rapid growth: founded in 2018, by 2022 its value had grown to $441 million.

Furthermore, the company's success is directly linked to *xka pastora's* fate. One of its subsidiaries, Revixia, focuses exclusively on salvinorin A to develop treatments for "substance use disorder, treatment-resistant depression, and pain" (https://atai.life/revixia-life-sciences/).

An Alternative Story of *Xka Pastora*: Confronting Discursive Violence

The second story I offer about *xka pastora* stems from my personal experience in the Sierra, where I have conducted research since the early 2000s. It is a second home for me and I return almost every year with my family. As a linguistic anthropologist, I was originally drawn to Oaxaca because it is one of the most linguistically diverse places on earth. Despite five centuries of oppression, people living there continue speaking their Indigenous languages. That is more than a demographic fact; Indigenous people across the region are actively working to defend and revitalize their languages. For several years, I lived in the Sierra to learn from and work with people who were using writing, music, and performance to strengthen and renew their languages (Figure 12.2).

Given the Sierra's long and troubled history with psychedelic tourism, when I first arrived there I went out of my way to avoid any talk about shamanism or "magic plants." When people asked, "You're here for the mushrooms?" I self-righteously insisted *no*. I was there, I said, to learn about their language. But over time, I realized that attitude was keeping me from hearing people when they told me that using sacred plants is essential to how they engage with their language. Many songwriters I worked with, for example, said they learned to write music because the mushrooms taught them.

Once I got better at listening, I began to understand how thoroughly interaction with sacred plants like *xka pastora* is embedded in social life in the Sierra. An important event in my dawning awareness of how deeply the plant and the Sierra's people are bound to each other occurred when I met *xka pastora* for the first time. The mother of the family I was living with, knowing I love spicy food, sent me into the garden for chili peppers. While I was poking around out there, I noticed that off to the side, hiding in the shadows, was a plant bent into an arc: a green rainbow of velvety leaves. In the Sierra, arcs mark things as sacred. Most homes have altars made with arcs of bamboo; during Day of the Dead, people make new ones and cover them with marigolds and seasonal treats. When loved ones die, people fan arcs of fresh palm leaves around their shrouded bodies as they spend one last night at home.

Suddenly, I understood: the family had bent the plant into an arc because she was sacred. She was also, I came to understand, linked to them through webs of reciprocal care: in caring for her, people care for each other, for their families, for their communities. There are places in the Sierra where *xka pastora* appears to grow

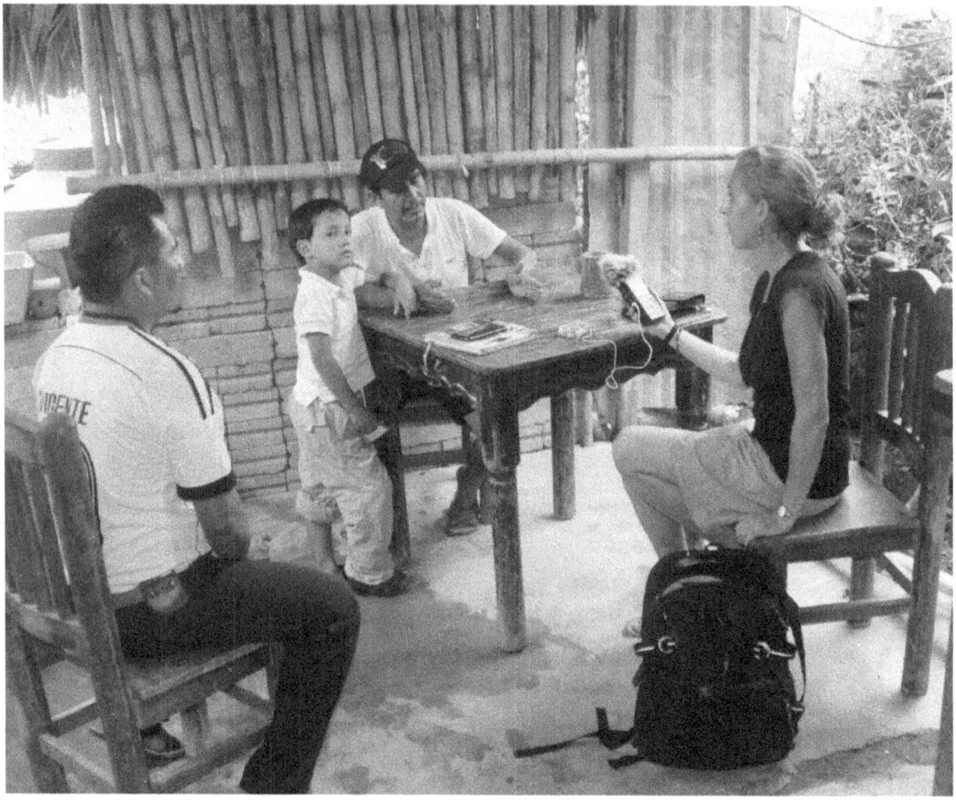

Fig. 12.2 The author conducting interviews in the Sierra with Vicente Zárate Baltazar.
Photo: Paja Faudree.

wild, but when she appears in gardens near homes it is because people have deliberately placed her there. They protect her not only from animals that might trample her but also from children who must be taught about her special status and from visitors who might inadvertently disrespect her if they trample her by mistake. It was no accident, for example, that the *xka pastora* plant I encountered that first day was on the edge of the garden, surrounded by protective trees and largely hidden from view.

People treat *xka pastora* with deep respect when they prepare her for rituals. They request permission to cut and use her leaves (the part used in ceremonies) by singing to her, saying prayers, and leaving offerings. They carefully remove the leaves in matched pairs—a reflection, people have told me, of the matched male-female pair necessary for the creation of life. People wash and bless the leaves, passing them through the smoke of burning copal resin, chanting and offering more prayers, before consuming the fresh leaves. In exchange, *xka pastora* opens channels of communication to earth spirits that saturate the Sierra but are inaccessible in daily life. People consider their guidance a source of great wisdom and insight that can help heal the sick, mend what is broken, find what is lost, set right what has gone awry. Furthermore, people not only talk *through* the plant; they also talk *to* her, "co-living" with her in ways that outsiders don't. In return, *xka pastora* takes people to hidden realms where they can find truth. She also helps them speak differently to each other as they build a depth of shared purpose closed off in everyday life.

But none of that can be found in YouTube videos, in articles touting the plant's medical potential, or in tales of the plant's "discovery." On the contrary, the discursive grooves of those narratives perpetuate discursive violence. They actively erase the perspectives of people who did so much to enable the plant's "discovery"—indeed, to make *xka pastora's* very existence and survival possible.

Those stories about what *xka pastora* means to people of the Sierra are not mine to share. What I can do instead is to help create space for the voices of the Sierra's people, to open a door for them, to invite them to share their perspectives if they choose to, on their own terms and in their own time. That effort involves encouraging people to reflect critically on the stories they are most likely to hear about the Sierra's "magic plants," to point out that the heroes of those tales are knowledge-seeking outsiders whose fantastic "discoveries" depend on hidden violence.

Occasionally, though, those writings offer fleeting and filtered access to alternative stories, as the suppressed voices of Sierra people break through and escape the confines of established discursive grooves. This passage from an article announcing the "discovery" of *Salvia divinorum* to the world narrates a 1961 encounter with a *curandera* (ritual healer):

> Maria Sebastiana Carrera had supplied us with many details about the use of the leaves … [but] declined to admit us to an actual ceremony because her neighbors (and doubtless she herself) would have considered the performance before outsiders a desecration and scandalous. Even as it was, when her session with us was drawing to a close, she burst into uncontrollable tears, and begged for forgiveness for what she had done. She had also given us valuable cosmological legends that are still believed in among the villagers, which I hope to publish elsewhere. (Wasson 1962:83)

The author's seeming indifference to the *curandera*'s anguish is astonishing in and of itself. Furthermore, by the time he wrote the article, he'd already learned a great deal about the price people in the Sierra were paying for the decision to announce news of the mushrooms to "the world"—*his* decision, as he was more responsible than anyone else on the planet for publicizing the "discovery" of the Sierra's "magic plants." But what I find particularly troubling is how he responds when confronted directly with such costs, as the *curandera* expressed her tortured qualms right in front of him. In a letter to him, another researcher who accompanied him on the trip stressed the *curandera*'s torment "she seemed to be terrified" (Johnson 1960). Nevertheless, the author remained fully committed to profiting, in one currency or another, from the information he had extracted from her.

This vignette makes clear that the extraction of secrets and sacred knowledge surrounding *xka pastora* was an excruciating process, and that the process of scientific "discovery" can cause great damage. The *curandera*'s visceral, deeply emotional response clearly signaled she was being coerced, that she had not given consent for the information to be extracted and used as she feared it would be. This interaction represents, in microcosm, a much larger pattern of violence through which not only individual researchers but entire companies' claims to advance science depend upon mining and exploiting Indigenous knowledge and resources, profiting from them financially while denying the theft upon which their claims depend. This encounter also demonstrates that the inequities structuring such cases are rooted in power discrepancies that are as much discursive as they are economic and political. As a man of great wealth and social status, the author's privilege stemmed not only from his ability to acquire and arrange whatever he wanted from people in the Sierra—which then, as now, is one of the most economically impoverished and politically marginalized regions in Mexico. His power also resided in his ability to shape the story of his encounter with people from the Sierra.[1] Seen through the lens of discursive grooves and the violence they promote, this interaction is no longer the site of an innocent ethnographic interview or scientific data collection. It becomes instead a scene of violation and theft.

Yet this vignette points to other possibilities, too; it offers a sparkle of hope. As Maria Sebastiana Carrera's suppressed voice pokes through, a competing story about *xka pastora* begins to emerge. The presence of the *curandera*'s voice even amid a discursive framework structured to silence her suggests that despite their systematic marginalization, people from the Sierra have nevertheless shaped public discourse about the plant. Perhaps more importantly, the inclusion of the *curandera*'s perspective, however limited, suggests new possibilities for those willing to listen for voices that escape the control of dominant discursive grooves. This case invites us to read claims of scientific "discovery" and the acquisition of scientific knowledge against the grain. It encourages us to eye such stories critically, looking harder for what—and who—their discursive grooves erase.

Doing so opens the door to the transformative potential of discourse. By telling different stories or telling stories differently we can create new realities. We can introduce new discursive grooves, new possibilities for recognizing and including people and perspectives that have been excluded, which can ultimately lead to the creation of new material realities.

Conclusion: Discursive Violence and the Possibility of Transformation

In my research on *xka pastora*, I embrace the transformative potential of discourse, using it to expose the established grooves in public discourses about the plant and to illuminate what those grooves distort and obscure (Faudree 2026). I show that the intimate familiarity that people from the Sierra have with *xka pastora* is born

[1] This includes the way the author's name is widely disseminated and lauded while those of Maria Sebastiana Carrera and others from the Sierra are rarely repeated; by avoiding the use of his name here I hope, in some small way, to promote discursive transformation and repair.

of many things—love, reverence, need, desperation, hope, ingenuity, persistence—but also from deliberate effort: labor. Furthermore, the knowledge that people from the Sierra acquired underpins and informs the scientific advancements that outside researchers claim in their tales of "discovery" and scientific achievement, even as the contributions of Sierra people are routinely erased by the discourses that consecrate knowledge creation. I aim to recover the stories erased by tales of *xka pastora's* "discovery," to provide a space for elevating stories that people from the Sierra can tell. Thus, I offer less an alternative to popular discourses about *xka pastora* than what I think of as ethnographic humility, an approach to ethnographic knowledge that opens doorways rather than providing answers by pointing to a larger set of stories that I welcome but cannot provide myself.

The discursive dynamics outlined here are not unique to *xka pastora*. Many psychedelic drugs are likewise derived from plants that exist today because Indigenous people created them through deliberate cultivation and intergenerational practices of care. They protected and continue to protect those plants from violent threats including not only colonial persecution but also capitalist extraction and ecological stress produced by escalating environmental crises. Yet that history and the interests of Indigenous people are largely excluded from public discourse. Indigenous people have given the world a wide range of plants, medicinal and otherwise, that revolutionized economies and cultures of nations across the globe—plants like tomatoes, potatoes, maize (or corn), vanilla, avocadoes, beans, tobacco, even my beloved chili peppers. Their centuries of experimentation revealed which plants are poisonous, edible, medicinal—or psychoactive. After those discoveries, Indigenous people began the long process of perfecting use of those extraordinary plants—adjusting the dosage, regulating the context, controlling their contact with other substances. Yet in common discourses about these plants—public stories about their history and their role in our lives today—the voices of Indigenous people are at best minimized and mostly absent entirely.

Such erasures, so common to tales of scientific "discovery," are a form of discursive violence. Furthermore, the consequences of these distortions are profound, not just ethically and morally but also economically, politically, socially. The erasures produced by discursive violence are directly tied to pervasive material realities that create and exacerbate extreme inequalities. Discursive violence naturalizes those inequalities, making it harder to subject them to critique let alone to change them. In the case of psychedelic plants like *xka pastora*, for example, Indigenous people have had hardly any input on policy and other political decisions about the plants. Almost all profits from the sale of those plants and drugs based on them go to pharmaceutical companies, merchants, and healthcare providers or institutions, whereas Indigenous peoples have received little to no economic compensation—despite their centuries of labor, even though they built the very foundations on which the "property rights" of others rest. While a few "tales of discovery" have been subject to rigorous critiques, most have been accepted uncritically.

This calls for a profound rethinking of how we understand histories of scientific knowledge and claims to scientific advancement. It demands a recognition of the importance of telling stories—not just by calling out the stories that advance discursive violence, but also by embracing reparative stories that can promote discursive transformation and reclaim narratives suppressed by dominant discursive grooves. Of course, in the face of the brutal, systematic injustices that haunt the story of *xka pastora* and other plants like it, changing the tales we tell is only part of the solution. But if we want the world to be different, we must begin by changing the stories we tell about it.

Questions for Reflection and Discussion

Reflection Questions

1. Had you heard about *xka pastora* before reading this chapter, and if so, what names had you heard people use for the plant? What connections do you see between this chapter and larger developments surrounding psychedelics and other drugs?
2. Why might it be challenging to identify discursive grooves in our own lives?

Looking In: Small Group Discussion Questions

1. Why does the author refer to the plant as *xka pastora* and use she/her pronouns (rather than referring to the plant as "it")? How are these language practices connected to discursive transformation? What is discursive transformation?
2. What is discursive violence? Explain the concept in your own words and give some examples, either from this chapter or elsewhere.
3. What are discursive grooves? In explaining the concept, use language that is comfortable to you and offer examples from this chapter, other chapters, or your own experience. How do discursive grooves enact discursive violence in stories of scientific discovery, whether those told about *xka pastora* or other scientific advancements?
4. What solution does the author propose to this sort of discursive violence? What is the role of language in this response? Are you convinced that the solution will be effective? Why or why not?

Looking Out: Large Group Discussion Questions

1. What is the relationship between discursive violence and structural violence in this chapter? What other readings from this volume explore this relationship and what do they show us?
2. What discursive grooves are present in other discourses about health and medicine? What kinds of discursive violence do these grooves perpetuate? How are they tied to structural violence?

References

Adams, Benjamin. 2023. These Three Drugs Could Make Up over Half of Forecasted Psychedelic Sales by 2029. Forbes, September 23.

Chuchiak, John, ed. 2012. *The Inquisition in New Spain, 1536–1820: A Documentary History.* Baltimore, MD: JHU Press.

Courtwright, David T., 2001. *Forces of Habit: Drugs and the Making of the Modern World.* Cambridge, MA: Harvard University Press.

Epling, Carl, and Jativa-M. 1962. A New Species of Salvia from Mexico. *Botanical Museum Leaflets, Harvard University* 20(3): pp. 75–76.

Faudree, Paja. 2015. Tales from the Land of Magic Plants: Textual Ideologies and Fetishes of Indigeneity in Mexico's Sierra Mazateca. *Comparative Studies in Society and History* 57(3): pp. 838–869.

Faudree, Paja. 2020. "Making Medicine" with *Salvia divinorum*: Competing Approaches and Their Implications. *Medical Anthropology* 39(7): pp. 582–596.

Faudree, Paja. 2026. *Magic Mint: Psychedelic Plants, Indigenous People, and the Violence of "Discovery."* Durham, NC: Duke University Press.

Hadar, Aviad, Jonathan David, Nadav Shalit, Leor Roseman, Raz Gross, Ben Sessa, and Shaul Lev-Ran. 2023. The Psychedelic Renaissance in Clinical Research: A Bibliometric Analysis of Three Decades of Human Studies with Psychedelics. *Journal of Psychoactive Drugs* 55(1): pp. 1–10.

Hayden, Cori. 2003. *When Nature Goes Public: The Making and Unmaking of Bioprospecting in Mexico.* Princeton, NJ: Princeton University Press.

Johnson, Irmgard Weitlaner. 1960. August 3. Letter to R. Gordon Wasson. Series II, Drawer W2.4, Folder 489. *The Tina & R. Gordon Wasson Ethnomycological Collection Archives.* ecb00001. Botany Libraries, Harvard University.

Johnson, Jean Bassett. 1939. Elements of Mazatec Witchcraft. *Ethnological Studies* 9: pp. 128–150.

Rukeyser, Muriel. 2006. *The Collected Poems of Muriel Rukeyser.* Edited by Kaufman, Janet E. and Herzog, Anne F., with Jan Heller Levi. Pittsburgh: University of Pittsburgh Press.

Siebert, Daniel. 1994. Salvia divinorum and Salvinorin A: New Pharmacologic Findings. *Journal of Ethnopharmacology* 43(1): pp. 53–56.

Wasson, R. Gordon. 1957. Seeking the Magic Mushroom. *Life* 42(19): pp. 100–110.

Wasson, R. Gordon. 1962. A New Mexican Psychotropic Drug from the Mint Family. *Botanical Museum Leaflets, Harvard University* 20(3): pp. 77–84.

SECTION 5

HEALING PRACTICES

Editors' Introduction

Many health disorders are incurable. These can include chronic conditions, chemical dependencies, severe injuries, and advanced states of disease. Yet even when a cure is not attainable, some kind of healing often is. Some healing interventions originate in the clinic, while others rely on non-biomedical forms of expertise. When people are contending with a serious ailment, turning to complementary and alternative medical practices is common, as is recourse to religious traditions, mental health practices and providers, and the succor of beloved friends, community members, and kin. All of these may be sources of vitally important, healing support.

The goals of healing practices can be diverse. Efforts may aim to manage or minimize symptoms, support natural processes of recovery, slow the advance of disease, alleviate mental or physical suffering, or help a person restructure life in an altered body. Healing can also extend beyond the individual to address difficulties in a family or social group. In some cases where physical healing is not possible, emotional, communal, and even spiritual healing can be achieved.

Language moderates all of these processes. Sometimes this is through the sharing of information. For instance, when a nurse shows a patient how to care for and dress a surgical site, the instructions are important for wound healing. But the role of language in healing exceeds merely describing procedures or even impacting a person's morale and investment in treatment. Some healing traditions are predicated on the provocative assertion that the act of talking itself can be therapeutic. Diverse strands of psychotherapy, for example, use language as the primary means of transformative healing.

Narrative is another critical tool in healing processes because humans imbue life events with meaning and sort out ways to persevere, in part through the telling of stories (Ochs and Capps 2002). Narratives about healing are often told collaboratively and shaped by medical cultures, from birth stories to addiction testimonies to diagnostic odysseys concerning rare conditions (cf. Mattingly and Garro 2001). Attending to these kinds of narratives can heighten physician empathy and skill (Charon 2006; Kleinman 1988), as well as revealing how people assert **agency** (the capacity to act intentionally), even when healing is protracted, partial, or uncertain.

The chapters in this section offer intimate ethnographic encounters that demonstrate the complex ways that language impacts healing. Abby Mack considers the role of embodied Charismatic Christian prayer practices in sustaining addiction recovery for a woman in Appalachia, one of the regional centers of the opioid crisis. Claudia Morales explores how migrants who are seriously injured while traveling through Mexico find themselves pressured to abandon cherished life plans and buy into a therapeutic narrative of recovery that ultimately leads to deportation. Finally, Candy Goodwin, Federica Raia, and Mario Deng share the story of Chuck Goodwin, whose experiences with terminal illness and death were profoundly shaped by frank, humane conversations with his cardiologist, and whose perspectives on dying rippled out to impact his extended community.

References

Charon, Rita. 2006. *Narrative Medicine: Honoring the Stories of Illness*. New York: Oxford University Press.

Kleinman, Arthur. 1988. *The Illness Narratives: Suffering, Healing, And The Human Condition*. New York: Basic Books.

Mattingly, Cheryl, and Linda Garro. 2001. *Narrative and the Cultural Construction of Illness and Healing*. Berkeley, CA: University of California Press.

Ochs, Elinor, and Lisa Capps. 2002. *Living Narrative: Creating Lives in Everyday Storytelling*. Cambridge, MA: Harvard University Press.

13

In the Spirit, in the Flesh

Performative Language, Embodiment, and Sustaining Recovery in Appalachia

Abby Mack

Introduction

Deborah Thumper was the first woman I met who experienced divine deliverance from polysubstance use disorder. Seventeen years later, she still gets goosebumps when she describes the night when it happened at a Christian tent revival in Central Appalachia, a mountainous region that spans North Carolina, Tennessee, Kentucky, Virginia, and West Virginia. After fifteen years of drug use, including years of habitual intravenous injections of methamphetamine and opioids, Deborah was set free from the bonds of her addiction. As others sang and prayed, Deborah was baptized in the Holy Spirit. She fell to the ground and began speaking in tongues. Powerfully moved by her experience, Deborah returned the next night and the night after, swooning in the Spirit every time. According to Deborah and the pastor who led the revival, many in attendance were similarly moved. Originally planned for a few days, the revival lasted for weeks.

In the years we have known each other, Deborah has often reflected on the miraculous and rare quality of her recovery. By her account, Deborah did not experience any physical symptoms of withdrawal. In the nearly two decades since, she has not relapsed. From a medical perspective, Deborah's recovery seems genuinely miraculous. Withdrawal from opioids and methamphetamine is dangerous and even life threatening. A quick cessation of these drugs is often accompanied by severe withdrawal symptoms, including excruciating pain, nausea, vomiting, intense cravings, and anxiety and depression. The potent effects opioids and methamphetamine have on the body can take years or even decades to overcome. Multiple relapses often characterize the path to recovery. Though Deborah and I frequently marvel at the story of her deliverance, lately, we talk about the work that has followed. As Deborah has explained it, that night under the tent canopy, she was called into relationships with God and her faith community. Since then, she has chosen to grow and maintain those relationships, skillfully cultivating a routine that involves constant prayer, regular church attendance, engagement with her faith-based recovery community, and attendance at conferences or revivals each year. This routine supports Deborah's

Abby Mack, *In the Spirit, in the Flesh*. In: *Language and Health in Action*. Edited by: Lynnette Arnold et al., Oxford University Press.
 DOI: 10.1093/9780198933953.003.0013

long-term recovery and has maintained her mental wellbeing through many difficult life experiences.

Deborah and I have traveled to revivals, attended recovery meetings, and shared many adventures exploring the beautiful Appalachian landscape (with a few visits to Dollywood for good measure). In time, I've come to see that language is a central part of her recovery routine. Deborah engages an **embodied, performative linguistic repertoire** that characterizes many Charismatic Christian worship practices. She has successfully engaged this repertoire to elaborate her spiritual life well beyond the confines of any church or tent revival. In doing so, Deborah draws upon the relational properties of language to maintain and deepen her relationship with God. When Deborah experiences anxiety or doubt, she calls upon a prayer practice that directs her attention away from the "natural" world to attend instead to God's will, a supernatural force that exceeds her human understanding. In the process, Deborah affirms a narrative about herself as a divinely loved member of her faith community whose recovery is secure, undeniable, and enduring.

Performative, Relational, and Embodied Language

Describing language as "performative" does not imply that it is inauthentic or manipulative. Instead, "performative" describes the material effects that language practices have on the world. It's helpful to break the word down, as J. L. Austin (1962) did when he coined the term in the 1950s. "Perform" means to carry out an action or "to carry into effect" (*Oxford English Dictionary*). The Latin-derived suffix "-ative" means of or related to. So, "performative" describes language that carries out an action. Language does more than describe the world. Under the right conditions, language *is* action that shifts the material reality of a person's world. For instance, a person changes their relationship and their marital status when they say "I do" in a marriage ceremony. In the years since Austin's work, other scholars have refined and elaborated his initial premise (see Searle 1989; Sedgewick 2003). For instance, Anna Corwin has documented how performative language practices in the form of ritual prayer function to elaborate and change the way elderly Catholic nuns engage God as a mediating presence in their relationships with each other, relationships with their own bodily mortality, and as a loving, active presence in their daily lives (Corwin 2012, 2021; cf. Luhrmann 2012, 2020). By highlighting the shifts in perception that occur in daily rituals of prayer and caretaking, Corwin's work shows the relational and embodied aspects of performative language practices. This triumvirate of adjectives—performative, relational, and embodied—will be critical in elaborating how language functions in maintaining wellbeing and long-term recovery in a case like Deborah's.

Opioids, Medical Care, Faith-Based Healing, and Narratives of Recovery in Central Appalachia

Since the early 2000s, Appalachia—Central Appalachia in particular—has outpaced the rest of the United States in rates of drug overdose and associated medical conditions like Hepatitis C and human immunodeficiency virus / acquired immunodeficiency syndrome (HIV/AIDS) (Schlakoff et al. 2020). From 2000 to 2019, people in Appalachia experienced death by overdose at a rate 65% higher than in the rest of the country (Meit et al. 2019). While the statistics have changed slightly since the onset of the COVID-19 pandemic and a dramatic shift in the availability of synthetic opioids like Fentanyl, Appalachia remains a statistical center for the opioid epidemic (National Center for Drug Abuse Statistics 2023). In recent years, methamphetamine use has been on the rise in Central Appalachia (Schlakoff et al. 2020). Some clinicians I have spoken to attribute the increase to the initial opioid epidemic, which reached its peak in the early 2000s (see, for instance, Macey 2018; Meier 2018). As state and federal restrictions and policing of opioid medications like oxycontin increased, many people avoided withdrawal by turning to "harder" illicit drugs, including heroin, black market fentanyl, and methamphetamines. The mixing of various illegal drugs—polysubstance use—makes recovery exceedingly difficult. However, despite serious gaps in medical care and social support, people in Central Appalachia can and do find paths to long-term recovery.

My co-researchers, China Scherz and Joshua Burraway (both medical anthropologists with experience researching substance use disorders in Uganda and the UK, respectively), were drawn to Central Appalachia to investigate how people living in the center of the nation's opioid epidemic achieved recovery in clinical and faith-based settings. I joined the team as a medical and linguistic anthropologist interested in how language practices inform how people achieve and maintain recovery from polysubstance use disorders over time. As a team, we wanted to understand how different language practices used in various recovery settings shaped a person's capacity to hope (for themselves, for others, for a future) and to act on such hopes, crafting new lives and discovering new possibilities for carrying on.

Since the 1990s, clinicians and recovery specialists have worked to reframe popular conceptions of addiction by shifting how it is described. Rather than a problem of willpower—where people struggling to recover are framed as criminals and morally deficient—these medical professionals advocate understanding substance use disorder as a "chronic, relapsing brain disease" (CRBD). This new explanatory model helps to destigmatize substance use disorder by drawing attention to the critical role an individual's neural circuitry plays in the addiction process, emphasizing that addiction is *not* a moral deficiency but a treatable biological process (Scherz et al. 2021).

While medical and public health professionals understand a "chronic" illness to be one that lasts a year or more, many patients understand it to mean a disease that can be treated but never cured. Indeed, the words "chronic" and "relapse" may have profound impacts on the culture of recovery programs and the people who participate in them. In their work on recovery from alcohol addiction in Uganda, China Scherz, George Mpanga, and Sarah Namirembe (2024) found that people seeking treatment where the CRBD explanatory model is dominant may adopt a self-narrative popularized in Alcoholics Anonymous: "Once an addict, always an addict." This narrative emphasizes the importance of self-responsibility in maintaining sobriety. Meanwhile, the authors found a different narrative and explanatory model of addiction in Ugandan Pentecostal Christian contexts. There, addiction was framed as a problem of demonic possession and spiritual warfare, where Christians were called to battle against the devil. Once delivered from demonic influence, people could tell a different story: that addiction was "not me." In this narrative of self, people in recovery could imagine a future where they would never be "addicts" again. Instead, they could focus on building a livelihood in a close relationship with God. Accountability, in this case, is centered less on the prospects of addiction than on protecting spiritual selfhood. As a research team, Scherz, Burraway, and I wondered whether we might find similar narratives in Appalachian clinical and faith-based programs.

Appalachian Historical and Regional Context

For many in the United States, the differences between biomedical and faith-based worldviews seem irreconcilable. One is based on natural, empirical (i.e., observable), scientifically informed observations about the world and the biological processes of the body. The other is founded in a worldview that allows for supernatural, spiritual explanations of ailments. The sense that such perspectives are opposed is exacerbated by the history of Christian politics in the US, including waves of legislation opposing scientific perspectives in the name of religious liberties. In addition, people who have experienced church-related trauma may, understandably, be resistant to taking faith-based forms of recovery seriously. Indeed, roughly a quarter of the people who participated in our research reported experiences of discrimination and abuse in church settings—particularly around sexual orientation—which contributed to their substance abuse.

At the same time, many in Appalachia are rightly suspicious of biomedical practice. Since at least the nineteenth century, government officials and popular culture have stereotyped the Appalachian region as "backward" and treated the people who lived there accordingly. In the early twentieth century, eugenicist policies resulted in the forced sterilization of Appalachians lasting well into the 1970s. These practices were founded on racist, classist, and ableist fears that positioned Appalachians (many of whom were considered by outsiders or identified themselves as mixed race with white, Indigenous, and Black ancestors) as a potential threat to the purity and success of the nation (Catte 2018; Pollard 2004). While a large percentage of Central Appalachians identify as non-Hispanic white (U.S. Census Bureau 2021), racial identity in Appalachia has been and remains historically, culturally, and politically fraught (Catte 2018; Smith 2004). Notably, these complexities undergird an enduring stereotype that continues to justify both medical and economic exploitation of the region.

In the late 1990s, Purdue Pharma marketed the opioid medication oxycontin as a non-addictive treatment for pain. The company targeted its marketing in regions like Central Appalachia, where the rate of occupational hazards was high as people engaged in physically strenuous and dangerous work such as coal mining and factory manufacturing (Macy 2018). Purdue Pharma's marketing strategies were remarkably effective, and before long, many Appalachians seeking relief from debilitating pain were treated with what was, in fact, a powerfully addictive opioid. Overprescription of oxycontin and other opioids by medical practitioners led to the diversion of these medications away from their intended use. In the years since many clinicians have sought to repair the harm caused but are often met with distrust. Justifiable suspicions, resentments, and traumas abound as people weigh options for recovery in faith-based or clinical settings.

Recovery Narratives

Without dismissing these important divisions, my ethnographic research revealed that the seemingly opposed worldviews of faith and medicine inform and often depend on each other. Indeed, many of the people I spoke with embraced the medical pluralism of the recovery care landscape in Appalachia and mixed and matched the various treatment models and approaches they engaged (see Arnold et al. ('Key Concepts in Language and Health') and Lee (Chapter 2), in this volume, for deeper engagement with "medical pluralism"). In the insurance-based clinic where I conducted fieldwork, for instance, clinicians used a CRBD model to intervene in the biological mechanisms of addiction via medication and cognitive behavioral therapy. Alongside these practices, they also engaged their clients in somatic processing, eye movement desensitization reprocessing (EMDR), and mindfulness meditation techniques that clients could use at home.

While clinicians taught their clients about the neural processes that informed their substance use disorder, they refrained from using the term "chronic, relapsing brain disease" because they recognized clients might be discouraged by the prospect of relapse. Instead, they encouraged clients to find their own language for recovery and engage in a mixture of therapeutic and group support programs. One clinician—in recovery himself—also led a faith-based support group. Meanwhile, pastors and peer mentors in faith-based programs adopted the CRBD model to understand the etiology of addiction. Faith-based support meetings frequently used colloquialized forms of cognitive behavioral therapy and somatic processing to address trauma and interrupt addictive habits. These practices supplemented a complex narrative of recovery in which people could become truly "free" from addiction. Although the potential for demonic interference was occasionally discussed, members of faith-based groups mostly focused on their own human fallibility (as compared to divine perfection). Rather than a "not me" narrative, this approach facilitated a "not me, anymore" account. Indeed, when Deborah was asked to share her story at an Alcoholics Anonymous / Narcotics Anonymous meeting, she began: "I'm Deborah. I am not an addict."

In the end, whether people adopted the "once an addict, always an addict" narrative as a helpful tool for accountability, the "not me" narrative as a means for overcoming shame, or the "not me, anymore" narrative as a means for self-forgiveness and accountability, most of the people in our study—regardless of their chosen recovery modality—told stories of qualified redemption achieved through intentional labor. They shared a story of hope for a life when they can and will do better, provided they continue working to maintain recovery. Critically, the labor of maintaining recovery is achieved through embodied, performative language practices that not only change how people describe their histories of addiction but actively shift how they perceive themselves, their bodies, and their social relationships. In the remainder of this chapter, I focus on the faith-based-language practices that characterize Deborah's lifeworld and experiences.

Run Up! Understanding Performative Language Practice In Charismatic Christian Contexts

"Run up!" Pastor Stephanie Harrison sang, "Run up!" Behind her on stage, a worship team member sang: "Spirit is coming!" Music swelled dramatically: piano, organ, and drums. "Run, run, run," Harrison sang on. Responding to the altar call, hundreds of women poured into the aisles of the church's massive sanctuary. Raising their hands, they sang. They swayed. They fainted—overcome by the power of the Holy Spirit. I was close to Deborah, who stood out among the crowd, tall and strong, her auburn hair pulled into a tight ponytail. "Glory! Glory! Glory!" a woman behind us sang, almost crying. Deborah bowed her head and began praying in tongues. The crowd soon separated us. Swaying with the women around me, I watched Deborah move toward the altar.

This was the Women of Fire conference, a massive and highly produced gathering, unlike the revival where Deborah experienced deliverance. The conference brought together an interracial, intergenerational, international, and interdenominational network of Charismatic Christian women at Redemption to the Nation Church. The sanctuary was a large auditorium that could—and did—seat thousands of people. The walls and columns of the church were covered with soundproofing material to mitigate the echo in the large space. Pastors and worship team members stood on a stage at the center of the sanctuary where giant LED screens projected song lyrics, Bible passages, and close-ups of people, captured by cameras mounted on long, sweeping cranes along the periphery of the sanctuary. This was my first experience at a Charismatic Christian worship event, and all my senses were on alert as I did my best to take it all in. Around me, thousands of women gathered with hopes of having new, healing—reviving—encounters with God.

"Glory! Glory! Glory!" the woman behind me sang, her voice a kind of punctuation to the crowd's collective whispers, shouts, and cries. A small woman fell beside me with a loud thud. I moved to stand behind her as I had seen others do the day before to protect her from being stepped on as she "rested in the spirit." Eyes closed, she smiled serenely as others stepped carefully to the side and continued toward the altar. After a long while, she stirred and opened her eyes. I helped her to her feet, we hugged, and she continued to worship, lifting her hands high. Relieved of my self-appointed duties, sensorily overwhelmed, and curious, I bowed my head and closed my eyes. Keeping my feet shoulder-width apart, I bent my knees slightly to avoid falling as the women around me danced in prayer. Without the LED screens and stage fog drawing my attention, I could tune in more clearly to my other senses.

Before long, I was surprised to feel someone's hand on top of my head. I opened my eyes to see a woman with salt and pepper hair teased high, praying over me. As I had seen other altar workers do, this woman pressed her hand on my forehead, directing my body backward. Recalling conversation with other women during our caravan to the conference, I knew authenticity was essential in this form of prayer. I did not want to be inauthentic, and I did not feel the Holy Spirit as Deborah said I might, so, I resisted the altar worker's direction and remained upright. She moved her hands to my upper abdomen and, suddenly and forcefully, pressed on my belly, knocking the wind out of me. I gasped as she finished praying over me before moving on. As I caught my breath, I wondered at my choice to resist. By staying "authentic" to my own understanding, had I missed an opportunity for deeper understanding?

Throughout the history of the religion, Christians have used the "laying of hands" or "handlaying" to engage each other in prayer, baptism of the Holy Spirit, and healing acts (Fatokun 2011). In his ethnographic work on Catholic Charismatic healing, Thomas Csordas (1997a, 1997b, 2002) describes how ritualized gestures like handlaying work alongside rhetorical strategies in sermons and prayers to engage Charismatic healers and their patients in "somatic attunement." These language practices redirect a person's attention to their own bodily experiences and senses as part of a collective that includes not only the people around them but also a divine presence. Together, sermons, singing, praying, and handlaying work performatively to change a person's relationship to the divine and create a new experience of the self as "sacred." The altar worker was facilitating a similar process for me.

As the altar worker quite literally took my breath away, her handlaying gesture referenced Pastor Stephanie Harrison's sermon on *ruach*, Hebrew for the divine, life-giving breath of God. As Harrison explained, *ruach* is the "unutterable, irresistible, undomesticated force that surges into history to remake, to heal, to transform." It is the God-given word, Harrison explained, that has allowed humans to begin speaking about "what we know but cannot say" of sublime encounters with the divine and the majesty of being alive. Pastor Harrison directed the audience to place their hands on their bellies and explained the difference between diaphragmatic and chest breathing. "This," she continued with her hand resting on her belly, "is where your spirit lives. This is where the *ruach*, the wind of the Holy Ghost, lives."

When the altar worker pushed on my belly, she shifted my attention away from the passive observational experience I was having and toward a direct, active encounter with my own body. Mimicking the pastor's gestural engagement with her belly and breath, the altar worker brought me into an embodied conversation. Her touch functioned as a form of phatic communication, opening a potential communicative channel like saying "hello" invites conversation in a phone call. Pressing on my belly in prayer, the altar worker created an opportunity for me to encounter, interact with, and engage the pastor's sermon, the broader community of worshipers, and the Holy Ghost—*ruach*—as described by Pastor Harrison. Certainly surprising, that moment was also one in which I was directed to experience the world around me as characterized by the potential for intimacy with my compatriots and the divine. Marjorie Goodwin (2017) describes this form of interaction as "haptic sociality," a linguistic and performative register achieved through touch that directs people to the potential for intimacy, engagement, and mutual attention toward a shared social action (see also Katila et al. 2020). In the following days and weeks, Deborah and others who attended the conference with us reported a feeling of joyful revival and renewal in their faith. I, too, experienced greater energy and exuberance, dancing—almost involuntarily—in my kitchen before breakfast as I listened to recordings of the songs and sermons.

In the Flesh or the Spirit? On Being Set Free and Quenching the Holy Spirit

In my efforts to understand the material changes that have occurred for Deborah in her process of recovery and how she maintains recovery through her spiritual practice, I have looked to scientific analyses of healing rituals. Several studies address the possible benefits of handlaying and prayer for people seeking healing from various illnesses. For instance, Pohl and co-authors (2007) investigate how intimate touch and communal bonds may provide powerful experiences of connection to therapeutic ends (though the study's conclusion is debated, for instance, see Ernst 2007). Clinicians and psychologists, aware of the powerful hallucinations and seizures that withdrawal from opioids may cause, might suggest that Deborah experienced her withdrawals at that first tent revival and interpreted the symptoms as divine. Noting my exuberance and joy after revival experiences, I am tempted to understand the back-and-forth swaying and dancing that characterizes Charismatic Christian worship as a mechanism that achieves a bilateral stimulation similar to somatic processing and EMDR. Some or all of these hypotheses may carry water. However, they also wholly disregard the testimony of people like Deborah, who attribute their healing to divine intervention and careful maintenance of an intimate relationship with

God. Rather than explain away Deborah's powerful account, I ask readers who might similarly privilege a scientific or "natural" worldview to sit with me in the humble place of not knowing for certain what may be happening for people like Deborah when they have encounters with the divine. After all, a scientific worldview is as culturally informed as any supernatural worldview; it just privileges different forms of evidence (cf. Kohn 2015; Holbraad and Pedersen 2017; Scherz et al. 2024).

Since that memorable conference, Deborah and I have reflected repeatedly on our shared and separate experiences. In refusing to bend as the altar worker directed me, had I performed ethically by remaining "authentic"? Or, had I "quenched" the Holy Spirit, shutting down an invitation for communicative engagement with God? Part of the tension may lie in what Deborah describes as the difference between being "in the flesh" and being "in the spirit." I stayed "in the flesh," bound by my body's needs and desires. I had been skeptical, or at least I had resisted engaging with what was not empirically observable. I was *thinking* naturally when I should have been *experiencing* supernaturally.

This tension was and has remained a struggle for me as a social scientist and an inquisitive person who wants a clear explanation. On the first night of the conference, I had almost quenched the Holy Spirit when I jokingly teased Deborah for singing a refrain, "great is your faithfulness to me," over and over. I could not remember hearing that song at the conference and demanded some kind of observable origin for Deborah's joyful expression of faith. It created a palpable tension in our relationship for weeks after, as Deborah wondered about my intentions and my understanding of the profound work of God in her life. Thankfully, Deborah is the kind of person who has been willing to forgive my limited understanding and engage my curiosities.

Almost a year after the conference, Deborah and I took a day trip to Asheville, North Carolina, where we floated in tubes down the French Broad River. On our drive, we recorded our conversation (as always). Deborah mounted the mic on my dashboard, and I reflected on what remained a puzzle for me: the difference between being in the flesh and being in the spirit. I was curious and in awe of how Deborah had reported "getting out of the flesh" and standing in the spirit to overcome fatigue, workplace injuries, and anxiety. Still thinking at a descriptive level, I asked about the transition from "flesh" to "spirit": "When you're shifting—that moment of shift—does it feel differently in your body?"

"Oh **ye: :s**," Deborah replied enthusiastically (for transcription conventions, see chapter appendix). "Huh. Yeah. Yeah. Like wor: :ds—I don't even know the words to explain." Deborah continued to meet me where I was—in the realm of the empirical—and describe the experience that, for her, exceeded language. She noted how nervous she often is to share her testimony—a genre of speech in which people share how God has intervened in their lives (cf. Hansen 2018), and that she didn't consider herself particularly "bubbly." "I've got **scars**[ ]I've got **all** these effects" from previous drug use. She reflected on these insecurities and her habit of planning what she might say.

"But," Deborah continued, "then I learnt over the years like, I prayed that the Lord would anoint me, the words that would come out of my mouth, that He would have me say what **He** wants me to say, not what **I** want to say. That I'm gonna be in the leading of the Holy Spirit and not what **Deborah** put together."

Deborah has shared a version of this account with me on different occasions. To get out of the flesh, a person must "die to self," let go of their anxieties or desires, and trust—profoundly—in the agentive and divine presence of God to guide one's speech, actions, and even capacity to attend to pain. In the process of praying, Deborah experiences a shift in perception. She continued, reflecting on her prayer practice and noting her goosebumps as she discussed God's presence in her life. Her voice and tone pitched upward with reverence and wonder.

(01)	Deborah:	You know, So I would start praying and learning how to pray that I would bind up the attacks of the flesh and loose the anointing of the Holy Spirit. And you start to gettin' that release of the pressure, and then a peace comes over you, like a calmness. Like you know how your body's hurtin'? and you get into that heat—in the sun—and we're like "ahhh"
(02)	Abby:	Yeah
(03)	Deborah:	It's like that, but there's a **bubbling**. Like a (.) bubbling that starts comin'—like I'll be at work and you know I run a machine so I'm by myself so I'm at my mind—And he'll lead me! You know how I do them outbursts with the songs? [Deborah's tone of voice changes here to more than just marveling. Now she is joking about my previous misunderstanding of her singing].
(04)	Abby:	[Laughs]
(05)	Deborah:	[Laughs] You know. That's that anointing flowing because I'm staying in the presence of God and it's like you know I'm putting the world just needs to **stop**—you know. And the presence of God needs to come in. You're—you're welcoming the presence of God. It's like an ongoing worship service, you know?

Over time, Deborah has learned to perform on herself the same kinds of embodied modifications I experienced at the conference to move her attention from her "fleshly" embodied experience and toward the presence of God. Having already allowed the Holy Spirit to dwell within her—having practiced that experience over the years—Deborah can hold her own "ongoing worship service." In this way, she overcomes the physical impact of her factory work in a dusty and un-airconditioned facility and her anxiety at speaking to an audience, feeling instead an "anointing flow;" the presence of God.

Conclusion

Deborah was "set free" at a revival seventeen years ago. But, as she will attest, that was not the end of her story. Motivated by her miraculous deliverance and the profound relationship with God her deliverance engendered, she has worked to engage a particular set of ritualized prayer and worship practices. In time, these *embodied* practices became habitual. In her everyday life, at home and work, she continues to mobilize the *performative* gestures and language practices she experiences in group worship settings to stay in near-constant contact with God. In the process, she materially shifts her perception of her body and her concerns toward a spiritual—not fleshly—worldview. Beyond resolving daily concerns, these practices build a narrative of the future that—while unclear—is not uncertain. Deborah knows in a way that exceeds language that her sobriety is certain, so long as she continues praying, speaking to, and feeling in *relational* communication with God.

Questions for Reflection and Discussion

Reflection Questions

1. Think of a time you felt a strong emotion at a concert, ceremony, or other similar crowd context. Why do you think you felt the way that you did? What role do you think language played in generating this feeling?
2. Before reading this chapter, what had you heard about how addiction and recovery work? How does your prior knowledge align with the CRBD model? In what ways does it align with the faith-based perspectives described in the chapter? In what ways does it differ from each of these models?

Looking In: Small Group Discussion Questions

A struggle ethnographers face when describing performative language practices is the common misperception that these practices involve inauthentic performance or even a form of manipulation. When observing or reading about the embodied performative language practices at the Charismatic Christian conference, for instance, a person might ask "were you pushed or did you fall?" The complicated answer from a perspective that takes language and interaction seriously is: "both." With this in mind, consider the following questions:

1. After reading this chapter, how would you define "performative language" to a fellow college student who is not in this class? In your explanation include at least one example from the chapter or a different context.
2. In what specific ways are Charismatic Christian language practices performative, relational, and embodied? Why is it important to distinguish these kinds of performative language from being "inauthentic" or "manipulative"?
3. How does the author's experience compare to Deborah's account of her own prayer practice? How does Deborah translate the performative aspects of group worship into her everyday life?

Looking Out: Large Group Discussion Questions

1. What do you make of the author's struggle with authenticity during her encounter at the Charismatic women's conference? How does this struggle inform her ethnographic research?
2. What considerations should ethnographers make in research and analysis when their own worldview differs from that of their research participants?
3. Most people in addiction recovery experience relapse. Deborah has not. What practices and forms of support have enabled Deborah to maintain sobriety and wellbeing during seventeen years, even in the face of difficult life experiences? What does this tell us about what is needed for people to sustain recovery from polysubstance use disorder and other forms of addiction?
4. What other healthcare experiences or interventions could be analyzed from a performative language perspective? How, for instance, do forms of meditation (e.g., transcendental or mindfulness) or ritual operate similarly or differently from the linguistic practice Deborah engages as she moves from "being in the flesh" to "being in the spirit"?

Appendix

Bold indicates some form of emphasis, which may be signaled by changes in pitch and/or amplitude.

: : colons indicate that the sound immediately preceding the colon has been noticeably lengthened

— a dash marks a sudden cut-off of the current sound

() visual and auditory information

(.) a micro-pause (less than a second)

[...] ellipsis

[] transcriber's note for clarifications for the reader

References

Austin, J. L. 1962. *How to Do Things with Words*. Oxford: Oxford University Press.

Catte, Elizabeth. 2018. *What You're Getting Wrong about Appalachia*. Cleveland, OH: Belt Publishing.

Corwin, Anna. 2012. Changing God, Changing Bodies: The Impact of New Prayer Practices on Elderly Catholic Nuns' Embodied Experience. *Ethos* 40(4): pp. 390–410. https://doi.org/10.1111/j.1548-1352.2012.01267.x.

Corwin, Anna. 2021. *Embracing Age: How Catholic Nuns Became Models of Aging Well*. New Brunswick, NJ: Rutgers University Press

Csordas, Thomas. 1997a. *Language, Charisma, and Creativity: The Ritual Life of a Religious Movement*. Berkeley, CA: University of California Press.

Csordas, Thomas. 1997b. *The Sacred Self: A Cultural Phenomenology of Charismatic Healing*. Berkeley, CA: University of California Press.

Csordas, Thomas. 2002. *Body, Meaning, Healing*. New York: Springer.

Hansen, Helena. 2018. *Addicted to Christ: Remaking Men in Puerto Rican Pentecostal Drug Ministries*. Berkeley, CA: University of California Press.

Ernst, E. 2007. "Laying on of Hands": Magic or Medicine? *Support Care Cancer* 15: pp. 121–122. https://doi.org/10.1007/s00520-006-0142-6.

Fatokun, Samson Adetunji. 2011. Laying on of Hands. In *The Encyclopedia of Christian Civilization*, ed. George Thomas Kurian, pp. 1331–1332. Oxford: Blackwell Publishing.

Goodwin, Marjorie H. 2017. Haptic Sociality: The Embodied Interactive Constitution of Intimacy through Touch. In *Intercorporeality: Emerging Socialities in Interaction*, Foundations of Human Interaction ed. Christian Meyer, J. Streeck, and J. Scott Jordan, pp. 73–102. Oxford: Oxford University Press. https://doi.org/10.1093/acprof:oso/9780190210465.003.0004.

Holbraad, Martin, and Morten Axel Pedersen. 2017. *The Ontological Turn: An Anthropological Exposition*. Cambridge: Cambridge University Press.

Katila, Julia, Yumei Gan, and Marjorie H. Goodwin. 2020. Interaction Rituals and "Social Distancing": New Haptic Trajectories and Touching from a Distance in the Time of COVID-19. *Discourse Studies* 22(4): pp. 418–440. https://doi.org/10.1177/1461445620928213.

Kohn, Eduardo. 2015. Anthropology of Ontologies. *Annual Review of Anthropology* 44: pp. 311–327.

Luhrmann, Tanya Marie. 2012. *When God Talks Back: Understanding the American Evangelical Relationship with God*. New York: Alfred A. Knopf.

Luhrmann, Tanya Marie. 2020. *How God Becomes Real: Kindling the Presence of Invisible Others*. Princeton, NJ: Princeton University Press

Macy, B. 2018. *Dopesick: Dealers, Doctors, and the Drug Company that Addicted America*. London: Little Brown and Company.

Meier, B. 2018. Origins of an Epidemic: Purdue Pharma Knew Its Opioids Were Widely Abused. *New York Times*, May 29. Accessed September 23, 2023: https://www.nytimes.com/2018/05/29/health/purdue-opioids-oxycontin.html.

Meit Michael, Heffernan Megan, and Tanenbaum Erin. 2019. Investigating the Impact of the Diseases of Despair in Appalachia. *Journal of Appalachian Health* 1(2): pp. 7–18. doi: 10.13023/jah.0102.02.

National Center for Drug Abuse Statistics (NCDAS). 2023. Opioid Crisis Statistics [2023]: Prescription Opiod Abuse. *NCDAS*. Retrieved July 23, 2025, from https://drugabusestatistics.org/opioid-epidemic/.

Pohl, Gudrun, Heidemarie Seemann, Niklas Zojer, Christina Ochsner, Christine Luhan, Michael Schwemper, and Heinz Ludwig. 2007. "Laying on of Hands" Improves Well-Being in Patients with Advanced Cancer. *Support Care Cancer* 15: pp. 143–151. https://doi.org/10.1007/s00520-006-0147-1.

Pollard, Kevin. M. 2004. A New Diversity: Race and Ethnicity in the Appalachian Region. *Demographic and Social Change*. Population Reference Bureau and Appalachian Regional Commission. Retrieved July 23, 2025 from: https://www.arc.gov/wp-content/uploads/2020/06/ANewDiversityRaceandEthnicityinAppalachia.pdf

Searle, John R. 1989. How Performatives Work. *Linguistics and Philosophy* 12(5): 535–585.

Sedgewick, Eve K. 2003. *Touching Feeling: Affect, Pedagogy, Performativity*. Durham, NC: Duke University Press

Scherz, China, Sarah Namirembe, and George Mpanga. 2021. Not You: Addiction, Relapse, and Release in Uganda. *Culture, Medicine, and Psychiatry* 46(1): pp. 101–114. https://doi.org/10.1007/s11013-021-09722-9.

Scherz, China, SarahNamirembe, and George Mpanga. 2024. *Higher Powers: Alcohol and After in Uganda's Capital City*. Berkeley, CA: University of California Press

Schlakoff, Christine A., Katheryn E. Lancaster, Bradley N. Gaynes, Vivian Wang, Brian W. Pence, William C. Miller, and Vivian F. Go. 2020. The Opioid and Related Drug Epidemics in Rural Appalachia: A Systematic Review of Populations Affected, Risk Factors, and Infectious Diseases. *Substance Abuse* 41(1): pp. 35–69. https://doi.org/10.1080%2F08897077.2019.1635555.

Smith, Barbara Ellen. 2004. De-Gradations of Whiteness: Appalachia and the Complexities of Race. *Journal of Appalachian Studies* 10(2): pp. 38–57.

U.S. Census Bureau. 2021. Central Appalachia. Accessed on July 23, 2025. https://www:census.gov/content/dam/Census/library/visualizations/2021/demo/central-appadlachia.pdf.

14

Caught between Stories of Healing and Migration

Rehabilitation Care for Migrants with Amputations in Mexico

Claudia Morales

La Bestia: A Desperate Last Resort

Every day, across Mexico, thousands of migrants wait with a mix of desperation and patience along the train tracks for La Bestia (the beast), the freight train that transports goods from Mexico's southern border with Guatemala to its northern border with the United States. Migrants carry only the essentials: a small backpack, a bottle of water, something to eat. Many also carry their small children in their arms. The metallic noise of the approaching train alerts them and they board in areas where the train slows; it does not stop for them. They stand on the couplings that join the cars together and then climb onto the metal roof, looking for a place to rest as they travel north. These journeys can last days, with migrants exposed to the elements and at risk of falling from the train as it picks up speed or sways around turns.

These migrants, people from around the world but mainly from Central America, rely on La Bestia because other modes of transportation through Mexico present dangers for them on their journeys north. The terrain they traverse is controlled by drug cartels, and migrants who cannot afford to pay the exorbitant fees to hire guides risk being kidnapped or worse. Buses and cars are monitored at checkpoints by Mexican immigration police and the National Guard, which have expanded their operations due to direct political pressure from the United States. In recent years, even local solidarity has come under scrutiny: civilians who offer transportation to migrants have been accused of human trafficking. This increased surveillance is part of broader efforts to keep migrants from reaching the United States. Under these conditions, La Bestia becomes the best possible option for many, despite the strenuousness of the journey and the high risk of accidents. People overcome by exhaustion can fall from the roof onto the tracks, crushed by moving wheels or between train cars that collide as the train brakes. The exact number of migrants injured by La Bestia is unknown and not recorded. Most accidents are fatal and those who survive often need amputations.

Claudia Morales, *Caught between Stories of Healing and Migration*. In: *Language and Health in Action*. Edited by: Lynnette Arnold et al., Oxford University Press. © Claudia Morales (2026). DOI: 10.1093/9780198933953.003.0014

In the past, migrants who suffered amputations were not guaranteed medical care and many were deported to their home countries before fully recovering from their injuries, resulting in life-threatening complications. In response to this situation, migrants with amputations organized with family members and other allies through organizations such as the Honduran National Commission to Support Returned Migrants with Physical Disabilities (CONAMIREDIS) and the Central American Regional Alliance of Migrants and Returnees. As a result of this pressure, Mexican immigration law now mandates that care be provided to people with life-threatening injuries, regardless of their immigration status. Migrants with amputations enter a special "amputee program" that mobilizes local and international humanitarian care systems to ensure that accident survivors have access to reconstructive surgeries, rehabilitation therapies, and free prostheses. Not everyone gains access to the program. Those who do are privileged in a context of abandonment where many do not receive care of any kind. However, once their recovery and rehabilitation is complete, migrants in the amputee program are deported back to their countries of origin.

Hospitals and international humanitarian care systems play an essential role in the recovery and care of migrants with amputations. Simultaneously, anti-immigration policies in force in Mexico and the United States utilize these institutions as deterrent mechanisms for migration. In this chapter, I explore the ambivalent and often overlooked role of medical institutions in immigration enforcement, focusing on the entanglement of healthcare and deportation and using the lens of language to gain deeper insights into how these forces work together. I focus on the story of Joe, a 19-year-old Honduran amputee, who exemplifies the multiple cases that I have followed during eight years of research. The ethnography of Joe's rehabilitation in Mexico illuminates how during this critical moment of physical recovery, he finds himself caught between two competing narratives: a **therapeutic narrative** and a **heroic migrant narrative**. The therapeutic narrative is focused on the patient's recovery after amputation, characterized by heroic efforts to overcome physical and mental obstacles to achieve physical healing and regain bodily independence. The heroic migrant narrative involves a journey to reach the United States, where the migrant achieves economic independence and fulfills symbolic responsibilities, such as becoming "a good example," often materialized through remittances (money sent home to support family).

I argue that, during the process of rehabilitation, the therapeutic narrative and the heroic migrant narrative collide in ways that at first seem to align, but later reveal deep disjunctures. I trace how Joe navigates the pressure to act as a hero in two different journeys at the intersection of healing and migration enforcement. I consider the coercion that the amputee program, and programs like it, exert on migrants to submit to policies that may conflict with their aspirations. Ultimately, I assert that narratives profoundly shape both therapeutic encounters themselves and migrants' responses to the pressures they face.

Competing Heroic Narratives

Central American migrants are guided and driven on their journeys north by the narrative of the heroic migrant. Lynnette Arnold (2024) analyzes the double representation of migrants in El Salvador: the "heroic migrant" and the "failed migrant." Heroic migrants support their families by working hard in the United States and sending remittances home to El Salvador, while failed migrants are those who are deported or suffer injuries during their journey. The Salvadoran state propagates these narratives to secure migrants' remittances while evading state responsibility for the political and humanitarian crisis in El Salvador that incubates forced migration. Beyond El Salvador, the narrative of the heroic migrant is widely embraced by many Central Americans as a coming-of-age story, a way to become a successful adult. As Marroquín Parducci (2019) describes, the successful migrant is one who, through effort, courage, and hard work, manages to prosper in a foreign country. To achieve this, migrants are called to embark on a heroic journey to transcend their material and social conditions.

Migrants who are injured and enter the amputee program in Mexico face pressure to embrace and embody an alternative narrative during their rehabilitation: the therapeutic narrative. This story emerges from the context of healthcare and functions independently of the heroic migrant narrative until the stories collide in the amputee program. Therapeutic narratives frame and shape experiences during clinical encounters, in this case physical therapy sessions that aim to help migrants regain physical mobility. The therapeutic narrative asks the patient to focus on recovery, which involves intense pain and requires immense physical and mental in efforts to regain mobility.

Despite the pressure to buy into the therapeutic narrative and abandon migration plans, many migrants with amputations have not given up on the heroic migrant narrative. They remain determined to embody the heroic migrant and do everything possible to avoid becoming a failed migrant. Their resistance to abandoning the migration journey does not go unnoticed by therapeutic staff. Rather, clinicians often feel they must compete with the heroic migrant narrative to keep patients focused on the effortful work that is required to recover from major injuries. Miriam Ticktin (2016) offers a critical examination of such care-focused humanitarian migration policies, highlighting how these policies, despite their intentions, may inadvertently cause harm to those they are designed to assist.

Although therapeutic and migration narratives have very different end goals—physical rehabilitation on the one hand and successful migration on the other—they both converge on the idea that advancing the plot requires the migrant to personify the character of the resilient hero. Since both narratives cast amputees in the role of the hero, they can seem to work together. But ultimately, these narratives create tensions for migrants with amputations as they weigh their limited options during a time of extreme vulnerability. Through collaborative research with migrant amputees in Mexico, I came to understand how these stories trapped migrants in a double bind of incompatible expectations.

As a Mexican medical anthropologist I am deeply interested in the role of language in healthcare within the context of migration. Over the course of several years, I worked to establish relationships with national and international migrant assistance organizations in Mexico. These relationships ultimately allowed me access to shelters and recovery facilities, where I was able to work with migrants in treatment. Over the course of three months at the rehabilitation center that I highlight in this chapter, I conducted interviews, engaged in participant observation, and attended and recorded therapy sessions with the participants' permission and cooperation. During this time, I worked alongside two other researchers—one from Mexico and one from the United States—who were researching similar topics. Together, we developed a collaborative methodology that included taking photographs and recording video materials of the therapy sessions and the interviews with both the medical personnel and recovering injured migrants. We gifted these materials to the center and the patients to showcase and preserve their work.

I met Joe, a young Honduran man, in November 2020 at a shelter in Central Mexico. He told me that his first attempt to reach the United States had been unsuccessful. He was apprehended while crossing Guatemala and deported back to Honduras. He was now in the midst of a second attempt. In February he had suffered an accident on La Bestia that required amputations above both of his knees and above the elbow of his left arm. By the time we met, Joe's wounds had healed and he was undergoing physical therapy in preparation for receiving prosthetic limbs. We went on to talk often, sometimes at the shelter where he was living, sometimes during therapy sessions, for example while the clinical staff took measurements for his prosthetics.

As we casually chatted, Joe shared his reasons for migrating. He told me about his origins, his shattered family networks, his personal struggles. He painted a canvas of his life colored by the grim nuances of poverty and orphanhood. As I listened to Joe, I recognized the heroic migrant narrative connecting the events of his life and giving them meaning. A coming-of-age story emerged, with a young orphan facing adversity and determined to free himself from poverty and escape violence. He saw only one option: migration to the United States. During these conversations, I could see Joe was struggling to adjust to his medical condition and his compromised life trajectory. His accident on La Bestia had introduced an "unexpected turn" (Ochs and Capps 2001) of events in his migration journey that he was struggling to resolve. In the following sections, I show how Joe became caught between two different versions of his hero's journey, each responding to the unexpected turn of his devastating accident. In one, he would be the heroic migrant who reaches the United States and finds a new life, while in the other, he would be the heroic patient who recovers from a life-changing accident. I consider how Joe navigated these competing narratives to make sense of his challenging circumstances and to find a way forward.

Emplotting Heroic Agency through Physical Therapy

Narratives are tools that health professionals use to shape interactions with patients, collaboratively constructing healing stories. The concept of **therapeutic emplotment** (Mattingly 1994) reveals how therapist-patient interactions can be used to create story-like structures that encourage patients to perceive therapy as a journey toward healing. The therapist invites the patient to embrace the healing plot, and advancing the plot means taking meaningful steps toward the goals set during the therapeutic encounter. Research on therapeutic emplotment (Crossley 2003; Kohn 2000), demonstrates that it is not just a storytelling scheme; it significantly influences the outcomes of care. Emplotment involves engaging the patient-protagonist in a plot: a sequence of events organized not just chronologically but meaningfully, in pursuit of a resolution. By closely examining Joe's therapy sessions, I witnessed how the physical therapist's instructions aimed to choreograph Joe's attention and actions, recruiting him into a plot that would advance him toward healing and recovery.

Joe arrived for his first therapy session at a rehabilitation center in Central Mexico on a windy November morning, pushed in his wheelchair by his case manager. Ana, the Mexican therapist in charge of Joe's rehabilitation, led them to the hospital's therapy gym, where she explained the first phase of Joe's treatment and got him started with strengthening exercises. Tiring midway through a set of sit-ups, Joe cracked a joke in order to gain a break. Recognizing the diversion, Ana encouraged him to persevere through the fatigue, "Andale, Joe, sin distracciones" (Come on, Joe, without distractions). At this first session, building rapport was important, but Ana did not hesitate to call Joe back to his role as patient, directing his actions and keeping him on task.

Later, when Joe experienced acute pain and dropped from a ladder during a climbing exercise, Ana paused the exercises and observed the stump of Joe's right leg with concern. She explained that if the bandage was not placed correctly, the stump would become deformed. "Debes de vendar bien, para que agarre resistencia. Debes de moldear el muñón" (You must bandage it well so that it generates resistance. You must shape the stump), she told Joe, touching the flesh and pressing specific points with her outstretched fingers. This interaction reminded me of what Joe's case manager had told me: the center that cares for migrants with amputations is one of the best of its kind in Mexico. The center is public but also receives private donations and focuses on physical rehabilitation, with support from psychology and psychiatry staff. This kind of attention and genuine care on the part of the staff is emotionally impactful for migrants, who have often experienced mistreatment at the hands of Mexican officials. Migrants also experience immense vulnerability being far from their family and friends, so their relationships with clinicians carry additional weight. I found that migrants sometimes interpreted the compassionate care of the staff as a sign they would be able to stay in Mexico after therapy. News that they would instead be deported often felt unexpected and disruptive to the therapeutic narrative. But this disruption was not always clear from the start because the therapeutic and migration narratives overlapped with a shared expectation of heroism.

This overlap was particularly noticeable in the early stages of physical therapy. For example, during the rehabilitation session, Ana explained to Joe that pain was normal in therapy and in daily life after an amputation. He should expect to feel pain as he builds muscle strength, but he should work hard to continue. She told him, "El dolor es normal, pero hay que ir más allá del dolor" (Pain is normal, but you have to go beyond the pain). This last phrase was delivered in a firm tone, almost like a motto, as if the therapist were a coach encouraging a runner to finish a marathon. By the end of his hour-long session, Joe lay down on the mats to recover from exhaustion. He promised Ana that he would practice his daily crunches at the migrant shelter where he was staying. Ana explained that to walk with a prosthesis, he would need a strong core to support his body. She jokingly added, "te van a salir cuadritos" (you're going to have a six pack), ending the session on a positive note.

As the above excerpts demonstrate, Ana encouraged her patient to play a heroic role. She framed efforts in rehabilitation sessions as a step toward overcoming the injury and advancing recovery. The therapeutic narrative was clear: Joe was asked to endure pain and overcome physical challenges through effort and persistence with the promise of eventual healing.

The theme of overcoming challenges is part of both the therapeutic narrative and the heroic migrant narrative. Both stories are centered around pushing bodies and minds to achieve an important goal, despite immense obstacles. This overlap was positive in some ways. According to Joe's care team, patients from the amputee program tended to exert themselves and regain strength more quickly than local, non-migrant patients "because they have a goal."

This therapeutic interaction exemplifies that at the early stage of Joe's recovery, the therapeutic and migration narratives seemed to align around the character of the hero. While the ability to overcome challenges is an essential part of the heroic migrant narrative, experiencing an amputation presents not only an obstacle to surmount but a new identity as a person with disabilities. Migrants must manage not only the physically painful experience of amputation but also negative perceptions around disability. Therefore, as migrants heal their physical wounds, they also struggle to reconcile this unexpected turn with the narratives they know.

Humanitarian Coercion and Agency

The last time I saw Joe in person, about a month into his therapeutic process, we were waiting outside the workshop where the hospital staff was designing his prosthetic. I asked him what he planned to do once he completed his treatment; I was confused about the process myself. I had seen that the government website for the amputee program was outdated and filled with jargon. Staff in the program only seemed familiar with the parts of the program in which they were directly involved. This was likely because the official network that provided care for migrants with amputations was made up of different organizations, with no one overseeing the overall process. Joe responded with deep anguish, looking away from me and toward a half-open door nearby. His answer was rambling and non-specific: perhaps he could return to the charitable Mexican family that helped him when his accident first occurred. Maybe something good would finally happen. He was clearly caught between stories, both of which demanded that he be a hero but did not provide him with concrete pathways for enacting this heroism as a person newly living with disabilities.

I continued to stay in touch with Joe via WhatsApp once I finished my time at the rehabilitation center. As the therapy sessions progressed, Joe learned about the reality of his limited possibilities in Mexico. He realized that if he completed his treatment, the result would be deportation. The more he regained his physical abilities, the closer he came to being deported. The disjuncture of deportation disrupted his trust in the therapeutic narrative. Ironically, the humanitarian process of rehabilitation had put Joe on an undesired path toward deportation that was structurally linked to the supposedly celebratory culmination of recovery.

The interrelationship between rehabilitation and deportation illustrates how humanitarian care becomes intertwined with immigration deterrence measures, where obedience and compliance are expected from migrants, even when this may conflict with their personal desires. During their interaction with humanitarian care, migrants are constantly pressured to demonstrate that they are "innocent" and "worthy of compassion," and their behavior is often judged and closely monitored (Ticktin 2016). Through this sort of **humanitarian coercion**, care institutions like the clinic force migrants to embody the role and responsibility of innocence imposed upon them, most notably by abandoning plans of unauthorized migration.

As a result of this humanitarian coercion, Joe became uneasy and stressed. Shelter staff where he was staying were increasingly unhappy with what they considered his "tantrums, entitlement and poor behavior." This scrutiny is part of how humanitarian coercion manifests and puts pressure on migrants. When Joe showed anger and dissatisfaction with a destiny that was not the one he wanted, the shelter staff decided he was "annoying" and needed to change his behavior. Since they knew of my close relationship with Joe, his case manager and the shelter staff asked me to encourage him to "cooperate" and complete his rehabilitation. After careful consideration, I decided not to intervene because I felt it was not my place to do so. Throughout our collaboration, I consistently aimed to listen to and respect Joe's wishes and self-determination. I communicated my decision to my fellow researchers, and we collectively agreed not to intervene.

In response to the increasing pressure he experienced, Joe decided to leave the amputee program and continue on his journey to the United States. The staff did not stop him, but advised him against leaving. They emphasized the dangers of crossing the border and reminded him that his injuries made him more vulnerable to violence. Ironically, in their efforts to get Joe to complete his rehabilitation, the staff cast him as a victim rather than a hero.

While Joe's decision may seem surprising, in my research I found that migrants with amputations often tried to continue their journeys north after amputation, some even starting again from their home countries after being deported. They are driven by profound economic difficulties in their home countries that are exacerbated by disability, adding to the burden of social stigma they face as "failed migrants." Due to their disabilities, not only do they become dependent on others, but their employment prospects, which were already limited before migration, are further reduced.

Up to this breaking point, the therapeutic narrative had aligned closely with Joe's interests, often intertwining with the heroic migrant narrative. However, the therapeutic narrative lacked solutions for the challenges he would face as a disabled man in Honduras. Conversely, until his accident, the heroic migrant narrative had been his guiding force, the story that directed, inspired, and motivated him. While the therapeutic narrative failed to offer hope for a prosperous future, the heroic migrant narrative provided him with a small but crucial sense of a future with possibilities. This is due to the connections between the heroic migrant narrative and the myth of the American Dream, which offers the tantalizing promise that anyone can achieve success in the United States. For Joe and other migrants with amputations, faith in the American Dream is often undergirded by a belief that the care system in the United States, including hospitals and social services, is more functional than the systems of care in their home countries. If he could make it to the United States, Joe felt sure that he would have a better life.

At this decisive moment, Joe resisted being displaced from the position of the heroic migrant to that of the failed migrant. He asserted his agency to continue his migration journey even if this meant not completing his treatment. **Agency** refers to an individual's ability to respond to social experiences and devise strategies for navigating challenges within constraining social systems. While people sometimes change dominant narratives and institutions through their agency, they also often reproduce these narratives and social structures (Giddens 1984). Seemingly left with no options, Joe acted agentively to draw upon the heroic migrant narrative and persevere on his journey to the United States.

To achieve this goal, he created and mobilized a network of solidarity and support as he moved north. I became part of this network, which existed outside of the hospital and the official care system. Participants in this network were motivated by the way that Joe framed himself as a heroic migrant. Just as this narrative allowed Joe to visualize and pursue future possibilities, it also helped members of his support network to imagine his path forward. (Of course, there were other stories at work too: members of the support network were also compelled by narratives emerging from religious beliefs or ideas about solidarity and humanism.) With the assistance of the Mexican family that had originally helped him at the scene of his accident,

Joe arrived at the border between Mexico and the United States. He undertook the challenge of crossing the desert but was unable to go far and had to return to Mexico. He found a shelter in a border town and there fostered the necessary connections among the shelter staff to contact a law firm in the United States. Thanks to their help, his legal case as a refugee was approved, and he was able to enter the United States with authorization and reunite with his extended family members who were living there. Once he had settled into his new life, Joe expressed admiration for the accessibility of his new city. For example, handicap doors made it much easier for him to get around in his wheelchair. “Things can only get better from here,” he told me, during a phone call, with optimism and hope. Against all odds, Joe had managed to embody the heroic migrant narrative, using it to propel himself forward and to build a support network that helped him reach his goal of building a new life in the United States.

Conclusion

Joes’ entrapment between narratives illuminates the role of health systems in networks designed to deter migration and the challenges for care in a global system that punishes and inflicts harm on migrants’ bodies. Through a close examination of Joe’s case, I explored the entanglement of healthcare and immigration enforcement by focusing on language, specifically the tension between the therapeutic narrative and the heroic migrant narrative. My analysis shows how, during their recovery, patients who suffer amputations are recruited by these competing narratives which have decisive implications for their healing process and migratory journey.

Both narratives offer a way of resolving the unexpected narrative turn of a near-fatal accident, and both are intertwined in the idea of overcoming obstacles and casting migrants as resilient heroes. The overlap can lead to confusion and disorientation among migrants who are trying to cope with their injured body while also finding a resolution to the unexpected turn of events. Migrants become caught between these competing narratives while striving to embody heroism. In the midst of this narrative tension, the therapeutic narrative was incapable of providing Joe with a desirable resolution that would go beyond physical recovery to address the larger question of how to survive and construct a life as a person with disabilities.

In the context of migration, institutions of care and clinicians themselves are also caught between narratives. The staff attending to Joe’s case recognized, like I did, the presence of a narrative competing with theirs. However, as employees within a system that had a narrow, specific definition of what care entailed, they emphasized the importance of their therapeutic narrative over the heroic migrant narrative, as the latter had initially led to Joe’s current suffering. Understanding that clinicians are also trapped in narratives is crucial to unravel the subtle ways in which healthcare and legal enforcement coalesce in the context of migration. Clinicians’ focus on healing can lead them to prioritize a therapeutic narrative that is disconnected from the actual realities of the people they are working with. Interrogating these institutionally imposed narratives might help practitioners to work more effectively with patients. More broadly, Joe's story and the findings from this study underline the need to change how institutions that provide humanitarian care operate within an international legal order that persecutes cross-border mobility, often resulting in harm and suffering for migrants, who are left seeking ways to recover from the long lasting marks of violence inscribed on their bodies.

Questions for Reflection and Discussion

Reflection Question

1. What stories about migration exist in your local context? How have you become aware of these narratives? How might your own or family experiences of migration influence your awareness of these narratives?

Looking In: Small Group Discussion Questions

1. What are the similarities and differences between the *therapeutic narrative* and the *heroic migrant narrative*?
2. How does the trope of the "resilient hero" function in both the heroic migrant narrative and the therapeutic narrative? How does this affect the healing journey of amputated migrants?
3. What is therapeutic emplotment? Provide a definition in your own words and identify some examples from the chapter or other contexts. How does this concept help us to see how narrative scripts are enacted through clinical encounters?
4. What is humanitarian coercion? Provide a definition in your own words and identify some examples from the chapter or other contexts.
5. What is agency? How do language and agency intersect, particularly when considering the role of language in shaping individual agency? What does the case presented in this chapter illustrate about agency and the role of language?

Looking Out: Large Group Discussion Questions

1. What do these two narratives and their overlap tell us about the relationship between care infrastructures and immigration enforcement? How are these two narratives shaped by and responsive to the structural violence that migrants like Joe experience? How are clinicians also caught between stories?
2. What are the ethical implications of conducting collaborative research? What would you have done in the position of the researcher: would you have

encouraged Joe to complete his treatment or supported him with his immigration project? Why would you make this choice and what would the implications be?

References

Arnold, Lynnette. 2024. National Heroes or Dangerous Failures: Mobilizing Gender in Salvadoran Migration Discourse to Create a Relational Neoliberal Personality. *Gender and Language* 17(4): pp. 412–432. doi.org/10.1558/genl.22687.

Crossley, Michel, L. 2003. Let Me Explain: The Narrative Plot and the Experience of a Patient with Oral Cancer. *Social Science and Medicine* 56(3): pp. 439–448. doi.org/10.1016/s0277-9536(01)00362-8.

Giddens, Anthony. 1984. *Constitution of Society, Outline of the Theory of Structuration.* Berkeley, CA: University of California Press.

Kohn, Abigail. 2000. "Imperfect Angels": Narrative "Emplotment" in the Medical Management of Children with Craniofacial Anomalies. *Medical Anthropology Quarterly* 14(2): pp. 202–223. doi.org/10.1525/maq.2000.14.2.202.

Marroquín Parducci, Amparo. 2019. Pedagogías lingüísticas y resistencias de la narrativa sobre migración internacional. *Chasqui* 14: pp. 161–176. Accessed August 8, 2024. https://dialnet.unirioja.es/servlet/articulo?codigo=7320762.

Mattingly, Cheryl. 1994. The Concept of Therapeutic Emplotment. *Social Science and Medicine* 38(6): pp. 811–822. doi:10.1016/0277-9536(94)90153-8.

Ochs, Elinor, and Capps Lisa. 2001. *Living Narrative: Creating Lives in Everyday Storytelling.* Cambridge, MA: Harvard University Press. doi.org/10.2307/j.ctv2d7x4pr.

Ticktin, Miriam. 2016. Thinking beyond Humanitarian Borders. *Social Research* 83(2): pp. 255–271. doi.org/10.1353/sor.2016.0030.

15

Learning to Experience Dying as a Part of Living

An Individual and Collective Journey

Marjorie Harness Goodwin, Federica Raia, and Mario Deng

I cannot escape death, but at least I can escape the fear of it.

(Epictetus. Discourses Book I, 108)

Introduction

On a gray, rainy Friday afternoon in March of 2018, Dr D., a cardiologist, picked up his patient, Chuck Goodwin, a linguistic anthropologist, to chat about an ongoing research project at a nearby Starbucks cafe. The real reason for the encounter was to get Chuck out of the house so that Candy, Chuck's partner, and co-author of this chapter, could prepare for a surprise party. Chuck had terminal cancer and only had a limited time to live.

For this occasion, friends, from various parts of the US and some from as far away as Singapore and Japan, had come to present Chuck with a book: a collection of writings of fifty authors all celebrating Chuck's influence on their own work. The book had been brought into print in a record three months' time, so that Chuck could read the articles while he was still alive. Chuck's cancer, which began in his eye, had spread throughout his body, and it was not known how long he would be alive.

Guests, some of whom had not seen him for a while, waited with apprehension at the house. Finally, Chuck arrived (see Figure 15.1). On opening the door and seeing the crowd, with his arms spread apart and smiling broadly, Chuck exclaimed loudly (for transcription conventions, see the chapter appendix):

Marjorie Harness Goodwin, Federica Raia, and Mario Deng, *Learning to Experience Dying as a Part of Living*. In: *Language and Health in Action*. Edited by: Lynnette Arnold et al., Oxford University Press. © Marjorie Harness Goodwin, Federica Raia, and Mario Deng (2026). DOI: 10.1093/9780198933953.003.0015

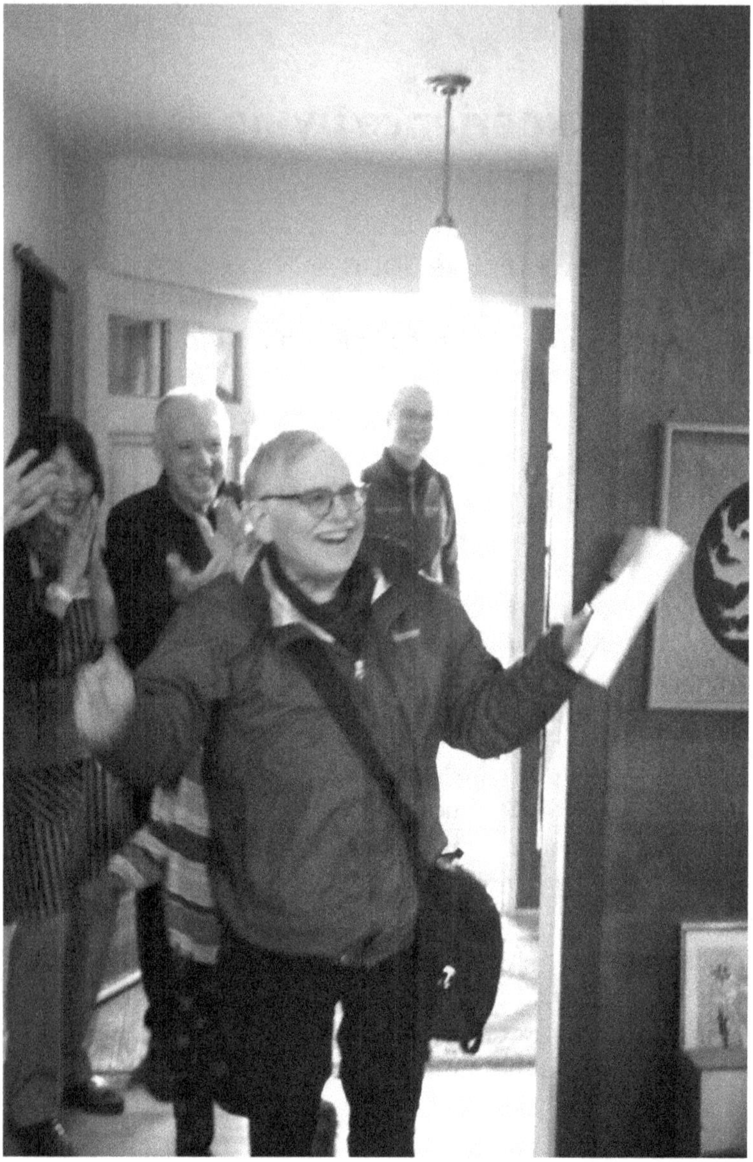

Fig. 15.1 Chuck arriving at the surprise party.

(01) Chuck: OH MY ***GO: :D***!
(02) Group: *((laughter))*
(03) Don: *((pointing))* And look. Everybody's here.
(04) Chuck: [OH ***WO: : :W***!
(05) Group: [*((clapping))* YEAH: : :
(06) Chuck: WOW WOW WOW!
WOW WOW OH ***WOW*** (.) ***WOW*** (.)
Oh ***WOW***! *((arms up))*
WOW! Oh my ***GO:***d. THIS IS IN***CRED***IBLE! Oh wow.

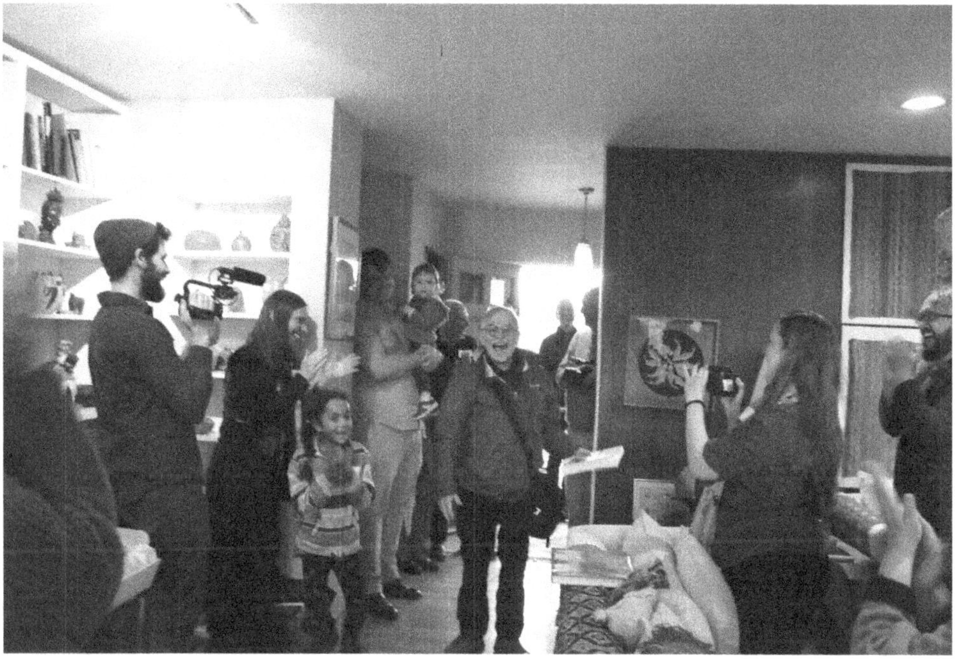

Fig. 15.2 Spontaneous applause at the surprise party.

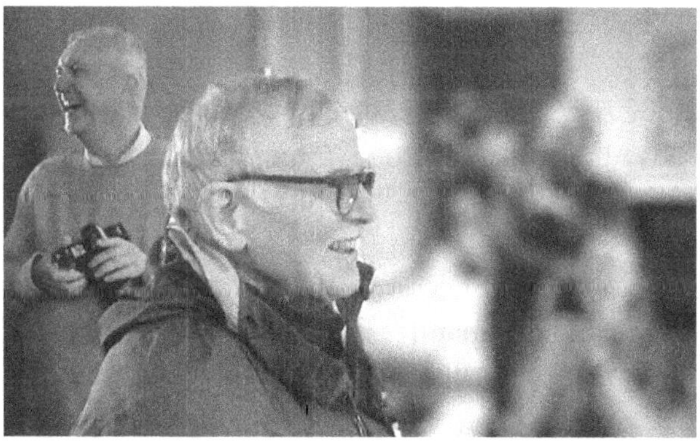

Fig. 15.3 Chuck expressing gratitude.

Chuck encountered a houseful of people who had come to celebrate him. Chuck's expressions of "OH ***WO:W***" were filled with joy, surprise, and excitement; his facial expression of widened eyes, raised brows, and dropped jaw contributed to his displays of wonderment.

Amidst his "oh wow" exclamations, spontaneous clapping emerged (Figure 15.2), a form of exuberance akin to what Durkheim (1926) calls "collective effervescence:" a feeling of emotional intensification and unity that can occur when a group of people participate in shared action, as during religious rituals.

A convergence of generosity and love filled the room. In response, Chuck expressed his gratitude (Figure 15.3):

Chuck: Oh ***thank*** you. ***Thank*** you. ***Thank*** you.
Oh: thank ***you.***
No. I said in all my e-mails and it's absolutely true.
You're the people that sustained me.
You ***are.*** And I realize
That with the book
And then when I sent out
That latest note about the thing.
I've been getting wonderful new e-mails back.
And it makes me feel in a way I never did before
Of being part of this community
That has grown through my lifetime.
And a lifetime of shared love of thinking
About human interaction and data.
And that leading to my warmest friends.
Who share my deepest feelings with me.
And that's all of you. And I am ***so:*** so happy.

Chuck's wide smile and exuberant thankfulness to his community of friends captured for Candy his uncanny ability to live in the present moment despite his imminent death. And as one friend expressed, his life was a "meditation on gratitude."

From the very outset of his cancer diagnosis, Chuck said that he felt intuitively that he had the absolute worst type of eye melanoma. He openly acknowledged rather than denied that he had this illness. In this sense, Chuck did not traverse the multitude of stages—denial, anger, bargaining, depression, acceptance—that Kubler-Ross (2014) delineated to describe the "emotional states seriously ill people commonly experience and the adaptive mechanisms they use to make sense of and live with incurable conditions" (Byock 2014:xiii). Instead, Chuck moved relatively swiftly into a mode of acceptance of death. This chapter explores how it was that despite impending death, Chuck was able to accept death with equanimity rather than denial.

To make sense of this question, we examine how Chuck's relationships and communication patterns with his doctor developed over time. Specifically, after (1) describing the methodology used in this study, we (2) describe what is entailed in the practice of Relational Medicine used by Chuck's cardiologist, Dr D., to socialize his patients to embrace dying as a part of living; (3) we examine a basic resource, the dyadic *encounter* (Goffman 1961), with its non-verbal and verbal communication dimensions including storytelling, that Dr D. makes use of to guide patients to accept dying as a part of living. During focused encounters participants maintain continuous engrossment in the official focus of activity (Goffman 1961:11). By examining the stories about illness Chuck exchanged with his doctor, we can investigate how one cancer patient came to embrace dying as a part of the cycle of life.

We organized the chapter chronologically to follow the temporal development through which Chuck learned to accept his impending death as part of life. To facilitate the reader in orienting to this development, we also include dates within each of the section's subtitles and provide here a brief sketch of his medical history. In the fall of 2015, Chuck experienced heart failure. He became so weak that his partner Candy needed to carry his laptop computer to his class. Exhausted from heart failure, he conducted one of his lab seminars lying flat on the floor. On December 17, 2015, Chuck had atrial fibrillation surgery. Candy was so terrified of the thought of losing her partner that she cried out to the interventional cardiologist, "When am I going to get my Chuck back?" Chuck had his first meeting with his new cardiologist Dr D., specialist in advanced heart failure, on March 2, 2016. In this meeting, Dr D. gave Chuck strict recommendations to change his diet, perform daily exercise, and take meditation classes while waiting for the diagnostic tests. These showed that Chuck suffered from coronary artery disease with a tight blockage in his right coronary artery, a condition which had led to Candy's father's death. To avoid surgery, Chuck needed lifestyle change and medication. Later that summer, on July 10, 2016, when he saw Dr D. again, Chuck had passed his stress test with flying colors. All was fine until February 6, 2017, when on a routine visit to the eye clinic, deadly choroidal eye melanoma was discovered in Chuck's left eye.

Study Methodology

This ethnographic report involves Chuck's cardiologist, Mario Deng (Dr D.), as co-author and researcher, along with Marjorie (Candy) Goodwin, Chuck's wife-caregiver, researcher, and co-author of this chapter, and Federica Raia, a researcher whose work focuses on care practices in medical and education contexts. The ethnographic project ("Living towards Dying"), a portion of which is presented in this chapter, is part of a much larger and multifaceted participatory research project (Raia 2020; Raia and Deng 2015; Raia et al. 2023), directed by Federica Raia, investigating the practices of teaching, learning, and patient care in high-tech medical practices of an "Advanced Heart Failure" program in a large US university hospital; the data include more than 500 hours of recorded medical encounters.

For the project, recordings of doctor-patient interaction were audio/videotaped over time, in the present case, for two years. Data consist of conversations between participants, rather than interviews. Participating healthcare practitioners, patients, and family caregivers also met to discuss the themes that emerged. These interactions were recorded as well. Researchers analyzed the recordings, using a micro-interactional method informed by studies of conversation analysis (Sacks et al. 1974), the study of talk produced in ordinary human interactions. Data were transcribed using an adapted version of the system developed by Jefferson, described in Sacks et al. (1974:731–733). In addition to talk, a host of other resources such as intonation, gesture, and touch, used concurrently by participants to frame their conduct (Goodwin 2018), were included in the transcripts. (See the chapter appendix for more details.) By closely attending to how these multiple resources are used conjointly in real time, we can analyze how social relations are achieved, moment by moment, during the conduct of social interaction. The stories we tell about illness and death not only describe but also shape our experience (see also Corwin 2021:9).

This ethnographic account details the journey that Chuck undertook with others in the process of "living towards dying." In email communication, Chuck spoke of his interactions with his students as a "continuing dialogue and exchange." His wish was that students would approach the lives of people they were studying "with a sense of awe and wonder and joy" at discovering the richness of what people were doing. Reflecting on these messages, one lab member wrote, "Chuck was showing us that by being part of an ongoing community that lives on without you, your own death becomes less tragic and final." She closed her email by saying, "As an academic mentor Chuck apprenticed us into the study of social interaction, but through these messages he became a mentor on dying." In this sense, the chapter challenges neoliberal biomedical myths of death as necessarily solitary, individuating, or heroic, in favor of a focus on "the communal and ongoing process of dying" (see Craig 2018:4).

Context of the Relational Medicine Experience

Chuck's dying experience differs from others in several ways. He shared a uniquely loving relationship with his wife, Candy, forming an existential dyad that supported both through facing death. Because of the specificity of his metastasized cancer, he also had a full year to prepare for the end of life, an invaluable stretch of time that many do not have. Furthermore, his long-standing friendship and medical relationship with Dr D. created an ideal context of care, combining trust, expertise, and empathy in a way that enriched his final months.

At the same time, Chuck received treatment from the same public university hospital and in the care of the same team that serves thousands of other patients from diverse socioeconomic and demographic backgrounds. Underpinning this care is the theory and practice of Relational Medicine (Raia and Deng 2015), consistently implemented at the main university hospital and a free clinic for the uninsured. A fundamental principle of Relational Medicine is that a person in need should not be alone but supported in developing their path of life that includes a path of dying as part of living.

Too often, the ability to plan, to touch one's family members, or engage in many of the small rituals that give life meaning are attenuated. Chuck was able to deal with his illnesses over a two-year period. He experienced first heart failure and then eye melanoma, from which he later died. Learning from his experience is important because many face diagnoses that force us to contend with our mortality. Indeed, people in the US have little experience of talking openly about death. Doctors, such as Atul Gawande, who write about their practice have said that their training seriously lacked any focus on how to talk about death. Gawande (2015:1) states:

> I learned about a lot of things in medical school but mortality wasn't one of them. . . . Our textbooks had almost nothing on aging or frailty or dying. How the process unfolds, how people experience the end of their lives, and how it affects those around them seemed beside the point. The way we saw it and the way our professors saw it, the purpose of medical schooling was to teach how to save lives, not how to attend to their demise.

While it is most common in medical encounters to avoid talking about death, Dr D., in the very first March 2016 meeting with Chuck, talked openly about his patient's fears and uncertainties: high blood pressure, shortness of breath, the closing down of his academic department. The doctor urged his patient to address what he called "living towards dying." By this he meant that because death is inevitable, it is important to live life to the fullest in the present moment, appreciating every day as it comes: in Dr D.'s words, "to be attentive to the 'here-and-now-ness of life.'" This type of openness in talking about death is not standard practice for doctors, nurses, patients, and caregivers, as most find it difficult to initiate talk about death. Maynard and colleagues (2015:92) state that discussions of quality and end of life "are at best infrequent and at worst nonexistent." Dr D. did not wait for his patient to initiate talk about death. Starting from the premise that death is inevitable, during the very first encounter with a patient, Dr D. offers advice on how to live toward dying.

The experience we report on, in which Chuck talks openly about death, differed in large part from others' experiences because Chuck came to be cared for by a doctor who practices **Relational Medicine** (Raia and Deng 2015). Relational Medicine is a way of practicing medicine that maintains the basic human right of "personhood," not only for the patient but for healthcare professionals as well. Dr D.'s understanding of being a doctor is that of "a healthcare professional supporting the patient on his/her journey from the land of dissimilitude (a situation of uncertainty) into self-determined life, accepting and incorporating the major changes of the body, in this person's life" (Raia and Deng 2015:111). Often functioning as a therapist or a counselor in addition to his role as a cardiologist, Dr D. seeks to create a safe space where the patient can convey his concerns and receive commentary.

For a doctor practicing Relational Medicine, care emerges in the dynamics of interactions with the patient (Raia 2020). Care is an activity; it is a way of supporting the patient to develop a new sense of self while undergoing disease. Care requires a continuous attunement to the dynamic situation of the encounter (Raia and Deng

2015:71). In this chapter we examine the conversational practices through which Dr D. closely attends to what his patient says, permitting discussion of patient fears and leading to discussion of what has ultimate meaning in his life.

Doctors practicing Relational Medicine often treat illnesses that require close coordination among family members for the patient's care, such as advanced heart failure; first medical encounters may last more than an hour (in contrast to twelve-minute primary care encounters). Forms of Relational Medicine depend on a range of material resources to which most individuals in the world including the US do not have access, which include not only time, but also trained physicians with whom we have relationships, health insurance, etc. In this chapter, we do not explore these structural resources which make the care of those practicing Relational Medicine possible, although they are important to keep in mind. Instead, we focus on the linguistic practices that are afforded both by the structural resources available to the interlocutors and by Relational Medicine training.

Storytelling and Relational Medicine

To explore Chuck's experience of living toward dying we examine language practices used interactively in storytelling, while narrating past, present, or future events. In institutional contexts, such as doctor-patient or counseling interactions, it is common for interactions to be formed out of paired question/answer sequences, initiated by the doctor or counselor (Peräkylä 1995). Such actions permit a relatively quick exchange of turns.

Storytelling is different. As conversation analyst Harvey Sacks (1995) notes, storytelling permits a teller an extensive unit of talk, typically containing multiple utterances. Dr D. structures his encounters with open-ended questions such as "How's life?" which invite the patient to develop their own story, rather than being constrained by a question requesting specific information. In interactions between Chuck and his doctor, storytelling provided a way for Chuck and his physician to develop a vision of living toward dying over multiple turns of talk, rather than units of question/answer pairs.

From the perspective of Ochs and Capps (2001:2), stories or personal narratives provide a way of using language "to imbue life events with a temporal and logical order, to demystify them and establish coherence across past, present and as yet unrealized experience." Here we examine how through storytelling Dr D. guides Chuck to develop a new sense of self and a meaningful sense of life while approaching an uncertain future. Through telling stories we not only relate chronological events or visions of events to come; we also relate our emotional life or moods, which are central to our being or dwelling in the world (Heidegger 1962).

Chuck's Story of Shellshock on Learning of His Cancer Diagnosis (February 8, 2017)

On February 6, 2017, on a visit to the ophthalmology clinic at University of California, Los Angeles (UCLA), a large, elevated lesion was found in the periphery of Chuck's left eye. It was diagnosed as choroidal eye melanoma with serious retinal detachment.

Two days later, after the diagnosis of eye cancer, on February 8, 2017, Chuck had a routine scheduled appointment with his heart doctor, who had been informed by Chuck of his cancer diagnosis. After first dealing with medical issues related to his heart, Dr D. inquired about the eye cancer. In response to Dr D.'s question "So what's the update?," Chuck presents his visceral reactions to what was going on, using metaphors alluding to the intensity of his emotional reaction. He provides the analogy of the "Phony War" to describe how he is feeling. The Phony War (October 1939–March 1940) defines the early months of World War II, after the German conquest of Poland, in September 1939, when, for a time, there were no open hostilities between the Allies and the Germans. For Chuck it means a time of waiting, anxiety, impatience, with little certainty about what is going to happen next:

Chuck: Okay. So about this? One way to say is—
I haven't looked on the web or anything.
The comparison and I think it's perhaps a good comparison,
Is the Phony War at the beginning of World War Two
When everybody knew the Germans were gonna attack
But there was that period in Paris when nobody did.
So I've just been sitting
Somewhat in a state of shell shock.
And not ye(h)t wan(h)ting to kno(h)w
Uh, the road (.) we're about to venture on.
I mean I'm concerned obviously in many ways.
I'm concerned about dying.
I'm concerned about the nature of the treatments.
Obviously I don't know if I'll lose an ***eye***,
If I'm gonna have an awful lot of chemo or something.
And also (.) I realize (.) I'm concerned (.) for Candy.

In response to Chuck's story (seven minutes later) Dr D. provides what Sacks calls a "second story." In his *Lectures in Conversation*, Sacks (1995:3–31) states that with a second story, the listener appears as a character in an event similar to the teller's. The telling of a similar experience can be a way of demonstrating or exhibiting understanding, confirming features of the told experience, with the meaning "you're not alone." The doctor's second story involves how his wife Federica felt when she discovered she had breast cancer. The news of cancer hit suddenly and destructively:

(01) Dr D.: Coming back to what ***you*** just said,
And thank you for sharing that.
It's just more on this—how it hits.
Kind of like a ***bomb***. Right?
(02) Chuck: [Yeah.
(03) Dr D.: [That's what I also felt.
And that's actually how Federica felt when she texted me
And when I called.
It was just this. It's the first uh thing.
And then you transform this into a plan and that's ongoing.
And obviously we're here, so 24/7 to talk about this.
To talk about that and uhm,
So I think this uncertainty time is really uh—is difficult.

The second story provides an empathetic demonstration of understanding of Chuck's narrative. Using a metaphor that paralleled Chuck's reference to war, Dr D. explained that news of his wife's cancer hit "kind of like a bomb." Then ending with "obviously we're here 24/7 about this," Dr D. provides the assurance that he will always be available for consultation.

Healing Guidance through Reframings of Patient Stories of "Emotionality" (April 21, 2017)

In this section, we will examine the ways the doctor guides his patient to envision a cohesive sense of self facing death through storytelling. By way of background information, after Candy's father had died in 1985, wanting to experience how death is celebrated in Mexico, the couple went to Oaxaca for the Day of the Dead celebration. During this holiday, families welcome back the souls of their deceased relatives for a brief reunion that includes food, drink, and celebration. Extended families come from distant parts of Mexico to gather by gravesites in the cemetery, decorated with fresh flowers, such as marigolds, to be with their loved ones. Small bands come to play favorite songs of the departed; children play dominoes on the gravesites. Altars in homes are lavishly decorated with flowers, candles, photos, and favorite foods and drinks of the departed.

Thirty years later, this experience formed part of Candy and Chuck's orientation to concepts about death and visions of how to die. This experience of how death is dealt with in Mexico forms part of the couple's existential past, important to their orientation to who they will be in their "path of becoming" (Raia 2020). In relating his present emotions regarding death to Dr D., Chuck speaks of the continuity between the living and the dead that the Mexican tradition supports. As he tells a story about the Day of the Dead, with its "healthy" interpretation of death by comparison with the US, he uses falsetto voice *((fal))* and begins to cry (as indicated by (h)—breathiness in the midst of words.)

(01) Chuck: And all the others. *((crying))* And in a way—
We shou(h)ldn't treat the ***dead*** as
So ***ter***rible. It made me think of The Day of the Dead in Mexico.
((fal)) Where people go and talk to a(h)ll their dea(h)d.
(02) Dr D.: Yeah. Yes.
(03) Chuck: And that ***seems heal***thier [uh
(04) Dr D.: [Yes.
(05) Chuck: 'Cause we have participated, with everybody.
(06) Dr D.: Yes.
(07) Chuck: And not that I believe in ***ghosts*** or afterlife,
But it should be that there's this continu(h)ity.
°Sorry° *((crying))* I didn't mean—

With his apologizing for crying and explanations that he's been attempting to "keep a tight grip" on things which have become "quite emotional," Chuck makes himself quite vulnerable. Such displays are only possible when trust is shared between participants, as is the present case. Dr D., closely attuned to the emotionality in Chuck's talk, comments "I'm very grateful that this is happening right now." He speaks of the importance of emotionality for the human condition and even challenges Chuck's idea that it's necessary to "hold a tight grip" on the emotions. Rather than emotionality being a problem, Dr D. reframes expressing emotion as appropriate to the situation. This commentary moves Chuck to articulate what really matters to him.

Dr D. imparts to his patients the importance of understanding the relationship of the body and mind to the health of the immune system. For him, "***E***:very moment of mind, soul, being in this world ... has its direct corollary correlate on the body level." Dr D. concludes with this statement: "So in other words it's all in one. There's nothing left out." Just at this moment, Chuck comes in with agreement: "Right. Right" and builds on Dr D.'s comments with his own perspective: "I'd ***on***ly wanna add, one other thing."

Chuck next elaborates his own version of what's important in life, speaking of his relationships with others rather than the abstract theory of Dr D. about the close entanglements of mind, soul, and body. Chuck, with great passion and while almost crying, describes how he has dedicated his life to his students and his wife. These people constitute "the present he can return to full of love and care and the greatest happiness." Chuck relates that he has no regrets in his life. Suddenly Dr D. reaches for Chuck's hand, and Candy gets out her cellphone (see Figure 15.4). She wants to capture this incredible moment in which touch is comforting and healing, which for her is like a parent's embrace of a child during trauma. Dr D. next elaborates how one's being can continue past death through other persons.

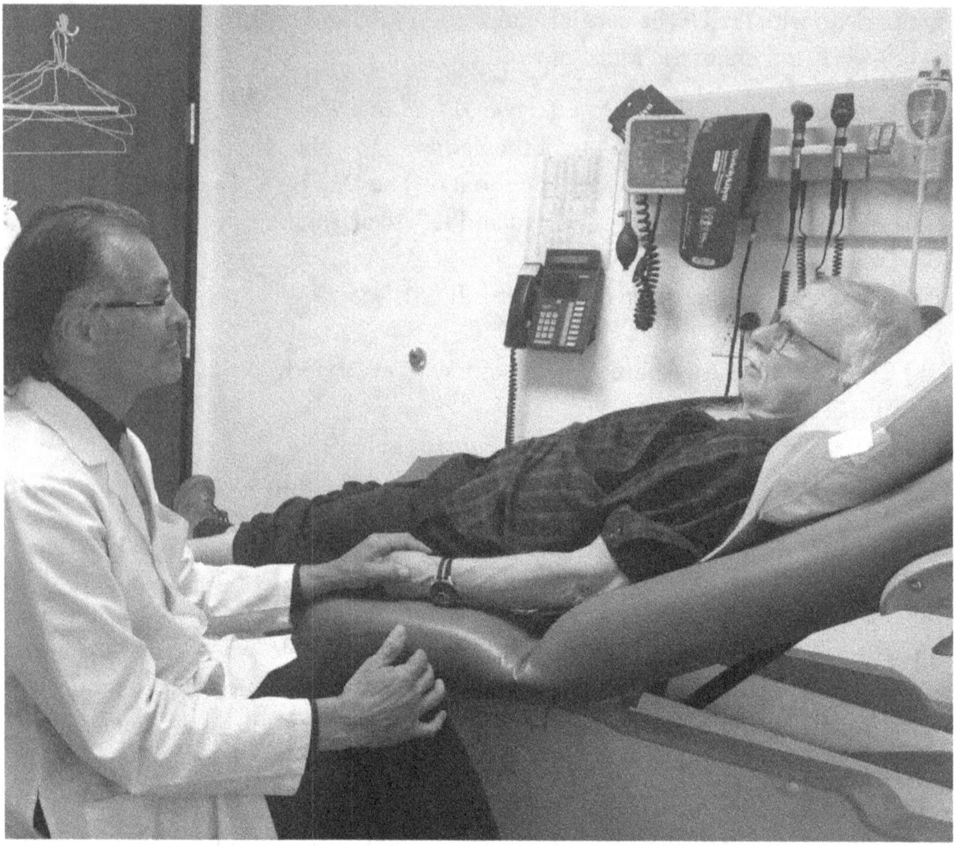

Fig. 15.4 Dr D. holding Chuck's hand.

(01) Dr D.: And that is where the question becomes

What is the—what are the entities of importance
In our living in this world, being in this world,

It's on ***one*** hand ***one***ness in the abyss of emptiness

(02) Chuck: [°Yeah,°

(03) Dr D.: [Of the irreversible
Uh absence of the potential of living.
On the ***o***ther hand, it's the dyadic oneness of two.=

(04) Chuck: =Right.

(05) Dr D.: In which all our transitory being is in a way e***ter***nalized.

(06) Chuck: uh huh,

(07) Dr D.: Because that other person carries me.

(08) Chuck: [Yeah.

(09) Dr D.: [As a dyadic unit.

(10) Chuck: Yeah. Yeah.

(11) Dr D.: I am ***be***ing in that other person

Dr D. transforms talking about a tight grip on emotions into an actual grip that anchors Chuck in a new space for facing and talking about death. Dr D. comments about the finality of death as "an abyss of emptiness of the irreversible uh absence of the potential of living." Next Dr D. provides a vision of living on past death as he states, "That other person carries me."

Chuck then continues the theme of how his life will persist in a transformed way after his death. After recounting how in the Mexican Day of the Dead tradition, the dead have a presence, he also invokes the figure of deceased anthropologist Gregory Bateson, whose ideas live on in his writings. Chuck adds that although he is about to retire, he feels he lives "through his students."

In response to Dr D.'s commentaries, Chuck begins to elaborate features of his life which affirm the continuity of his person in the past and future. The sense of being at peace with his life, which Chuck narrates here, is possible because Chuck exists within a large community of people who together, through their daily interactions, provide webs of love and continuing affirmation of the person he is.

Dr D. engages Chuck in building a narrative about the future where Chuck has a continuing presence. Dr D. achieves this by carefully listening, recruiting what is relevant in Chuck's life, and anchoring the story in possibilities for a cohesive sense of self facing dying as part of living. We see through the ways in which patient and doctor tell stories and respond to them how language is used to "establish coherence across past, present and as yet unrealized experience" (Ochs and Capps 2001:2). In realizing that his ideas will persist past his lifetime in the work of his students and through his own writings, Chuck is able to reach a form of equanimity. Future generations of scholars will build upon the enduring insights Chuck provided, leading to continuous innovation and transformation of ideas, making him live on through this work.

In December 2017, the stories Chuck told to his doctor and friends no longer expressed the kind of angst or despair that Chuck initially felt when he found out he had cancer. When asked how it was that he was able to cope, Chuck said that he had learned from the experience of losing his dog that there was "no way to fight death." He recalled that when his father had a stroke that left him unable to speak, his father "didn't waste his time hoping he'd get his speech back" and "accepted where he was at all those points." Commenting on his own situation Chuck said, "I'm in the mind set where not only all life, but the universe itself is very mortal. So there is no way to hold back time. You just have to live with what's happening and make the best decisions." Chuck accepted that his life, as the entire universe, is ephemeral. When Chuck came to terms with the finality of life, he was at peace.

Chuck's Toast to Life and his Legacy (March 2, 2018)

On March 2, 2018 (a month before he died), the surprise party that opened this chapter was held in Chuck's honor. Chuck expressed gratitude to people who had come. He drew from his experience of the Day of the Dead to talk explicitly about his own ideas about how to die. In a toast to his guests he stated:

Chuck: And the other thing I really wanna say,
I'm so happy to see the children here today too.
Because—I envision—I told you this and I'm not trying to be dark.
But instead of my life fading out
All by myself.
Like in a hospital room,
I envision when my life finally fades out, It's fading out in a scene like this.
That's filled with the life of others.
With all sorts of generations.
That seems to be the world we inhabit.
Rather than a private world of pain and death.
But a world that is sustained through the richness of other people.
And their care, concern, intellectual stimulation,
And it's the most wonderful thing.

Chuck's vision was of his final days being "filled with the life of others." He continued to meet with his seminar toward the last week of his life, though it was in the bedroom rather than the lab. Neighbors and friends came to visit him. His sister Pat, a hospice nurse, stayed with Chuck and Candy before and after the death.

Concluding Thoughts

We began this chapter asking how it was that Chuck, a patient with terminal cancer, was able to accept death with equanimity. We examined the forms of communication used by a doctor who practices Relational Medicine. Through engaging in storytelling with Chuck, Dr D. was able to deeply understand the concerns and fears of his patient. The doctor's responses were carefully attuned to the patient's narratives, displaying empathy in second stories or providing instructive commentaries leading to new ways to envision the meaning of his life. The themes of Chuck's stories changed over time. Chuck's initial stories in February 2017 were of anxiety, fear, and feeling a sense of hopelessness. With his doctor's guidance, in April, Chuck came to understand that his ideas would live on with his students' work and his own writings. By December of that year his stories spoke of accepting death as a part of the natural life cycle. Chuck considered Dr D. "a healer" who could guide him "to live in the shadow of death."

The openness with which Chuck spoke to his doctor and community is uncommon among those approaching death in biomedical settings. By sharing his experiences, Chuck mentored others on how to approach death, supporting the notion of dying as a "community responsibility" (Aoun 2022).

In sharing stories, we provide temporal "images" that account for our past and future possibilities of being ourselves. When the future possibility of being was taken away from Chuck because of his terminal cancer diagnosis, Chuck responded with what he called in a conversation with his doctor getting a "tight grip" on his emotions to avoid giving in to panic and losing control over what was meaningful in his present life. Indeed, Raia (2020) shows that to make sense of who we are and our actions in the present we must have a cohesive sense of not only who we were in the past, but also our future possibilities of existence. In this sense the doctor's advice to concentrate on his life with his wife Candy, which Chuck felt was the "most important advice" he could have received, had an important function. It provided Chuck with the possibility of seeing himself in a dynamic unit with the people he loved while facing death. This projection into future possibility reestablished the cohesive sense of Chuck's past in relation to his future possibilities of being.

Just as he had hoped, Chuck's writings have continued to be well recognized as impactful after his death. In 2019, a year after his death, Chuck was honored by receiving the Sapir Book Prize for the best book in linguistic anthropology during the last two-year period, as well as the Distinguished Book award from the Ethnomethodology and Conversation Analysis section of the American Sociological Association. Chuck's lab continues to meet, transitioning to Zoom at the onset of the pandemic, with Candy leading the group. With weekly exchanges, new possibilities for collaboration across five continents keep emerging. Chuck's ideas live on in both the writings and presentations of numerous scholars who view his work on cooperative action as foundational for studies of human interaction. Writing this chapter and having others respond to it is part of the continuity of his life and legacy.

Questions for Reflection and Discussion

Reflection Questions

1. What was it like for you to read about Chuck's end of life? What past experiences or thoughts about the future did it bring up for you?
2. How comfortable are you talking about the process of dying with friends or family? From your own perspective, to what degree do you think death should be a private matter or something that is shared with others? Why?

Looking In: Small Group Discussion Questions

1. Define Relational Medicine in your own words. What is distinctive about a doctor who practices Relational Medicine?
2. The authors recorded doctor-patient interactions across several years. Based on the example of Chuck's medical experiences, what do we learn from this

type of longitudinal approach and why are longitudinal approaches important to studying language and health?
3. The authors pay close attention to micro-interactional moments in their data. How is the close analysis of interaction important to the argument in this chapter?
4. Dr D. and Chuck use storytelling as a part of Chuck's medical care. What role do stories play in this chapter and what other roles do stories play in doctor-patient interaction?

Looking Out: Large Group Discussion Questions

1. What were the results of Chuck's willingness to talk openly about death and dying with his doctors, his family, his colleagues, and his friends? What practical implications might this have for terminally ill individuals, their families, communities, and care providers?
2. The authors of this chapter were intimately involved in Chuck's life. Comparing this chapter to other chapters in the book, how do you see evidence of the authors' closeness to Chuck in their methods, analysis, and writing?

Appendix

Transcription Symbols
Talk is transcribed using a modified version of the transcription system developed by Gail Jefferson (Sacks, Schegloff and Jefferson 1974:731–733).

1. **(°)**: A degree sign (°) indicates that the talk on either side of it is low in volume.
2. **Cut-off**: A dash (—) marks a sudden cut-off of the current sound.
3. ***Bold Italics*** indicate some form of emphasis, which may be signaled by changes in pitch and/or amplitude.
4. **Overlap bracket**: a left bracket ([) marks the point at which the current talk is overlapped by other talk.
5. **Colons** indicate that the sound immediately preceding the colon has been noticeably lengthened.
6. **Intonation**: Punctuation symbols are used to mark intonation changes rather than as grammatical symbols:

   A period indicates a falling contour.
   A question mark indicates a rising contour.
   A comma indicates a falling-rising contour.

7. An **(h)** indicates an inbreath or aspiration; here it indicates crying in the midst of talk.

8. **(.)** indicates a micro-pause in the midst of an utterance.
9. **(=)** indicates latching; there is no interval between the end of a prior turn and the start of the next utterance.
10. **Comments**: Double parentheses enclose material that is not part of the talk being transcribed, indicating talk being spoken in some special way, such as *(fals)* meaning falsetto.

References

Aoun, Samar M. 2022. Supporting the Dying Is a Community Responsibility. *Palliative Care and Social Practice* 16: pp. 1–4.

Byock, Ira. 2014. Foreword. In *On Death and Dying*, Elisabeth Kubler-Ross, pp. xi–xv. New York: Scribner.

Corwin, Anna. 2021. *Embracing Age: How Catholic Nuns Became Models of Aging Well*. New Brunswick: Rutgers University Press.

Craig, Megan. 2018. Learning to Live with Derrida and Levinas. *Graduate Faculty Philosophy Journal* 39(1): pp. 3–36.

Durkheim, Emile. 1926. *Elementary Forms of Religious Life*, transl. Joseph Ward Swain. New York: Macmillan.

Gawande, Atul. 2015. *Being Mortal: Illness, Medicine, and What Matters in the End*. London: Profile Books.

Goffman, Erving. 1961. *Encounters: Two Studies in the Sociology of Interaction*. Indianapolis: Bobbs-Merrill.

Goodwin, Charles. 2000. Action and Embodiment within Situated Human Interaction. *Journal of Pragmatics* 32: pp. 1489–1522.

Goodwin, Charles. 2018. *Co-Operative Action*. Cambridge: Cambridge University Press.

Heidegger, Martin. 1962. *Being and Time*, transl. J. M. E. Robinson. New York: Harper & Row.

Kubler-Ross, Elisabeth. 2014. *On Death and Dying: What the Dying Have to Teach Doctors, Nurses, Clergy, and Their Own Families*. London: Simon and Schuster.

Maynard, Douglas W., Dogoberto Cortez, and Toby C. Campbell. 2015. "End of Life" Conversations, Appreciation Sequences, and the Interaction Order in Cancer Clinics. *Patient Education and Counseling* 99: pp. 92–100.

Ochs, Elinor, and Lisa Capps. 2001. *Living Narrative: Creating Lives in Everyday Storytelling*. Cambridge, MA: Harvard University Press.

Peräkylä, Anssi. 1995. *Aids Counselling: Institutional Interaction and Clinical Practice*. Cambridge: Cambridge University Press.

Raia, Federica. 2020. The Temporality of Becoming: Care as an Activity to Support the Being and Becoming of the Other. *Mind, Culture and Activity* 27(3): pp. 1–21.

Raia, Federica, and Mario Deng. 2015. *Relational Medicine: Personalizing Modern Healthcare: The Practice of High Tech Medicine as a Relational Act.* Hackensack, NJ: World Scientific.

Raia, Federica, Murray Kwon, and Mario Deng. 2023. *Uncertainty, Decision-Making and Team Work in High-Tech Healthcare: PERSON-SoulMindBody-HOOD and Relational Medicine.* Singapore: World Scientific.

Sacks, Harvey. 1995. *Lectures in Conversation II*. Cambridge, MA: Basil Blackwell.

Sacks, Harvey, Emanuel A. Schegloff, and Gail Jefferson. 1974. A Simplest Systematics for the Organization of Turn-Taking for Conversation. *Language* 50: pp. 696–735.

Afterword

The Case for Narrative Competence in the Clinic and Beyond

Mara Buchbinder

This book offers a broad look at the many intersections between language and health.

As a medical anthropologist based in an academic medical center who studies and works alongside physicians, as well as teaches medical students, I have spent much time reflecting on why thinking about language and health should matter to clinicians. On one level, the answer may seem obvious. Language is a fundamental tool of both representation and interpretation. It is the bridge between the patient's subjective experience of illness and the treatment tools of medicine. It mediates all aspects of clinical interaction, from diagnosis to treatment uptake to the way that bad news will be received. And, just as language can be a bridge, it can also be a roadblock, constituting an important hurdle for access to health care, as Section 2 of this book, "Language Access," explores. From this perspective, language holds enormous power over the clinical encounter.

Yet one of the most important and least acknowledged reasons for clinicians to think about language is that doing so can help them to become analysts of, rather than mere participants in, clinical interaction. Section 1 of this book, "Clinical Interaction," demonstrates that clinicians may sometimes bring harmful cultural and moral assumptions into interactions with patients. Approaching the clinical encounter as an analyst would, with intellectual curiosity, can help clinicians to better understand patients' lives and stories on their own terms.

The physician and literary scholar Rita Charon is the founding director of the program in Narrative Medicine at Columbia University. Twenty years ago, Charon introduced the concept of **narrative medicine** to frame narrative as a clinical competence (Charon 2001). She proposed that the ability to "recognize, absorb, metabolize, interpret, and be moved by stories of illness" could enrich clinical practice and patient care (Charon 2007:1265).

The important insight here is that narrative is not just a container for important information about the patient—as Kleinman's (1988) *The Illness Narratives* might suggest—but a set of analytic skills that can be taught clinically. Such skills stretch beyond the basics of communication and listening imparted to all beginning physicians to include foundational principles of textual analysis. Charon (2004:862)

Mara Buchbinder, *The Case for Narrative Competence in the Clinic and Beyond*. In: *Language and Health in Action*. Edited by: Lynnette Arnold et al., Oxford University Press. © Mara Buchbinder (2026). DOI: 10.1093/9780198933953.003.0016 recounts how she employs these strategies within the course of an ongoing clinical interaction:

> I listen not only for the content of his narrative, but for its form—its temporal course, its images, its associated subplots, its silences, where he chooses to begin in telling of himself, how he sequences symptoms with other life events. I pay attention to the narrative's performance—the patient's gestures, expressions, body positions, tones of voice.

For Charon, **narrative competence** entails textual skills like perspective taking, charting a story's underlying structure, and identifying literary devices like metaphor, as well as creative and affective skills like imagining possible endings and cultivating empathy for the story's characters. Such skills have long been familiar territory for psychotherapists but arrived relatively later to medicine.

The benefits of narrative competence are multiple. By better understanding the patient's story, Charon contends, clinicians can better understand the disease itself. Additional impacts that have been documented empirically include stronger communication and collaboration skills, self-awareness and self-reflection, and empathy (Arntfield et al. 2013). Narrative competence also upholds the tenets of patient-centered care, a foundational framework for contemporary US medicine.

Granted, not all clinicians have the capacity to develop narrative competence. Doing so requires time and material resources not afforded to all clinical trainees, particularly those in the Global South (Street 2014; Wendland 2010). Moreover, narrative competence must be paired with **structural competence** to truly change the patient's story. Structural competence is a term coined by the physician-social scientists Jonathan Metzl and Helena Hansen (2014) as a complement to **cultural competence**—the notion popularized in the 1990s that clinical professionals can enhance patient care by developing fine-grained, contextual understanding of cultural variables such as race, ethnicity, class, and religion (Hunt 2019). Structural competence, by way of contrast, puts the emphasis on social determinants of health that lie much further upstream, such as public transportation, infrastructure, housing, zoning laws, and food delivery systems.

It's not hard to make the case that today's clinical trainees need exposure to structural competence. In recent years, it has been promoted in every clinical specialty from dentistry (Alarcon et al. 2022) to nursing (Waite and Hassouneh 2021). Section 4 of this book, "Language and Environment," can enhance these pedagogical efforts by showing how language mediates the processes by which structural inequalities shape social, political, and material environments and human health.

Yet training in narrative competence, though perhaps less fashionable, is just as important as structural competence to equipping future clinicians for success. Narrative competence is in some ways a prerequisite to structural competence: narrative tools can help clinicians to elicit patients' stories and grasp details about the structures that shape their lives. Narrative thinking can also draw attention to the biographical imprint of structural inequalities—and, importantly, a possible future in which things might be otherwise.

The University of North Carolina School of Medicine, where I have taught first and second year medical students for the past fourteen years, recognizes these competencies and strives to promote them through our unique curriculum in the humanities and social sciences. Through multidisciplinary courses taught in small group settings, we introduce students to social science and humanities perspectives on medicine. Narrative competence and structural competence are both featured in the course lexicon. Our goals for students are to develop skills in critical thinking and analysis, which they must exercise in both oral and written forms, and to cultivate a capacity for uncertainty and ambiguity. (Unlike their basic science curriculum, in our humanities and social science curriculum they frequently encounter questions to which there are no clear answers.)

Our first course assignment is for students to write their own personal illness narrative. Over the years, I have had students reflect on everything from childhood bedwetting to orthopedic surgery to mental illness, often bringing a unique, refreshing perspective to these common experiences. One student in our course eventually published her personal illness narrative in *Current Psychiatry*, under the title "The Doctor Is Sick":

> Yes, the doctor is sick. Who is she anyway? She is not even a doctor! She is just a third-year medical student who is fighting, fists up, her descent into madness. Has she won? She is trying to find a way to accept what she is. Does that mean she is a winner or a loser? It is chronic, but manageable, bipolar madness. There are lots of other people like her. But it is still overwhelming, and she is not even sure she wants to join anybody else. (Anonymous 2016:46)

Inviting students to begin their critical studies of biomedicine with self-reflection accomplishes two goals. It enables them, first, to consider—often for the first time—how their family, cultural, and socioeconomic backgrounds shape their experiences of health and illness; and, second, to confront some of their taken-for-granted assumptions about illness, medicine, and healing. The personal illness narrative is followed by a visit to a patient's home and an essay that situates the patient's medical history within a broader biographical framework. For this exercise, we ask students to spend as much time on the contextual details of their patients' lives and home environments as they do on their medical treatment.

Together, these assignments teach our first semester medical students that being analysts of health, illness, and healing is a cornerstone of medical practice. Our hope is that by refining these analytic skills early on, students will retain the practical knowledge to infuse their future clinical practice with analytic tools. Writing their own illness narratives and listening deeply to patients' stories also encourages students to consider how language constructs and mediates healing practices, as explored in Section 5 of this book, "Healing Practices." This is our brand of narrative competence, one that we have been collectively honing for over forty years.

Another way of being a narrative analyst is to take on new concepts for framing experience. The notion that health concepts circulate and travel outside of clinical medicine into other communities is central to the chapters in Section 3, "Community and Communicability." In a similar vein, humanities and social science concepts can travel outside of academia to enrich, inform, and reframe clinical practice. This is another important way in which scholarly work on language and health can be valuable to clinicians.

In 2010, sociologist Stefan Timmermans and I introduced the term "patient-in-waiting" to describe a liminal state between normal health and pathology that we had documented in our research on newborn screening for genetic disorders. We described how technological advances in medicine had made it possible for patients to hover between sickness and health for a prolonged period, due to new diagnostic technologies and clinical uncertainty about the significance of their results (Timmermans and Buchbinder 2010). The concept has since been widely adopted and cited, yet what has been most surprising for us has been the positive reception by the geneticists we studied, who started using the term in clinical communication with families. For these geneticists, using this language was a way of acknowledging the collateral damage of newborn screening, which sometimes marked an otherwise healthy baby as potentially seriously ill.

This, then, is another form of narrative competence: welcoming new language to describe clinical phenomena when it can bolster meaning and understanding of patients' experiences. The chapters in this volume can do the same kind of work for clinicians. I hope that clinician readers will embrace this volume in this spirit. They have much to learn from its authors.

References

Alarcon, Bertha, Lucian O'Conor, Sean Rowan, Bradley S. Henson, Anne E. Doan Van, Paul Simeteys, and Marisa K. Watanabe 2022. Bringing Structural Competency to the Forefront of Dental Education. *Journal of Dental Education* 86(9): pp. 1083–1089.

Anonymous. 2016. The Doctor is Sick. *Current Psychiatry* 15(5): pp. 42–46.

Arntfield, Shannon, Kristen Slesar, Jennifer Dickson, and Rita Charon 2013. Narrative Medicine as a Means of Training Medical Students Toward Residency Competency. *Patient Education and Counseling* 91(3): pp. 280–286.

Charon, Rita. 2001. Narrative Medicine: A Model for Empathy, Reflection, Profession, and Trust. *JAMA* 286(15): pp. 1897–1902.

Charon, Rita. 2004. Narrative and Medicine. *New England Journal of Medicine* 350(9): pp. 862–864.

Charon, Rita. 2007. What to Do With Stories: The Sciences of Narrative Medicine. *Canadian Family Physician* 53: pp. 1265–1267.

Hunt, Linda. 2019. Beyond Cultural Competence: Applying Humility to Clinical Settings. In *The Social Medicine Reader*, Volume II: Differences and Inequalities, ed. J. Oberlander, M. Buchbinder, L. Churchill, et al., pp. 127–131. Third edition. Durham, NC: Duke University Press.

Kleinman, Arthur. 1988. *The Illness Narratives: Suffering, Healing, and the Human Condition*. New York: Basic Books.

Metzl, Jonathan, and Helena Hansen. 2014. Structural Competency: Theorizing a New Medical Engagement with Stigma and Inequality. *Social Science & Medicine* 103: pp. 126–133.

Street, Alice. 2014. *Biomedicine in an Unstable Place: Infrastructure and Personhood in a Papua New Guinean Hospital*. Durham, NC: Duke University Press.

Timmermans, Stefan, and Mara Buchbinder. 2010. Patients-in-Waiting: Living Between Sickness and Health in the Genomics Era. *Journal of Health and Social Behavior* 51(4): pp. 408–423.

Waite, Roberta, and Dena Hassouneh. 2021. Structural Competency in Mental Health Nursing: Understanding and Applying Key Concepts. *Archives of Psychiatric Nursing* 35(1): pp. 73–79.

Wendland, Claire. 2010. *A Heart for the Work: Journeys through an African Medical School*. Chicago: University of Chicago Press.

Index

For the benefit of digital users, indexed terms that span two pages (e.g., 52–53) may, on occasion, appear on only one of those pages.

The manufacturer's authorised representative in the EU for product safety is Oxford University Press España S.A. of el Parque Empresarial San Fernando de Henares, Avenida de Castilla, 2 – 28830 Madrid (www.oup.es/en or product.safety@oup.com). OUP España S.A. also acts as importer into Spain of products made by the manufacturer.

www.ingramcontent.com/pod-product-compliance
Lightning Source LLC
Chambersburg PA
CBHW082158130526
45079CB00010B/508
9780198933922